THE **TOP 10** LYME DISEASE TREATMENTS

A battle to fight

Conventional medicine alone is not enough. Alternative medicine alone is not enough. The Lyme Disease infection is just too stubborn, resilient, and survival-driven.

Together, as a team, conventional and alternative medicine have a chance. Fighting Lyme Disease requires that we draw from all available resources—our very survival depends on it.

Healing from Lyme Disease is an intense battle, not a casual undertaking. When treated casually, healing stagnates. When attacked with vigor and determination, armed with information and strategy, healing progresses and excels. Let us remember that healing Lyme Disease is a battle—and let us fight strongly, with unwavering resolve.

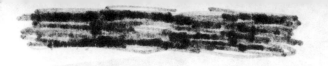

THE **TOP 10** LYME DISEASE TREATMENTS

DEFEAT LYME DISEASE WITH
THE BEST OF CONVENTIONAL AND
ALTERNATIVE MEDICINE

First Edition

By
Bryan Rosner

Foreword by
James Schaller, M.D.

Editors
Julie Byers, M.A.
Michael Huckleberry, M.A.

For more resources, including free online discussion groups, visit:
www.lymebook.com/resources

BioMed Publishing Group
P.O. Box 9012
South Lake Tahoe, CA 96158
www.LymeBookStore.com

ISBN 10: 0-9763797-1-6.
ISBN 13: 978-0-9763797-1-3.
Copyright © 2007 Bryan Rosner.
Cover image before modification © 2004 Jeffrey Nelson.
Cover design by Erika Farmer—www.WowDesignServices.com.

Lyme Disease books, videos & resources: www.LymeBookStore.com

Disclaimer

The author is not a physician or doctor, and this book is not intended as medical advice. It is also not intended to prevent, diagnose, treat or cure disease. Instead, the book is intended only to share the author's research, as would an investigative journalist. The book is provided for informational and educational purposes only, not as treatment instructions for any disease.

Lyme Disease is a dangerous disease and requires treatment by a licensed physician; this book is not a substitute for professional medical care. Do not begin any new treatment program without full consent and supervision from a licensed physician. If you have a medical problem, consult a doctor, not this book. If you are pregnant or breastfeeding, consult a physician before using any treatment.

Many of the treatments presented in this book are experimental and not FDA approved. Some of the book's content is speculative and theoretical. The author and publisher assume no liability or responsibility for any action taken by a reader of this book—use of this book is at your own risk. The statements in this book have not been evaluated by the FDA.

The author offers no guarantee that the treatments in this book are the best Lyme Disease therapies; instead, they were simply the treatments that the author found (through research and experience) to be most helpful. Do not rely on this book as the final word.

The Foreword for the book, written by James Schaller, M.D., is for informational purposes only. It is not intended as medical advice. The Foreword expresses Dr. Schaller's opinions only.

Acknowledgments

This book would not have been possible without the enduring, selfless, enthusiastic work of Julie Byers, M.A. Julie took the book from an unpolished state to a finished project.

Mike Huckleberry, M.A., proved yet again that his editing skills are invaluable. Mike has a sharp eye for editing manuscripts. His knowledge of my first book and understanding of my writing goals allowed him to have unique insight.

James Schaller, M.D., showed genuine interest in the project and extended an encouraging and supportive hand, as well as a visionary, hopeful outlook.

The following people reviewed the book prior to publication. Nenah Sylver, Ph.D., gave freely of her time, spending hours on the phone with me. Scott Forsgren provided a helpful critique. Tracie Schissel was very encouraging as the book neared completion. Andrew Cutler, Ph.D., has offered great advice and mentorship during the writing of my books. Mary Brescia, R.N., was encouraging, caring, and helpful. Jeff Mittelman gave excellent content suggestions and his contribution as moderator of the Lyme-and-rife group served to free up my time to write this book.

Doug MacLean provided much of the inspiration and research (a rare combination) for my books and continues to be a tremendous asset to the Lyme Community.

Julie Anderson, A.R.N.P, continues to be the healthcare provider with whom I am most impressed, both for her broad knowledge base and her pioneering strategy for healing disease.

Linda Heming, and her desire to help Lyme sufferers by spreading information and hope, showed me that there are a few good people left in the world.

Erika Farmer, who designed the cover, was much more creative than I could ever be.

My family was supportive as usual, especially Leila, my wife.

A story of hope and healing—Kay's saga continues

In my first book (*Lyme Disease and Rife Machines, 2005*) you will find Kay's story, as written by Kay in 2001, on the page immediately following the Disclaimer. Many readers have since asked for an update on how Kay is currently doing. Here it is, as written by Kay in 2007.

I f you are reading this with interest, you are probably dealing with Lyme Disease in your life. I'm writing this as a survivor of Lyme Disease, which is the most devastating health issue I've ever experienced. My Lyme Disease went untreated for years. Here is a recap of my story:

When the Lyme bacteria crossed the blood brain barrier, my husband became highly motivated to find help. We had a port surgically inserted to transport heavy duty antibiotics, antiprotozoals, and antifungals into my body. While this was helpful, as were all the pharmaceuticals I used, the effects of the drugs took their toll on me and were never effective enough.

If you have read my first story, you will remember that I prayed for a miracle and received it. My miracle came in the form of Doug's electromagnetic frequency machine [this is a type of rife machine, as discussed in Chapter 5]. Being too sick to even worry about "how it worked" or "what if it doesn't work," I began treatment on the machine. As you may recall from my first story, it took me at least 18 months of severe herxing (a result of Lyme bacteria die-off) before I began to feel significantly better.

Now, my update. Today, finally, praise God, I am leading a full and exciting life again! It was a long and painful path, but, in my opinion, it was the only path that slowly and surely brought me back to better and better health. I have some residual damage (mostly in my digestive tract) but I do not believe it is from Lyme Disease; instead, I think it is from all those heavy pharmaceuticals I used.

The Doug Machine was by far the most helpful treatment I have used. Throughout my recovery, though, there have also been various other helpful treatments and supplements. My supplementation regimen has changed countless times over the years. Currently I am taking several supplements which are helping me: ImmuAll made by Natural Care, Epicore made by Vitamin Research, and HMF Replete made by Genestra. Also, I have always found it helpful to take vitamins and minerals and stay away from white flour products and sugar.

Recently, I was tested and informed that my testing results showed no sign of active Lyme Disease. What a blessing. My prayer is that you would receive your miracle, too. A special thanks always to Doug, Dan from NY, and to Bryan; all people who so selflessly gave of their time and energy to help others.

God's Blessings To Each of You.

-Written by Kay in 2007

Also by Bryan Rosner

When Antibiotics Fail: Lyme Disease and Rife Machines, With Critical Evaluation of Leading Alternative Therapies

Available from www.LymeBook.com

Dedication

This book is dedicated to the Lord Jesus Christ,

And to my parents, Doug and Diane, without whose support my books would never have been written.

Table of Contents

Chapter 2: The Marshall Protocol 97

Chapter 3: The Salt / Vitamin C protocol 133

Chapter 4: Detoxification 141

Foreword

New millennium treatments for Lyme Disease
By James Schaller, M.D.

One of the unfortunate truths of current treatment practices in tick-borne illness is the simple reality that many patients do not fully recover. In my practice, this occurs for many reasons, including such culprits as indoor mold toxin exposure, patient genetic limitations in the removal of Lyme Disease biotoxins, and, quite often, undiagnosed new Babesia and Bartonella strains.

As a practicing physician, I have the opportunity to observe firsthand the intricacies of Lyme Disease and its co-infections. I have found that Borrelia Burgdorferi is rarely the only active infection present. Ticks pass on many infections which have the ability to quickly reach all body cavities and tissues—from the brain to the teeth and everywhere in between—and to release surface biotoxins that dysregulate numerous hormones including thyroid hormones, fertility hormones, testosterone, DHEA, and leptin. The latter is usually too high and is associated with treatment resistant obesity. These surface biotoxins hijack many lesser known hormones, proteins, and inflammatory chemicals, resulting in widespread pathology throughout body systems and organs.

Additionally, my experience is that 99% of Lyme Disease patients have psychiatric or subtle neurological findings, which are often missed by sincere health care workers. Clinical manifestations include diagnoses as varied as depression, obsessive-compulsive disorder, rages, schizophrenia, brain fog, memory loss, a profound decrease in reasoning abilities, poor insight, panic attacks, agitation, confusion, personality changes, mania, seizures, strokes, and many more.

These are just a few of the many obstacles facing modern health care practitioners who treat Lyme Disease. As a result of these complexities in tick-borne illness, eradicating Lyme Disease is virtually never simply a matter of using high dose antibiotics for a month or a year. Successful treatment is far more involved. I make these comments because, in 2007, it is naive to think that all new, important treatment information for Lyme Disease or its co-infections will come from a few infectious disease physicians or family doctors. We need an expanded approach, one that encompasses a wide array of treatment methodologies and options. The antibiotic-only approach, whether applied for a short time or a long time, is simplistic.

Into this arena, Bryan Rosner offers an exceptionally broad, important and clearly written book that is sure to be a top medical resource for this decade. This author is unusually gifted at clearly presenting newly emerging treatments or revised treatments. This book allows you to actually understand important and fascinating new information without having to strain your brain.

The topics he has chosen are very broad and relevant and offer easily understood lessons to both Lyme Disease illness veterans and those new to this profound disease. He offers hope in the context of a wide range of options beyond merely expecting your physician to cure you in once-a-month appointments largely limited to antibiotic adjustments. Bryan Rosner thinks big. He offers big solutions. He offers diverse and varied answers to the problem of chronic Lyme Disease treatment.

He is also a big listener. He has been listening to many of the top minds in innovative medicine and has successfully prepared a fine, educational read that leaves one satisfied and encouraged. He has tried very hard to study deeply, and to be balanced and humble. Yet he offers information any author would be proud to write.

Bryan Rosner is a passionate explorer willing to sweat the extra miles. And to the good fortune of Lyme Disease sufferers, he is not exploring space or the deep oceans or foreign lands. Instead he is exploring breakthrough treatments that offer hope to those suffering from this devastating affliction. Wisely, each of his top 10 interventions stands alone, since he knows Lyme Disease is never treated with a cookbook approach, but only with highly individualized, closely supervised care.

Lastly, and most importantly, Bryan Rosner is one of us. His passion to learn and heal the suffering that he himself has defeated, is the passion of one connected to those still left behind with incomplete healing. He studies and writes with the zeal of one who cares for his readers. His tone is neither cold nor detached; instead, it is that of a friend.

To help you achieve a complete recovery, he offers this exceptionally creative and fascinating book with many new and clearly described options for hope.

James Schaller, M.D.
www.personalconsult.com

Author of 16 books, including:
- The Diagnosis and Treatment of Babesia
- Suboxone: A Revolutionary New Medication for Pain and Detoxification
- The Use of Artemisinin for Cancer, Malaria and Babesiosis
- 100 Commonly Missed Causes of ADD, Irritability and ODD in Children
- Mold Illness and Mold Remediation Made Simple

Author of articles in 25 medical publications, including:
- The Journal of the American Medical Association
- Medscape
- The Journal of Clinical Neurosciences
- Journal of the American Society of Child and Adolescent Psychiatry
- Internal Medicine News
- Family Practice News
- Townsend Journal
- American Journal of Psychiatry

Disclaimer: This Foreword is not intended as medical advice. These statements have not been evaluated by the FDA. If you have a medical problem, see a licensed physician.

Preface:
The Lyme Chronicles

A personal perspective

When perceived by naïve eyes, modern medicine gives no hint that something is amiss. The medical establishment has all the appearances of authority and proficiency. From new, opulent hospital buildings complete with gray-haired, confident doctors on whose walls hang official credentials, to medical web sites created by the best web designers, the statement is clear: Western medicine knows its stuff. Furthering this perception is, of course, the assurance from medical professionals that everything health can be measured and manipulated and made right.

Clearly, current medical practice has done much good for humankind. In our age-old battle to maintain and restore health, we have celebrated great victories in healing. Broken bones and crooked teeth yield quietly to modern medicine. Critical car accident victims enjoy incredibly optimistic odds as a result of helicopters and advanced emergency rooms. Most bacterial infections cause us no more trouble than the nuisance of a trip to the doctor's office and then the pharmacy. I am grateful for, and I personally benefit from, modern medicine in its many forms.

INTO THE WORLD OF LYME DISEASE

Despite progress in medicine, some maladies continue to plague us. Worse, some medical conditions are even wholly disregarded by the conventional medical community because they do not fit the prevailing paradigms of diagnosis and treatment. When I discovered I had Lyme Disease and subsequently sought treatment, it became obvious that Lyme Disease is such a condition. The longer I was sick, the harder it became to ignore the many clues that Western medicine really didn't have room for Lyme Disease. The complex diagnostic process and dynamic treatment procedures necessary to get well are too different from what doctors are taught in medical school to be widely recognized and applied. The disease simply does not fit the system. Of course, ideally, the system should be flexible to fit the disease—but that doesn't always happen. Most of the conventional-minded doctors I sought for help either denied the existence of the disease altogether, at least in its chronic form, or treated me with therapies which I later discovered to be antiquated and wildly irrational.

Conventional medicine is not the only subsection of healthcare which has difficulty diagnosing and treating Lyme Disease. Most of the arena of alternative medicine is also confused and misled. Although generally more open-minded, acupuncturists, herbalists, homeopaths, alternative MDs, and unconventional healers all tripped over each other and contradicted one another about what I should do. Generally, they recommended roughly the same approaches that conventional doctors recommended, but instead of drugs, they encouraged me to use herbs, essential oils, or homeopathic remedies. Some of the treatments of both conventional and alternative medicine helped me, but none gave me back my health. Most of the health care practitioners I encountered lacked a solid understanding of Lyme Disease pathogenesis.

In the instances when I found a treatment that did help, results were so slow to manifest (due to the hardiness of the infection) that I could never tell if I was using the best available treatment or wasting time with marginally effective approaches. Either way, inevitably, any help I received from a treatment would dissipate and be replaced by increasing and resurgent symptoms.

The truth, the disturbing, authentic truth, is that none of the more than 40 conventional and alternative practitioners I saw really knew what to do. They all wanted to help, but the resources just weren't there. Months of research led me to the discovery that Lyme Disease occupies a dark corner of humankind's medical knowledge base, denied adequate research and funding and even acknowledgment. As a result, Lyme Disease to this day remains a mysterious illness. This is why most Lyme doctors are persecuted as fringe renegades and most of the best books on the subject are written by lay people who were forced to educate themselves by exhaustively searching the annals of medical research and patient experiences.

Despite my worsening Lyme Disease infection and frustration with the medical resources available to me, I continued to seek help from various doctors for many years. That is, until fall of 2002. The following is an account of the events which finally forced me to internalize the reality that Lyme Disease sufferers are on their own.

THE REVELATION

It was a cool, autumn evening in Nevada. I patiently sat in the office of the medical director of a world renowned "underground" (translated: not condoned by Western medicine) Lyme Disease clinic. This clinic was allegedly one of the most competent Lyme Disease treatment facilities on the planet. This was the top of the ladder of treatment options: expensive, proficient, and well-known, with a patient base that includes people who travel from all around the globe. I felt that I had separated the wheat from the chaff and finally found a valuable way to spend my treatment dollars and time.

And, dollars and time I did spend. After staying at this clinic for three weeks and spending over $15,000, I wasn't really any better, and I wanted to ask someone what the next step was. I didn't know I would actually secure a meeting with the medical director of the clinic himself; in the past he had been elusive and cryptic and I always wound up seeing one of the staff physicians. The clinic was large, with over 50 employees, and the director busied himself with important meetings and lectures. Naturally, I was elated to see this respected and successful alternative-minded physician in person, and I was certain he would have answers and a new path for me to try. After all, a toolbox with useful therapies and suggestions is something you expect from someone who is arguably the world's leading expert on alternative treatments for Lyme Disease, right?

When, in response to my desperate pleas, he offered no new path but instead shrugged and apologized flatly while writing me a prescription for the most antiquated and ineffective chronic Lyme Disease therapy in history (a two-week course of doxycycline), a light went on in my head. As my previous years of struggle in the medical community finally came into focus, I realized that I was truly *on my own*. There were no more specialists to go see. No more second opinions to be had. I climbed the ladder of medical professionals all the way to the top, and I still did not find what I needed. I left the clinic, depressed and broke and hopeless, with a nagging thought repeating itself over and over in my mind: no one in the world knows how to handle chronic Lyme Disease.

OUT OF THE WORLD OF LYME DISEASE

Under normal circumstances I would not choose to take my health into my own hands. The near-infinite resources available in the arena of modern medicine render it silly for people without a medical education to poke around and try to figure out new ways to solve health problems. The probability of a non-medical person finding a medical breakthrough is about as high as that of a business person waltzing into NASA with a correction in the formula used to calculate the shuttle's reentry path.

And, I really didn't have a desire to explore new solutions to medical problems. Before I got sick (although now I believe I have had chronic Lyme since birth), I was happily engaged in a successful business career. I wasn't looking for new, low-probability-of-success projects. But after that fateful evening in Nevada, it appeared I had no choice but to go it on my own. Conventional and alternative medicine just didn't work for me despite years of treatment and over $100,000 in medical bills. Where would it end? How much more of my life would I waste waiting, hoping for something to change?

I reluctantly concluded that I would either figure this out myself or I wouldn't get better. Ironically, I later learned that one of the most significant discoveries in Lyme Disease treatment history was achieved by a businessman with no medical training—Doug MacLean, who pioneered modern rife technology as a treatment for Lyme Disease. NASA, indeed! Out of options, I now had only one option, so I jumped in head first and committed to doing my absolute best to research, understand, and beat this disease.

What ensued was a none-too-glamorous journey in which I traveled through years of experimentation and endless hours of research. I talked to hundreds of Lyme Disease sufferers and physicians, and even founded an internet-based Lyme Disease support group which now has over 2,000 members. I compared notes with patients and health care practitioners alike. I experimented with countless herbs and pharmaceuticals—many of which were purchased without a prescription from online and overseas pharmacies (do not try this at home!). Using my body as a guinea pig, I had some pretty scary experiences. The worst was when I went to Italy and spent $20,000 on an experimental treatment during which time the patient in the room next to me actually died due to complications of the treatment. Italy didn't heal me.

Many people told me I was crazy and asked how I could take such risks with my own life. The answer was quite simply that I had no other choice. Most people do not understand this concept; most people do not know what it is like to be pressed up against a wall like that. All people who suffer from chronic Lyme Disease do know what it is like. It was crazy, what I was doing. But crazy is better than sick and miserable or dead. Many significant discoveries in history were made by people who took risks they would not normally take simply because they had no choice. A good friend and research partner once said, "you can always identify the pioneers because they are the ones with the arrows in their backs."

I kept detailed records of how I responded to different therapies, and spare mental energy was used to continuously pour over and rehash unsolved issues and unanswered questions. Even when I was not researching, my brain was engaged, processing, contemplating. I corroborated my experiences and conclusions with those of other Lyme Disease sufferers. I found that my discoveries were indeed common among dozens, even hundreds of people afflicted with chronic Lyme Disease who had been doing their own research and guiding their own treatment programs. The information on how to get well was out there, it just wasn't organized. Nothing was very complicated, just obscure. And worse, conventional medicine didn't seem to be interested in helping.

Ultimately, after struggling for several years, I found my way back to an enjoyable, healthy quality of life. Looking back, the therapies and protocols I used to get better are actually not very complex or extreme. Simplicity often goes hand in hand with value. One of the most interesting discoveries I made was that the toolboxes of conventional and alternative medicine actually have the right tools. The problem is that the right tools are either used incorrectly, ignored when they are needed, or esoterically buried deep beneath more commonly used yet less useful tools. In fact, most of the time I spent researching was not dedicated to examining beneficial treatments but instead, trying to navigate through the distraction of hundreds of worthless treatments. Although one of the goals of this book is to introduce you to what I believe are the best conventional and alternative Lyme Disease therapies, a goal of no less importance is to also help you save time by sparing you the monstrous task of sorting through the tools that don't work.

If you have reservations about listening to a non-medical person talk about a medical subject, I don't blame you. You should be wary. I do not ask you to accept this book as scientific fact or proven data. I do not ask you to take my word as gospel. However, let me be the first to break the news to you: if you have chronic Lyme Disease, you don't have many great options staring you in the face. What modern conventional and alternative medicine has to offer you is far short of the mark. "Scientific fact and proven data" leave much to be desired in the area of Lyme Disease treatment. The discoveries and experiences of pioneering Lyme Disease sufferers will be at least as useful to you as the medical textbooks on which your doctors base their decisions and statements. Quite likely, as time goes on and research continues, better options will become available. Until they do, you have much to learn from those who have gone before.

Lyme Disease sufferers are all pioneers, on the frontier of medical discovery—including you! You are a pioneer, and it is your right, actually your responsibility, to sift through the available information and come to your own conclusions. Failure to do this can have dire consequences simply because the alternative is often continued suffering. So think of my book not as your final answer, but instead one of many resources, a roadmap to get you started. If I did my job well in writing this book, I can save a few pioneers from unnecessary arrows in their backs.

Roadmap of this book

Lets take a brief look at what you can expect from this book.

Information for the Reader, the next section of the book, provides some important facts and tips that you should be aware of prior to reading the book.

The *Introduction*, which follows *Information for the Reader*, offers background information about Lyme Disease, including obstacles in the diagnosis and treatment processes, and also examines some key issues affecting patients and practitioners. In addition, the *Introduction* compares conventional and alternative medicine and challenges you to re-examine your current thinking and paradigm with regard to Lyme Disease treatment.

After the *Introduction*, the book dives right into the 10 most effective conventional and alternative Lyme therapies. *Part I* of the book, comprised of *chapters 1-5*, presents the five core treatment protocols, or ideologies on which a foundational treatment plan can be based. These five protocols are the guts of the book—they constitute the main components of successful Lyme Disease treatment.

Part II of the book, comprised of *chapters 6-10*, presents five nutritional and herbal supplements that can be used in a supportive capacity alongside the five core protocols of *Part I*. These supplements must be understood as supportive and not foundational. In other words, they do not work toward a cure, but instead, they provide accelerated healing and symptom reduction as the five core protocols work toward a cure.

After we have seen the top 10 Lyme Disease treatments (5 core protocols and 5 supportive supplements), *Chapter 11* describes how to integrate them into a comprehensive treatment program. *Chapter 11* gives you a basic framework for setting up your treatment plan. You may wish to skip ahead to this chapter before reading the book. Scanning it first can give you an idea of where we are going, how we are getting there, and what the final goal is.

INFORMATION FOR THE READER

Early-stage (acute) vs. late-stage (chronic) Lyme Disease

The therapies and strategies on which this book focuses are intended for the treatment of late stage, chronic Lyme Disease. It is important to recognize that treatment of newly acquired, early-stage Lyme Disease is an entirely different endeavor.

Treating late stage Lyme Disease is accomplished by carefully analyzing and balancing various treatments as part of a comprehensive, long-term treatment plan. Developing such a treatment plan is the focus of this book.

In contrast, treatment of early-stage, acute Lyme Disease requires immediate, aggressive antibiotic therapy. The probability that acute, early-stage Lyme Disease will progress into chronic Lyme Disease increases dramatically the longer antibiotic therapy is postponed. Therefore, if you were just recently bitten by a tick and you are in the early stages of Lyme Disease, it is critical that you find a Lyme Literate Medical Doctor (LLMD) immediately to initiate antibiotic therapy. LLMDs are much more qualified to treat Lyme Disease than are general practitioners or infectious disease doctors. You can get a referral to an LLMD at www.lymenet.org and also at www.lymediseaseassociation.org. The "LLMD" title is not an official credential or designation, but instead indicates that a given physician is willing and qualified to work with Lyme sufferers.

The Lyme community: your greatest asset

Neither conventional nor alternative medicine has all the answers about Lyme Disease. As sufferers of Lyme Disease, we must stick together, share information, and move ahead as a united group, helping one another sift through the endless books, articles, and websites available. Lyme Disease is set apart from other medical conditions because breakthroughs in Lyme Disease treatment often result from collaboration, cooperation, and research conducted by the Lyme Disease community itself, in comparison with breakthroughs in other areas of health research, which are often attained via outside research organizations such as pharmaceutical companies and universities. We can all learn from one another and in many cases, our personal experiences with helpful or harmful treatments can provide road-maps for one another.

One of the best methods by which to communicate with Lyme Disease sufferers is the establishment of Lyme Disease support groups. Historically, these support groups have involved actual in-person meetings. Now, because of technology, internet-based discussion groups are becoming more and more popular and accessible.

Internet discussion forums provide a gathering medium in which Lyme Disease sufferers can get together for the purpose of making new friends, sharing treatment information, supporting one another, and building a database of Lyme Disease information. Internet discussion groups have several advantages over regional, geographically organized support groups that meet in individual cities and towns. Although local support groups obviously foster deeper interpersonal relationships, internet support groups provide these advantages:

1. These groups are accessible to everyone, even people who live in remote, rural locations where local support groups may not be

available. What's more, internet discussion groups are accessible from your own living room so the travel time, expense, and inconvenience involved in attending local support groups is avoided.

2. When participating in an internet discussion group, there is no need to block off a certain evening of the week to meet with the participants. Internet discussion groups are available at all times, day or night. You can post your own messages and read other peoples' messages whenever you like. Participants can read your messages and respond to you whenever it is convenient for them. It is easy to integrate participation in internet discussion forums into your daily life. You can access an internet group for a few minutes on your lunch break, at night before you go to sleep, or on a leisurely Sunday afternoon.

3. Much of the current research on and information about Lyme Disease is being distributed on the internet instead of in newspapers or printed publications. Obviously, the internet is becoming more and more influential in the flow of information in dozens of industries. Participants on an internet discussion group can easily share with each other recent online news articles by simply posting links. In comparison, in order to share information at a local support group, someone must print the information, make copies, and remember to bring them on the actual night of the meeting.

4. Most internet discussion groups have storage archives where past messages are indefinitely retained. Search functions utilizing keywords make it quick and easy to go back through months or years of discussion history to isolate topics you are interested in or researching. In this way, resources and discussions are effortlessly organized into a useful, continually growing database of information. In comparison, local support group meetings are not recorded, and, once the meeting is over, the information exchanged and discussions had will be soon forgotten forever and will become inaccessible to people who could not attend. Even if the meeting was recorded or videotaped, specific discussions or topics will be difficult to recall quickly without cumbersome fast-forwarding and re-

winding of audio or video tapes. On an internet discussion group, in a matter of seconds, you can find specific topics discussed over a wide range of time.

5. Local support groups have attendance of anywhere from five to 50 people on average. Many of the larger internet discussion groups focusing on Lyme Disease have hundreds or thousands of members. While local support groups are small gatherings, internet support groups are large conventions. Internet discussion groups allow you to not only benefit from the experiences, knowledge, and contribution of a few people who live in your hometown, but also to enjoy access to thousands of Lyme Disease sufferers and researchers all around the world. Information exchange becomes centralized instead of decentralized.

Naturally, internet discussion groups will never replace the interpersonal interactions that occur when people meet together in person. However, as you can see, participation in online discussion groups can be beneficial in numerous ways. And an added bonus is that the vast majority of the groups are available absolutely free of charge.

There are dozens of online Lyme Disease support groups—three of the most useful and informative are the Lyme-and-Rife group, Lyme Community Forums, and LymeNet.

The Lyme-and-Rife group. This group was established in April of 2003 and has over 2,000 members. It focuses on using rife machine technology to treat Lyme Disease. Access the group at www.lymebook.com/resources.

Lyme Community Forums. This group was established in November of 2006. It is the primary discussion forum for numerous Lyme Disease topics. You can access the group at www.lymecommunity.com.

Lyme Disease Network. The Lyme Disease network was established in 1994 and offers numerous resources, including a large online discussion group with over 11,000 members! Visit the group at www.lymenet.org.

Lyme Disease and Rife Machines

This is the second of two books I have written on the topic of Lyme Disease. My first book (*Lyme Disease and Rife Machines*, 2005) focused on the subject of treating Lyme Disease with rife machines (see Chapter 5 for an explanation of rife machine therapy). It established the fundamental, essential concepts pertaining to successfully fighting chronic Lyme Disease with rife machine technology. If you have read my first book, you may be wondering whether or not I still believe, even after writing a second book, that rife machine therapy is useful and effective. For those of you who have not read my first book, it presented rife machine therapy as the best known primary treatment for chronic Lyme Disease.

The answer is yes—research and user reports still indicate that rife machine therapy is the most effective core treatment—my stance on this issue has not changed. In fact, additional evidence since my first book was published solidifies rife machine therapy's place not only as a promising solution to the problem of treating chronic Lyme Disease, but also, to the best of my knowledge, a non-toxic solution. To date, I am unaware of any other therapy which rivals rife machine therapy in terms of effectiveness, affordability, convenience, and overall usefulness.

The book you now hold in your hands, my second book, is not intended to replace *Lyme Disease and Rife Machines*, but instead, to complement it. Neither book will replace the other because each has unique content. Not only will this book not replace my first book, it will also hopefully not contradict it. In other words, the concepts presented in this book should seamlessly integrate with those presented in *Lyme Disease and Rife Machines*. This is because the information in the first book is, in my opinion, still highly accurate. The two books should fit together like puzzle pieces. In instances where they do not, it is probably a reflection of lack of established information, speculative concepts, or a lack on my part of complete understanding of the information—after all, this entire area of research and writing is cutting-edge and not fully understood.

Quite a few people have asked me if/when a second edition will be available for *Lyme Disease and Rife Machines*. When I tell them that there are no current plans for a second edition, I am often met with surprise. In this day and age, information moves at a very rapid pace and people expect updated information all the time. The truth, however, is that not much has changed regarding the principles of treating Lyme Disease with rife machines (to the best of my knowledge) since I wrote the earlier book. *Lyme Disease and Rife Machines* was based on 20 years of information compiled by the Lyme Disease community—information which has been tested, verified, and re-tested numerous times. In the past two years, nothing of great significance has occurred in terms of research and findings.

The good news about this stability of information is that those of you who understand the concepts set forth in *Lyme Disease and Rife Machines* will not have to relearn or change your current understanding as would be required if a second edition were published. *Lyme Disease and Rife Machines*, in my opinion, is still as accurate and applicable as ever. The book you now hold in your hands will not require you to relearn anything but instead will simply broaden your existing knowledge base.

Of course, we still have a lot to learn about treating Lyme Disease with rife machines. This is still a very experimental field. There are several reasons why new information is hard to come by. Most significantly, very few resources in the forms of both money and man-hours have been dedicated to the study and improvement of electromagnetic therapies in the treatment of Lyme Disease. Not only are rife machines unstudied by well-funded research organizations, Lyme Disease itself is also largely ignored by conventional medicine and does not receive adequate funding and attention. In fact, shortly before I released this book, The Infectious Disease Society of America, an organization crowned with the authority of determining nonnegotiable guidelines for treating Lyme Disease, released their new treatment guidelines that basically state that there is no such thing as chronic Lyme Disease and that doctors who treat this fictitious disease may be subject to discipline and possibly loss of license. This new development will only serve to stifle, not augment, new Lyme Disease research.

An additional reason for lack of new information on the subject of treating Lyme Disease with rife machines is the fact that the Lyme Disease community remains fairly decentralized and fragmented and has not yet established an efficient and productive means by which to develop and present new information and findings. The community has come a long way thanks to the efforts and dedication of dozens of Lyme Disease sufferers who share in the vision of progress, healing, and community. In the past three years, numerous informational resources have become available to Lyme sufferers using rife technology. One example is the Lyme-and-rife internet discussion group which, at the time I write this, has over 2,000 members and offers an excellent forum through which people can centralize information and updates. However, we still have a long way to go to reach the goal of efficient and timely news updates and distribution.

With all that said, despite the rather discouraging lack of forward progress in the research of Lyme Disease treatment with rife technology, I still believe that the concepts set forth in *Lyme Disease and Rife Machines* are quite worthwhile and accurate. I am not aware of any other treatment program that offers such dependable and beneficial results as the treatment program presented in *Lyme Disease and Rife Machines*.

The "herx reaction" and other vernacular terminology

Throughout this book, I will make reference to the reaction that occurs when Lyme Disease bacteria are killed, and subsequent inflammation and toxin release occurs. This reaction is known as the Jarisch-Herxheimer reaction, named after the two doctors who first discovered it. In this book I will refer to this reaction as the "herx reaction." It is also commonly referred to as "bacterial die-off", a "healing crisis," and "getting worse before you get better." This book will not provide a detailed explanation of what the reaction is, why it occurs, and how to deal with it. This information is provided in Chapter 4 of *Lyme Disease and Rife Machines.* You can also locate information about Lyme Disease herx reactions in dozens of internet and printed Lyme Disease resources.

Additionally, other terms used in the book may be unfamiliar to you. When you encounter a word or phrase with which you are unfamiliar, the best course of action is to simply look up the meaning of the word. This is often not possible in standard dictionaries due to the specialized content of this book. A few strategies for looking up unfamiliar terms are the following:

1. Google them, meaning, go to www.google.com and type the word or phrase in question into the search box, then explore some of the search results. When searching for a phrase (two or more words), use quotes in the search. For example, if you are searching for the phrase *antibiotic resistant bacteria,* then the search would read "antibiotic resistant bacteria." Some of the search results you acquire through Google (or any other search engine) will not be scientifically credible. Therefore, be selective in which results you read.

2. Use www.wikipedia.com, a user-authored, massive online encyclopedia which has definitions of numerous specialized words and phrases. Again, some results in this venue may not be credible, so be discerning.

3. Ask your doctor about words or concepts you do not understand.

4. Ask people at Lyme Community Forums, which can be accessed at www.lymecommunity.com. Lyme Community Forums is an online Lyme Disease community where you can make friends with other Lyme Disease sufferers, receive support and encouragement, and learn about new treatment options. Members of the group can help you understand terminology you are unfamiliar with.

What is (and is not) in this book

I would like to provide a brief description of what is (and is not) in this book before getting too deep into the material. By doing this, readers will have a good idea of what to expect. They will know which topics they can rely on the book for, and which topics they should learn about by seeking other resources.

There are already dozens of books, websites and resources that provide what I refer to as "Lyme Disease 101." In the interest of parsimony, this book is *not* intended to offer a basic Lyme Disease education. Examples of basic information that this book does not provide include:

- Information about ticks, including a description of various types, where they're most likely to be found, how to prevent bites, proper technique for their removal, and which animals harbor them.

- Where to get tested for Lyme Disease and which tests are most reliable.

- Which antibiotics are most efficacious in the treatment of early-stage Lyme Disease.

- Current health insurance policies with regard to Lyme Disease.

- A thorough description of the pathology of Lyme Disease.

- Adequate coverage of current happenings in the arenas of Lyme Disease legislation, patient activism, and treatment guidelines.

- Various other entry-level Lyme Disease concepts.

Instead of basic information, this book focuses on complex topics, difficult debates, treatment breakthroughs, and cutting-edge Lyme Disease research. In particular, we will examine advanced treatment solutions for stubborn, antibiotic-refractory Lyme Disease infections. I chose to focus on advanced rather than simple topics because, as mentioned, there is already an abundance of entry-level Lyme Disease information. The last thing the world needs is another book on removing ticks and recognizing bulls-eye rashes.

In contrast, there is not much out there that delves into some of the more pressing, practical, and complicated issues facing Lyme Disease sufferers. Basic Lyme Disease information (Lyme Disease 101) leaves people with a great need for answers to more difficult questions. For example, most of the available Lyme Disease resources basically state the following:

- Lyme Disease bacteria look and act in these ways.

- It gets into the human body by these processes.

- It makes you really sick.

- Conventional treatments are effective some of the time.

- If conventional treatments do not work, which happens quite often, then no one really knows what to do, and you will probably be sick forever—oh, and by the way, most conventional medical researchers and practitioners do not even acknowledge chronic Lyme Disease.

This book picks up the trail where Lyme Disease 101 leaves off: what to do about cases of Lyme Disease that have failed to be resolved by standard (or even "aggressive") antibiotic treatment. The book offers practical, broad, and user-friendly discussion of cutting-edge treatment options which have been found to be beneficial for difficult or chronic cases of Lyme Disease. The book is based on thousands of patient experiences, numerous published studies, and the wisdom and clinical observations of dozens of health care practitioners. It offers you information that you can actually use.

Although the book does not focus on basic Lyme Disease principles, I believe you will find it worthwhile because it offers advanced, critical information not found anywhere else in print or on the internet.

The internet: a double-edged sword

In modern times, the internet plays a critical role in the flow and transfer of information. Hence, many parts of this book will refer you to the internet for additional information on the topics discussed. One of the benefits of the internet is that you can easily access it, anytime you like, to get the information you need.

One of the disadvantages of the internet is that I cannot ensure that the sites I recommend in the book will indefinitely remain the same. Some of the web sites I recommend will inevitably change or disappear over time.

When this occurs, you may be unable to acquire the additional resources which I intended for you to have access to.

Thus the double-edged sword that is the internet.

Because I believe it is critical for you to have access to additional resources beyond this book, I will provide updates for my readers as the internet evolves and changes. You can find these and other updates at www.lymebook.com/resources. If you notice that a web site I recommend is no longer available, check the resources page mentioned above for new links and information.

Bryan Rosner's Lyme Disease E-Newsletter

In addition to the website mentioned above, I also edit an email newsletter designed to keep readers up-to-date in areas that evolve and change too quickly to be adequately covered in printed books.

This newsletter is only published 2-6 times per year, so you do not need to worry about receiving superfluous email on a weekly or monthly basis. In addition to news and information updates, the newsletter also notifies you of new Lyme Disease educational resources, such as books, videos, DVDs, and software.

To subscribe to the newsletter, visit www.lymebook.com/newsletter. At this website you can also read the archives of past newsletters. Subscription is free and you can unsubscribe at any time.

Introduction: Welcome to the World of Lyme Disease

Medical freedom and how it impacts you

There is a disturbing and dangerous dynamic currently playing out in the arena of Lyme Disease treatment policy. In the first few pages of Stephen Buhner's new book, *Healing Lyme*, he talks about the "Lyme wars," which refers not to the battle between your body and Lyme Disease bacteria but, instead, the battle between two factions of the medical community with polar opposite views about what Lyme Disease is and how to treat it. At the center of this conflict is a disagreement about whether the chronic form of Lyme Disease is a real medical condition caused by a dangerous, insidious bacterial infection or a fictional disease resulting from psychological factors and paranoia. Mr. Buhner observes that "the intensity of the conflict has regrettably reached almost religious levels amongst the different proponents ... caught in the crossfire are those with Lyme Disease who are trying to understand what is happening to them and to discover how best to deal with it."

So deep and polarizing is the disagreement about whether or not chronic Lyme Disease is a real condition that there has come to be a high, insurmountable, dividing wall between parties on either side of the debate.

Relations are hostile. Physicians who believe in the existence of chronic Lyme Disease and who are willing to help patients suffering from it are known as Lyme Literate Medical Doctors (LLMDs). LLMDs are compassionate, supportive, and understanding when dealing with chronic Lyme Disease sufferers. They are also willing to prescribe aggressive antibiotic therapy to fight the entrenched bacterial infection. LLMDs are willing to use antibiotic therapy because they observe that, time and time again, chronic Lyme Disease sufferers actually get better with antibiotic therapy. Additionally, LLMDs are aware of the mounting scientific evidence indicating that chronic Lyme Disease is indeed caused by the persistent presence of Lyme Disease bacteria in the body, instead of hypochondria or psychological problems. To an LLMD, such scientific evidence is more than just abstract theory—it is something they observe day-in and day-out in their clinical practices. To Lyme Disease sufferers, LLMDs are heroes, offering the hope of health to the sick and hopeless.

Physicians on the other side of the debate, those who do not recognize the existence of chronic Lyme Disease, see LLMDs as quacks. The vast majority of physicians specializing in infectious disease ascribe to the position that chronic Lyme Disease is "all in your head." When dealing with chronic Lyme Disease sufferers, doctors of this belief are typically arrogant, condescending, and belittling. They will often refer Lyme Disease sufferers to a psychologist or worse, send them walking out of their offices empty-handed and demoralized. They attribute alleged symptom improvement from antibiotic therapy to the placebo effect.

The beginning years of the debate about chronic Lyme Disease were mostly academic, and physicians on either side of it simply ignored each other and continued practicing medicine to the best of their ability. During this initial time, the government basically stayed out of the argument and allowed room for freedom of medical practice, similar to the freedom enjoyed by doctors of various disciplines who treat cancer in numerous ways.

But lately the stakes have been raised considerably. The last few years have seen many of the nation's Lyme Disease doctors persecuted and even disciplined by state medical boards. This has happened as a significant segment of the governing authorities have, despite glaring and mounting evidence to the contrary, settled into the camp that does not recognize the existence of chronic Lyme Disease as a real medical condition. Hence, almost overnight, physicians who treat chronic Lyme Disease went from being respected and left alone, to being persecuted and disciplined. So adamant have the medical authorities become that some physicians have even lost their licenses, or in less severe cases, been frightened enough to close their doors to Lyme Disease patients.

A new development that has led to even higher stakes in the debate was the recent release of new Lyme Disease treatment guidelines by the Infectious Disease Society of America (IDSA), an organization generally recognized as the authority on infectious disease. These new guidelines have been accepted and implemented by the Centers for Disease Control (CDC). Here is an excerpt from the new guidelines:

> *There is no convincing biologic evidence for the existence of sympto-matic chronic B. burgdorferi infection [the pathologic agent in Lyme Disease] among patients after receipt of recommended treatment regi-mens for Lyme Disease. Antibiotic therapy has not proven to be useful and is not recommended for patients with chronic ($\geq$6 months) subjec-tive symptoms after recommended treatment regimens for Lyme Dis-ease (E-I).*

These new guidelines threaten your access to therapies which have his-torically been available at the discretion of licensed physicians. The guide-lines have been cause for outrage among Lyme Disease patients, practitioners, and researchers. In fact, the State of Connecticut Attorney General, Richard Blumenthal, has even launched an official investigation into whether the IDSA has violated antitrust laws in setting these guide-lines. This investigation may lead to a lawsuit. According to Richard Blu-menthal, as quoted in the November 17, 2006 issue of the Hartford Courant, "the new guidelines were set by a panel that essentially locked out competing points of view."

Because of the authority of the IDSA, and the CDC's adoption of the new guidelines, treatment of chronic Lyme Disease has become more than just controversial—it has become illegal, or at least, questionably legal. What does this mean to you? The result of this recent shift toward persecuting and disciplining LLMDs is that it is becoming increasingly common for Lyme Disease sufferers to be denied the medical care they need.

In the early years of the debate, although many doctors turned chronic Lyme Disease sufferers away, there was always a safe haven to be found in the office of an LLMD. Not so anymore. The safe havens are increasingly in short supply, and in danger of disappearing altogether.

Additionally, well-funded Lyme Disease research is becoming increasingly rare. Ironically, many diseases far less prevalent than Lyme Disease are actually receiving a higher level of funding. As a result, the outlook for breakthroughs in Lyme Disease treatment is rather discouraging.

The current state of affairs with insurance companies does not help the situation—many companies have followed suit behind the regulatory authorities and now deny coverage to chronic Lyme sufferers. Richard Blumenthal notes that "one of the common complaints we've received relates to denials of insurance coverage … it's a very chilling economic effect."

Admittedly, both sides of the debate have some justification. Because I have personally endured chronic Lyme Disease and benefited tremendously from treating it, and because I have observed many other cases in which the same thing has happened, I reside in the camp that recognizes chronic Lyme Disease as a real condition. My position is further solidified by the plethora of scientific evidence indicating that Lyme Disease bacteria can persist in the body even after antibiotic treatment. However, despite my experiences and despite the available evidence, I can acknowledge that there is in fact a debate taking place, whether I like it or not.

The real question here, however, is not whether or not chronic Lyme Disease exists. That debate will likely still be raging at the time this book is published. The real question is whether or not people should have a right to exercise medical freedom of choice in an area of medicine that is not clearly defined, in the same way that cancer patients have the right to choose which type of treatment to use. Do Americans, living in a country founded on personal freedom and rights, have the right to choose which medical treatments to pursue? The government has answered this question with a resounding "no." The unproven hypothesis that chronic Lyme Disease is not a real condition has been accepted by the government as proven fact, and it has been decided by the government that you should also accept this unproven position as fact. The government not only believes that you should passively accept their conclusion—they also force you to do this by limiting your access to treatment. This is quite possibly one of the most un-American pronouncements in American history. According to the law, you have a right to freedom of medical choice, yet, according to the law, you cannot exercise that right.

It is a grave error and travesty that the regulatory agencies are attempting to curtail your freedom to choose medical treatment. According to the new IDSA guidelines, future Lyme Disease sufferers will only have access to, and will only be educated about, treatments and resources which are accepted and condoned *only by one side of the debate*. The mounting scientific evidence supporting the existence of chronic Lyme Disease combined with the overwhelming symptom reduction experienced when it is treated justifies chronic Lyme Disease treatment as a medical freedom which should be available to everyone, as it has been available for decades past.

Unfortunately, despite the efforts of patient activism groups and other voices for the cause, there is nothing to indicate that the government will soon change its stance on this issue. So, sufferers of chronic Lyme Disease have three choices: they can give up and remain sick, fight the uphill battle of attempting to secure treatment in the mainstream medical community, or take matters into their own hands and try to get well on their own.

The latter of these options is the approach this book takes. If the mainstream medical community is unwilling to provide assistance with the treatment of chronic Lyme Disease, we have no choice but to seek treatment elsewhere, on our own. Of course, it is still a valuable use of time to petition the government for a change in treatment policies. Due to the mounting evidence supporting the existence of chronic Lyme Disease, it is probable that the government will change its position eventually. However, in the meantime, sick people still want to get well. Given the desperate, debilitated condition that many chronic Lyme Disease sufferers are in and the constriction of medical freedoms currently taking place, there needs to be an immediate solution that is not dependent on changing government policies. Lyme sufferers must be made aware of both sides of the debate and educated about the full range of treatment options available.

To that end, this book was written. The treatments chosen for this book were selected because of their effectiveness, established by reports from patients using them, and available scientific research. However, a consideration of no less importance was the extent to which they allow patients to remain independent and make their own decisions. Most of the treatments in this book can be used autonomously, without a prescription from a physician, and without the government's permission. They are affordable with or without insurance. They are convenient and can be used whenever they are needed without advance planning. The therapies can be done at home, and the time and money required to make long trips to treatment clinics and doctors offices is spared. These treatment characteristics allow someone sick with Lyme Disease to still live a relatively normal life during the recovery process, without becoming a slave to doctors appointments, waiting rooms, and large medical bills. Most importantly, the treatments in this book allow you to circumvent the immutable decrees passed down from the medical powers that be. In short, this book presents therapies that you control.

In addition, most of the treatments presented in this book are relatively non-toxic. Although they are on the cutting edge of Lyme Disease research, the known side effects associated with their use are minimal. In fact, in comparison with most pharmaceutical drugs, the treatments in this book have a relatively low level of inherent risk. Many of the approaches presented do not use drugs at all. In the instances where drugs are presented as treatment options, drug doses are kept to a minimum, and breaks are recommended between courses of drugs.

A note of caution is in order to ensure that this message is not misinterpreted. If possible, sick people without medical training should still rely on a licensed physician before using any therapy. A trained doctor is a far better treatment supervisor than a layperson. The services of an LLMD are invaluable to the recovery process. Many LLMDs are still open for business and accept new patients. I am by no means suggesting that treating yourself based on the information in this book is a superior option to receiving professional medical care. However, with the future of LLMDs in question, and your medical freedom under fire, the point here—and the basis of this book—is simply that the final decision about your treatment should be made by you, not the government. This is called freedom. In a country where freedom is the cornerstone of our security and prosperity, this book offers you the freedom to research the available treatments for yourself and make your own decisions rather than blindly relying on what your government says is best for you.

What is Lyme Disease and why are new treatments needed?

Lyme Disease is a bacterial infection caused by Borrelia Burgdorferi, an elongated, spiral-shaped bacteria transmitted to humans through the bite of a tick. Known as spirochetes, these bacteria are unusual, not well studied, elusive and difficult to cultivate in the laboratory, and capable of advanced survival activities more commonly found in larger, more intelligent organisms.

Most Lyme Disease literature erroneously reports that Lyme Disease was first documented in Lyme, Connecticut, in the late 1970s. Actually, record of the infection dates back to 1883 when a German physician named Alfred Buchwald observed a degenerative skin condition which is presently hypothesized to have been a Lyme-related ailment. Subsequently in the United States, as early as 1920, physicians began correlating what are now known to be Lyme Disease symptoms with tick bites. By 1950, doctors had already discovered that antibiotic therapy provided relief for the symptoms in question. Although it was not until the 1970s that the disease got its name, evidence from various sources makes it apparent that Lyme Disease is much older than popularly believed.

First, the good news—in many cases of acute, recently acquired Lyme Disease, pharmaceutical antibiotics (the standard treatment of choice) are effective in completely eradicating the infection or at least, permanently alleviating symptoms. Someone who goes hiking or camping, gets bitten by a tick, and rushes to their doctor with a bull's-eye rash and flu-like symptoms has a chance of getting completely cured. The generally accepted rule is that if antibiotic therapy can be initiated within 24 hours of a tick bite, Lyme Disease is preventable.

Now, the bad news—there are dozens of reasons why it doesn't always happen this way. Unfortunately, the current mainstream medical procedures for diagnosing and treating Lyme Disease can fail at many points in the diagnosis and treatment process, leading to prolonged suffering and frustration. The odds are stacked high against people suffering from Lyme Disease. First we will examine obstacles in diagnosing Lyme Disease and then we will look at problems with current treatment practices.

OBSTACLES IN DIAGNOSIS

Despite the vast and increasing prevalence of Lyme Disease in the United States and other countries, many doctors are still not trained to look for the disease. Lack of training results from the misguided belief among mainstream medical colleges that Lyme Disease is actually not a prevalent, rapidly spreading infection but instead a rare and uncommon condition.

Some doctors will tell a sick person returning from a camping trip to take some Pepto-Bismol after diagnosing them with food poisoning from camping food. Other doctors will suggest Giardia, as a result of drinking contaminated stream water, and proclaim that the telltale bull's-eye rash is just a harmless insect bite or an allergic reaction to some grass or pollen or other irritant found in nature. Still other doctors will recommend watching symptoms for a few weeks to see if they improve on their own, after which time, if a person really had contracted Lyme Disease, antibiotic therapy would be too late anyway. If the bacteria are allowed to survive in the body unchallenged by antibiotic therapy for more than a couple days, treatment becomes much more complicated and protracted because the bacteria invade and colonize many organs and tissues. For this reason, early detection and treatment are critical—yet they often do not occur because Lyme Disease is not on the forefront of most physicians' minds.

If a physician is actually trained to look for Lyme Disease and he/she orders a Lyme Disease test, the next obstacle in the way of accurate diagnosis is the high probability of inaccurate, false-negative test results. As many as 60% of people infected with Lyme Disease will actually produce a negative test result! This can happen because the antigens and antibodies which the tests look for are not present (or at least not detectable) in the body during a large part of the bacterial life cycle. Therefore, anyone who receives a negative Lyme Disease test result in the presence of clinical symptoms should be suspicious and consider a therapeutic trial of Lyme Disease therapy, a procedure in which a person suspecting Lyme Disease is given a course of Lyme Disease treatment to see if clinical improvement results.

An additional problem with laboratory tests is the processing period. Because processing a Lyme Disease test can take a couple weeks, even if a positive result is received, it may be too late for antibiotic therapy to eradicate the infection.

Timing of symptom onset also contributes to missed diagnoses, even when dealing with a competent physician. Since symptoms often do not appear until several weeks or months after the infection is acquired, a person coming down with a mystery illness may not suspect Lyme Disease even if they vaguely remembered a tick bite, because there may be no apparent association between the tick bite and the new symptoms. This confusion makes it difficult for even a good physician to sort out what is going on.

To make matters worse, in many cases, symptoms of Lyme Disease may be delayed even longer than weeks or months. In some cases, symptoms may not appear until years after initial infection, leading to an even smaller probability of proper diagnosis. In addition, initial symptoms can be so subtle as to be mistaken for "growing pains" or "being out of shape". In these cases, tests would not even be ordered unless a shrewd physician or patient pieced together the puzzle. And, even if tests were ordered, the looming risk of a false-negative result creates more confusion.

New evidence has also identified other possible routes of transmission for the infection, including mother to child during pregnancy or breast-feeding, mosquito to human, and sexual intercourse. These routes of transmission are not recognized or acknowledged by most of mainstream medicine. This denial is in the face of glaring evidence to the contrary and is a cause for additional confusion when diagnosing Lyme Disease. Because some Lyme Disease sufferers have never spent much time outdoors, they will automatically be disqualified from Lyme Disease screening—even if, in reality, they are subject to other risk factors such as a mother with Lyme Disease.

Adding to the already stacked odds that a Lyme Disease sufferer will not be diagnosed properly is the elusive and variable nature of the disease presentation itself. Lyme Disease can and does manifest as dozens of different diseases and conditions which are conventionally believed to be incurable and unrelated to Borrelia Burgdorferi infection. Examples of such diseases include Parkinson's, ALS, depression, arthritis, chronic fatigue syndrome, fibromyalgia, Epstein-Barr virus, candida, schizophrenia, multiple sclerosis, obsessive-compulsive disorder, and others. Because of its ability to mimic so many seemingly unrelated conditions, Lyme Disease is known as the "great imitator." The ability for the disease to manifest in so many ways is a result of the spirochetes' capability of infecting each and every major organ system in the body. Unfortunately, most physicians do not suspect Lyme Disease when dealing with one of these other conditions even though, in a significant number of cases, Lyme Disease is the root cause.

As if the situation weren't bad enough already, many doctors do not acknowledge that Lyme Disease exists in more than a few isolated parts of the United States. Chances are a person with a newly acquired Lyme Dis-

Medical Proficiency: A Double-Edged Sword

Western medicine excels at diagnosis. We have MRIs, CT scans, x-rays, biopsies, echocardiograms, urine tests, hair tests, stool tests, and of course, hundreds of ways to test the blood.

You will not need to be convinced that Western medicine's ability to effectively diagnose saves lives. All of us have been, or know someone who has been, greatly helped by having a mysterious health ailment properly identified and labeled.

Unfortunately, however, our complete reliance on and blind faith in Western medical diagnosis can result in suffering equal and opposite to the healing we receive from it. Western medicine's proficiency in diagnosis is a double-edged sword: on one hand, it saves thousands of lives and contributes to an ever-increasing life expectancy, but on the other hand, its smashing success often leads to overconfidence in areas of less proficiency. If a diagnosis we receive is accidentally wrong, we may never find out because of our unwavering confidence in modern medicine. Most physicians will not help us challenge the verdict because they too have unshakable confidence in the ultimate proficiency of their profession.

Lyme Disease is one affliction which does not amiably submit to the diagnostic procedures of Western medicine. Many people who are actually suffering from a Lyme Disease infection are walking around in circles having been misdiagnosed with a plethora of seemingly unrelated health conditions which mimic Lyme Disease, including multiple sclerosis, obsessive-compulsive disorder, arthritis, fibromyalgia, schizophrenia, and many others.

If you or someone you know has a mystery disease, you should consider the possibility that it may actually be Lyme Disease—even if the mystery illness was diagnosed by a doctor and has an official label, and even if past Lyme Disease tests have produced negative results.

ease infection will encounter a physician who does not believe the disease is native to the area in which they live. In reality, Lyme Disease has been documented in every state in the United States and many countries throughout the world.

As you can see, diagnosing Lyme Disease is a complicated task. Having awareness of this complexity is the first step toward healing those suffering from this affliction and toward ensuring that future diagnostic procedures become more reliable.

OBSTACLES IN TREATMENT

The diagnosis process is unfortunately not the end of the obstacle field confronting Lyme Disease sufferers. Even if diagnosed early and accurately, a Lyme Disease sufferer faces sizable challenges in the treatment process.

Current antibiotic guidelines set forth by the Centers for Disease Control are vastly inadequate and based on antiquated, inaccurate, and unreliable data. While some people do get well by following these guidelines, a significant percentage do not. Many people remain sick despite a two or three week course of doxycycline or penicillin—the length and choice of antibiotic therapy which the Centers for Disease Control dogmatically and ignorantly insist is adequate treatment. Recent estimates suggest that up to 30% of Lyme Disease cases do not get resolved after following these CDC guidelines.

A preponderance of research establishing the necessity of extended courses of antibiotic therapy for the unlucky 30% has been completely ignored by medical regulatory agencies. As a result, symptoms and misery can continue for the unlucky 30% even though the "right treatment" was given. People who are still infected despite antibiotic therapy have what is referred to as chronic Lyme Disease. The chronic form of the disease is becoming an epidemic in the United States and abroad.

Or is it? A significant percentage of doctors and regulatory agencies do not recognize the existence of chronic Lyme Disease. The prevailing belief is that if someone has Lyme Disease and is treated with a several-weeklong course of antibiotics, they must, by definition, be cured. This belief fails to take into account the last 20 years of scientific research, as there have been numerous studies which evidence that Lyme Disease bacteria are often still present in the body even after antibiotic therapy. In fact, some studies show that common antibiotic regimens have very little effect on the bacterial infection.

Doctors and researchers who do not acknowledge chronic Lyme Disease have invented a bogus label for people who still have symptoms after a short course of antibiotics: "Post-Lyme Syndrome." Patients abused with this diagnosis are either told that nonliving bacterial toxins are keeping them ill, or worse, that remaining symptoms are psychiatric in nature and they should see a shrink who treats hypochondria and paranoia. So, many patients end up attempting to treat a raging bacterial infection with talk therapy. The truth is that chronic Lyme Disease is in fact a real condition, caused by an active bacterial infection, and largely disparaged by conventional medicine.

The conclusion that chronic Lyme Disease is not a valid medical condition is so preposterous, so irrational, so unscientific that one can't help but question whether the presiding research organizations are actually pursuing truth or instead, acting as puppets beholden to a political or medical agenda. There is simply too much research to ignore. And as time goes on, instead of behaving rationally and slowly examining new research and moving toward adoption of chronic Lyme Disease as a real condition, the regulatory agencies seem to be going in the opposite direction and becoming more adamant about their erroneous conclusions.

The doctors who recognize chronic Lyme Disease, and are willing to treat it, are few and far between. LLMDs use extended courses of very powerful antibiotics, sometimes in combinations of two or three drugs simultaneously, at much higher than FDA approved dosages, to try to help people with chronic Lyme Disease. Doctors who treat chronic Lyme Disease are heroes with good intentions, coming to the rescue when no one else will.

But even if patient and LLMD are able to connect, there are still additional obstacles. Unfortunately, LLMDs who do step out on a limb and actually try to help people with chronic Lyme Disease by reading the literature and implementing rational treatments are often persecuted, sued, disciplined by state medical boards, ridiculed, and at risk of losing their medical practice, as we have discussed in the previous section of the book. Increasing persecution and legal danger has led to the decision by many doctors not to treat Lyme Disease patients, or at least, to adhere to the inadequate treatment guidelines established by the government.

Although it is becoming increasingly perilous, many LLMDs are willing to brave the legal climate because some people with chronic Lyme Disease do recover by using extended courses of antibiotic therapy. In these cases, people who would have otherwise not recovered at all owe their lives to LLMDs. Offering hope to hopeless patients is the daily business of a Lyme Disease doctor.

Unfortunately, there are some very significant drawbacks to long-term antibiotic therapy. Patients receiving long-term antibiotic therapy often face grueling battles with insurance companies as a result of skyrocketing medical bills. Because official government standards indicate that only a short course of antibiotics is necessary in the treatment of Lyme Disease, many people are not able to get their extended treatment covered.

Another significant drawback to long-term antibiotic therapy is side effects. Because antibiotics are given in very high doses for long periods of time, side effects can be devastating. In some cases, the side effects can be worse than the disease. Many people end up with permanent damage to various organs caused by extended-course, high-dose antibiotic therapy.

The most significant drawback to long-term antibiotic therapy, though, is that it does not always work. The best antibiotics, given at high doses for months on end, often fail to eradicate the elusive and survival-oriented Lyme Disease bacteria. In these cases, symptom improvement can be fragile and relapses are common. "Open ended" antibiotic therapy is frequently required to keep some people stable. My first book, *Lyme Disease and Rife Machines*, has an in-depth explanation of exactly how and why antibiotics can fail.

The above treatment obstacles do not just exist in theory. The reality is that there are thousands of chronic Lyme sufferers who continuously live a miserable existence despite having attempted to get help from dozens of doctors.

As you can see, the situation can be quite hopeless. Lyme Disease sufferers are left to try to find answers on their own between doctors' appointments where they are given anything from a diagnosis of paranoia to an inadequate course of antibiotics to a denial of insurance coverage. At every step in the diagnosis and treatment process, Lyme Disease sufferers encounter an uphill battle which often leads to prolonged sickness, financial ruin, and unimaginable stress. Many Lyme Disease sufferers live their lives in complete despair, having tried every antibiotic under the sun without lasting relief.

The bottom line on diagnosing and treating Lyme Disease is that there are many ways to end up with the infection but not many ways to get rid of it. This, as you may have guessed by now, is why we need breakthrough therapies for Lyme Disease.

Now you can see why a book on new Lyme Disease treatments is useful. This book was written because there is a need for this book. People who have failed to get well by using aggressive antibiotic therapy, or people who wish to avoid aggressive antibiotic therapy, will find alternatives on the following pages. After reading about the alternatives, Chapter 11 will provide practical guidance on how to integrate them into a complete treatment plan. Although there is no easy cure for chronic Lyme Disease, there are valuable treatment options which have improved the lives of thousands of people and in some cases, provided complete remission of symptoms. Yet, many of these treatments remain largely unknown. Hopefully this book will change that.

Conventional vs. alternative medicine

In this day and age, you would have to live in a cave not to notice the raging battle between conventional and alternative medicine. Twenty years ago, alternative medicine was barely more than a casual club, not to be taken seriously, not solid enough to rely on for real health problems. Today, alternative medicine has gained acceptance and respect on a much larger scale, even among the mainstream media. What's more, many Americans are coming to actually trust alternative medicine more than conventional medicine, heading to the health food shop or acupuncturist before the family doctor.

Usually at odds with each other, conventional and alternative philosophies differ not only in how they treat disease, but also in their explanation of why disease develops in the first place. As the interest in and acceptance of alternative medicine continues to grow, so does the intensity of the debate. Advocates of both positions can be quite hostile to the other side. The debate has recently reached a boiling point, involving the passions, fears, biases, personal experiences—and let us not forget, financial interests—of those involved. Amidst the inferno, it has been largely forgotten that the goal of health care is not to establish exclusive, single-minded medical truths, but instead, to utilize all available medical treatments that cure disease—regardless of which paradigm they belong to.

The simple fact, irrespective of declarations by hotheads on either side of the debate, is that both conventional and alternative approaches have equal value in treating disease. Where conventional medicine fails, alternative medicine often succeeds, and vice versa. The most logical strategy for evaluating available treatments is to ignore whether a given therapy is conventional or alternative, and focus instead on whether or not it actually works. Alternative and conventional medicine should not be viewed as opposing forces but instead, teammates. No one should have to choose between a hammer and a screwdriver—each should be kept in the toolbox for the appropriate time and place—and so it should be with conventional and alternative medicine.

This philosophy is what separates this book from others on Lyme Disease treatment. Most available books side heavily with either conventional or alternative medicine. In contrast, this book doesn't care about the label of a given treatment—whether it be conventional or alternative—but instead, only, whether or not the treatment works. The effectiveness of numerous treatments was evaluated based on scientific research and hundreds of user reports, not passionate opinion or theoretical models of medicine.

It's a good thing both conventional and alternative medicine are available, too. The Lyme Disease infection is so pervasive and resistant that we need all available resources, not half of them. As you read this book, you will encounter a variety of approaches: antibiotics and herbs, drugs and nutrients, specialized and holistic. This balanced perspective is not just helpful when treating Lyme Disease, it is mandatory.

A specific example of how a balanced approach is played out in this book can be seen in how the book addresses the topics of treatment with antibiotics and treatment with rife machines. Common belief is that these two treatments are in direct opposition to each other, and in many ways they are. Antibiotics are a conventional treatment, while rife machines are an alternative treatment. Each treatment works by a completely different method of action. However, in this book, these two treatments are viewed as teammates instead of enemies. The book presents ways in which each treatment can be used to complement the other.

Doctors have a hard time successfully treating Lyme Disease because, especially in modern times, they are very specialized in what they do. Doctors are qualified experts in the narrow cross-section of medicine in which they were trained, board certified, and practice. Because the successful treatment of Lyme Disease requires a multifaceted and multidisciplinary approach, drawing on a broad range of medical resources, no single doctor is equipped to develop and implement a comprehensive treatment plan. That is why it is so difficult to obtain complete treatment from your physician. Some physicians are highly proficient in administering antibiotic therapy but are unaware of or unable to recommend rife machine therapy. Other physicians are experts in acupuncture but would not prescribe a drug if the patient's life depended on it. You get the point.

This book was written to evaluate, consolidate, and summarize the most effective conventional and alternative Lyme Disease treatments, drawing from a broad, interdisciplinary perspective, without regard to whether or not the given treatments are based in conventional or alternative medicine.

It's time to shift your paradigm

Because the immune system's normal responsibilities include fighting off dangerous infections, we get used to having the right to stay occupied with our lives while our body wards off our colds and flus. We go to work, go to the movies, watch TV, read the newspaper, and go about life's business when we are sick because we know that our trusty immune system will take care of the problem. If we get really sick with a bad flu or bronchitis or some other illness, we may take some "downtime" for sleep and chicken soup, but we do not typically go out of our way to help our body recover.

Get ready for a wake-up call! Lyme Disease is different than your average winter flu. Because Lyme Disease bacteria can effectively evade and defeat the human immune system, the infection can persist inside your body for months, years, and decades. This is what we refer to as chronic Lyme Disease. The bacteria are successful in short-circuiting immune system activities so you stay sick—even after taking antibiotics.

People with chronic Lyme Disease, if they want to actually get better, must step in and give their immune system a hand. Colonies of Lyme Disease bacteria entrenched deep in the body will not be eradicated by the efforts of the immune system alone. Strategically fighting the Lyme Disease infection must become a part of your daily routine just like brushing your teeth, walking the dog, making dinner, and going to work.

Thus illuminated is the reason many people do not recover from chronic Lyme Disease. Either they do not know that they must play an active part in defeating the infection, or they know this but are unwilling or unable to muster up the energy necessary.

At this point some readers will squirm in their seats with disappointment and dread at the prospect of having another obligation to squeeze into their already overloaded lives. "I just don't have the time or energy to actively participate in Lyme Disease treatment," many will be thinking. "Isn't there some magic pill I can take or something?"

No. There is no magic pill.

If you were expecting a book about 10 overnight cures for Lyme Disease, I am sorry to disappoint you. There is no such magic formula yet. To beat Lyme Disease, it will be necessary to adjust your current paradigm. I'm talking about the paradigm by which you assign value to your daily activities. Modern culture teaches us to be obsessively concerned with our exterior circumstances, obligations, image, and prestige, while ignoring our inner health (physically, psychologically, and spiritually).

We feverishly pursue a clean, well-maintained car, manicured yard, wrinkle free wardrobe and the next level of achievement at work. Not to mention our obsession with information—checking e-mail multiple times per day, reading the paper daily, watching our favorite television show (or recording it so we can watch it later).

In short, we don't lack the time to play an active role in the healing process, but we do lack discernment in how to spend our time. Is beating Lyme Disease and getting your health back more important than television? Or maybe you don't watch TV, maybe you occupy yourself with more dignified activities like golf or the stock market. Is recovering from Lyme Disease more important than these? Only you can answer this question. But the fact remains—if you want to get better, you will need to take action on a daily basis.

Fortunately, the time and energy it takes to actively participate in eradicating Lyme Disease from your body is not overwhelming or superhuman. It is feasible even if you have low energy and are very sick. Establishing a daily routine which includes anti-Lyme treatments and lifestyle activities requires only a few hours of thought and action per week. The treatments and routines in this book, while definitely requiring time and discipline, were chosen due to their unrivaled effectiveness but no less important, their convenience and affordability. Most of the treatments in this book can be done on your schedule, at home, in a short amount of time.

The first step to beating Lyme Disease is not a treatment or supplement. It is adjusting your paradigm and preparing yourself to actively participate in the recovery process. Beating Lyme Disease can be almost as easy as brushing your teeth and taking your car in for an oil change. The issue is more about you and your priorities, and less about whether or not the treatments are available.

The best treatment of the 10

I bet that got your attention! Let's just get down to business and talk about the most effective of the 10 treatments. Great idea, in theory. In reality, it is impossible.

For a long time, I believed that a single treatment could be identified and separated from the others as being "the" treatment. My experiences and communications with dozens of patients and practitioners, however, ultimately convinced me that at the present time, no such treatment can be singled out. There is a large amount of evidence indicating that rife machine therapy (Chapter 5) is the best treatment, but the fact remains that some Lyme Disease sufferers get more benefit from other therapies than they do from rife machine therapy.

There are several reasons why no single treatment can be identified as the best treatment. First, and most importantly, the Lyme Disease complex and associated co-infections cause numerous forms of dysfunction in the body. No single therapy currently in existence can address all of the problems created by Lyme Disease. For example, rife machine therapy successfully kills spirochetes and prevents the spread of the infection throughout the body, but it does not address certain hormonal imbalances that cause immune system dysfunction, nor does it attack the cell-wall-deficient form of the bacteria—only the Marshall Protocol can accomplish these two goals. Similarly, while the Marshall Protocol is tremendously beneficial, it does nothing to detoxify the body. Other therapies are necessary for detoxification, including exercise, saunas, liver detoxification therapies, etc. In the same way that a car cannot function without an engine, wheels, and a

steering wheel, Lyme Disease recovery typically requires multiple intercon-
nected treatments.

The second reason why no single therapy can be deemed best is that
each individual suffering from Lyme Disease experiences a slight (or sometimes profound) difference in how the disease presents and manifests.
Variation in the disease can be due to numerous factors. Although we do
not know precisely why Lyme Disease can manifest so differently among
different individuals, we do have a few solid explanations:

1. There are many different types of Lyme Disease bacteria, and possibly even other types of bacteria capable of establishing infection in
   the body that mimic Lyme Disease bacteria. Each of these different
   types of bacteria may be susceptible to completely different methods of antibacterial therapy.

2. Current Lyme Disease tests do not offer 100% accurate results. In
   fact, the accuracy of Lyme Disease tests may be as poor as 50%.
   Therefore, determining exactly what is causing symptoms is part
   science and part speculation. So, people who think they have Lyme
   Disease may in fact have some other problem that requires different
   treatment.

3. Different people, with different body chemistries and different genetic constitutions, may respond differently to chronic infection.
   Biochemical changes in the body as a result of infection most likely
   vary significantly between individuals. Therefore, the appropriate
   biochemical interventions may also vary between individuals.

4. Concomitant health problems in people suffering from Lyme Disease are most certainly different. For example, some Lyme Disease
   sufferers are also affected by obesity or diabetes. Others may have
   mercury poisoning or co-infections. These variations in accompanying health disorders change the way people respond and react to
   various treatments.

5. The people affected by Lyme Disease live in very different climates
   and environments. Some people live in brand-new houses at high

elevation. Others live in older houses at lower elevation. Variations in climate and living environment mean very significant differences in nutrients and toxins to which the body is exposed. There is more oxygen available at lower elevations, and less at higher elevations. Newer homes expose people to different synthetic toxins than older homes. Some homes are infested with toxic mold, while others are not. These environmental variations quite possibly have a profound effect on how Lyme Disease manifests, and consequently, the treatments that work best.

6. Co-infections, such as Ehrlichia, Babesia, and Bartonella, can have a tremendous impact on the overall disease picture. Resent research has shown that up to 90% of people infected with Borrelia Burgdorferi (the causative Lyme Disease bacteria) may also be harboring co-infections, which may have been acquired at the time of the tick bite along with Borrelia Burgdorferi (ticks are hosts to many types of pathogenic microbes, not just one). Since the recovery process stagnates if co-infections are not detected and treated, it is critical that every Lyme Disease sufferer address co-infections—please do not miss this important point. An LLMD is an essential resource and can help you deal with co-infections.

These are only a few examples of variables that can lead to differing responses to Lyme Disease treatment. The bottom line is that what works for one person does not always work for another. The problem is not that available treatments are lacking, but instead, that each person with Lyme Disease has different needs. While one person may be cured by a certain treatment, another person may not see results, or worse, may be made sicker by the treatment.

These principles came into undeniable focus in mid-2006, while I was researching to write this book, when a research partner and I engaged in a debate about the benefits and risks of two different Lyme Disease treatments: the Marshall Protocol and the Salt / Vitamin C protocol (both presented in this book as top treatments).

Why Are The Treatments In This Book More Beneficial Than Other Lyme Disease Treatments?

Well, it depends on what your definition of "beneficial" is. You're probably thinking, "that's simple, 'beneficial' refers to a treatment's ability to kill Lyme Disease bacteria." Unfortunately, it's not that simple. Although killing Lyme Disease bacteria is important, and should even be considered the core of any anti-Lyme treatment protocol, there are other factors to consider. Does the treatment have side effects? Is it affordable? Is it convenient? Due to the long treatment time frame in eradicating chronic Lyme Disease, affordability, convenience, and lack of toxicity are extremely high priorities.

Various exotic therapies available in specialized clinics across the world may provide a more acute, intense antibacterial effect than the therapies in this book. IV antibiotics may accomplish this as well. However, based on extensive experience and research, these types of treatments usually do not lead to long-term healing. The treatments that provide long-term progress are those that can be done little by little, in the privacy of your home, over the course of months or years, to slowly and consistently reduce bacterial load and change the biological terrain in the body. This requires a different kind of Lyme Disease treatment—one that is gentle, holistic, effective, and sustainable—not a short-term, expensive, intense treatment. Such therapies comprise the top 10 treatments in this book.

Also, killing bacteria is not the only task to be accomplished. Detoxification and immune system support are very important, as is preventing Lyme Disease bacteria from converting to dormant, entrenched forms. Hormonal issues must be addressed. Killing bacteria is only the beginning. Again, various clinics in the United States, Europe, and Mexico offer intense "balancing" and "detoxifying" programs, participation in which typically requires thousands of dollars and a several-weeklong stay at a clinic. However, balancing and detoxifying the body is not something that can happen overnight. Results attained at fancy clinics are typically short-lived. True results come from long-term lifestyle changes and therapeutic modalities that can be conveniently and affordably integrated into daily life. Developing a sustainable, long-term treatment strategy is far more effective than using a quick-fix, overnight cure. One Lyme Disease researcher said accurately that recovering from Lyme Disease is a marathon, not a sprint.

So, a successful Lyme Disease treatment campaign has two foundational tenets. First, it must include not only bacterial load reduction, but also detoxification, immune system support, and other cooperative healing modalities—and these tasks must be accomplished effectively and efficiently. Second, a successful Lyme Disease treatment program must be sustainable (convenient, affordable, and non-toxic) for long-term use.

The 10 therapies selected for this book are based on these criteria, and that is what sets them apart from other more common, less valuable approaches to treating Lyme Disease.

My research partner expressed the belief that the Salt / Vitamin C protocol is superior to the Marshall Protocol in terms of safety and effectiveness. I, on the other hand, tend to conclude the opposite. Both of us arrived at the conclusions we did based on our own personal experiences with the protocols, scientific evidence we have encountered, and communication with dozens of Lyme Disease sufferers.

I consider this research partner to be one of the most knowledgeable experts in the field of Lyme Disease treatment. Debates such as these are the fuel that powers the fire of innovation, ultimately leading to newer and better paradigms in Lyme Disease treatment. Yet, as our friendly debate unfolded, I became increasingly shocked by the fact that our conclusions could be so different. In the past, we had seen eye to eye on so many issues. So what happened here? Why the not-so-small discrepancy?

It would be easy to conclude that one of us is simply wrong, and the other right. And, this may in fact be the case. However, in my opinion, available evidence indicates that we are both right and both wrong. Some Lyme Disease sufferers experience dramatic improvement with the Marshall Protocol and do not experience the same benefits with the Salt / Vitamin C protocol, while other Lyme sufferers experience the opposite. In addition, some Lyme sufferers actually say they were harmed by the Marshall Protocol, while others say they were harmed by the Salt / Vitamin C protocol. Further, some Lyme Disease sufferers experience benefit from *both* protocols. These statements are not just speculation, they are based on actual reports from real Lyme Disease sufferers.

The only logical conclusion is that both protocols are intrinsically valuable. Each addresses a different component of the Lyme Disease complex, and therefore neither protocol could replace the other. Since every Lyme Disease sufferer has different circumstances and a different disease presentation, the value of each protocol will be different for each individual. It is inaccurate to conclude that one therapy is better than the other. For a *specific* individual, one of the two therapies may hold comparatively greater benefit. But for the entire population of Lyme Disease sufferers, comparative benefit cannot be established. This is why my research partner and I drew such different conclusions about the same treatments and the same disease.

Another example of individuality in treatment effectiveness can be seen with sauna therapy. There has been an intense debate about which type of sauna is more beneficial: dry heat or far infrared. Proponents of both types of sauna are absolutely convinced that their type is most effective. It requires a shift in thought process to get to the bottom of the issue; the reality is that neither type of sauna is "better" than the other. Instead, the preferred method of sauna therapy depends on individual tolerance and results. For some people, far infrared saunas provide better results, but for other people, dry heat saunas are more suited. The key here is to recognize the importance of individual differences. This dynamic is not limited to sauna therapy but is equally applicable to all facets of Lyme Disease therapy from antibacterial modalities to deoxidization to supplementation.

What does this mean to you? It means that a book can only take you so far. Books are written for the masses. You are an individual. No book can possibly have perfectly accurate information for every individual. This book can help you narrow down the field of available treatments to a handful of highly beneficial options. But you must adapt and modify the information in this book to your own individual circumstances. Your own intuition, logic, detailed records / treatment diary, and other personal tools will ultimately determine your course of action. You have to read this book through the lense of personal knowledge of your body and circumstances. In most cases, identifying your individual needs can only be accomplished via trial and error, so you will be doing a lot of that.

In addition, you should employ a trusted physician to help you navigate through the waters of available Lyme Disease treatments. Not only should your selected physician be intelligent and up-to-date on the latest treatment options, he/she should also be willing to spend the time and thoughtful energy necessary to provide you with a one-one-one relationship in which the two of you are able to develop a truly individualized, customized, and targeted treatment plan. Your physician/patient discussions should include more than just which Lyme Disease therapies to use. These discussions should also address other unique aspects of your situation, including other health problems you may be dealing with, co-infections (such as Babesia or Bartonella), possible mercury toxicity, candida, emotional stressors, indoor mold exposure, etc. Dr. James Schaller refers to this type of one-on-one connection as an 'augmented' patient/physician relationship. Physicians willing to participate in the lengthy office meetings necessary to build a customized treatment plan are few and far between, so you may need to search for a while in order to locate one.

In the future, as additional research is conducted in Lyme Disease treatment, comparative effectiveness of different protocols may become less ambiguous, and individualized treatment plans may be less necessary. However, that may never happen. Time will tell. In the meantime, each Lyme Disease sufferer must still move forward and decide which treatments to use, taking into account individualized circumstances and needs. This point cannot be overlooked as you start contemplating and developing your own treatment plan. Do not take a cookbook, one-size-fits-all approach, but instead, be flexible and open to variations in treatment models.

Time: The treatment of all treatments

With all that said, if I were forced to choose one treatment that stands out above the others (even with recognition of the need for individualized treatment planning), it would be *time*. Is time a treatment, you ask? Yes, it is. It has been said that "Time heals all wounds." With regard to Lyme Disease recovery, that famous statement is more than just a figure of speech—it is a reality. Over time, assuming that you use some of the right treatments and avoid most of the wrong treatments, you will get better and better and better. Time is the currency by which Lyme Disease treatment is measured. Recovering from chronic Lyme Disease typically takes from 6 months to 5 years.

Why is the recovery process so long? The best answer is simply that at the present time, Lyme Disease remains a very difficult illness to beat. While the treatments in this book often do lead to substantial healing progress, their downfall is that they require a lot of time. If given enough time, in my opinion, remission from Lyme Disease is possible in even the worst cases. But unfortunately, success is not possible in a short period of time. Some of the specific reasons for the long recovery process include:

1. Every effective Lyme Disease treatment relies to some extent on the bacterial lifecycle process. Most bacterial infections that humans acquire, such as strep throat, have very short lifecycles (1 minute to 10 days), so effective treatment can be accomplished in a short amount of time. Lyme Disease bacteria, on the other hand, have a very long lifecycle. Medical textbooks describe the Lyme Disease lifecycle as being between three and 30 days long. New research indicates that some parts of the lifecycle are six months to a year long, or even longer. Because successful treatment requires passing through at least several bacterial lifecycles, the healing process can require several years. One of the components of the long bacterial lifecycle is the process by which cyst-form bacteria convert to active, spirochete-form bacteria, which can be quite drawn out.

2. Lyme Disease bacteria group together inside the body in dense colonies. In some cases, lone bacteria may be isolated and infect cells of the body in low numbers, but in most cases, the bacteria form tightly-packed colonies that have multiple layers of bacteria. Treatments in use at any given time will only affect outside layers of bacterial colonies, while inside layers remain safe and shielded. This is one of the characteristics of Lyme Disease that make it so insidious and treatment-resistant. Because bacteria group together in colonies that have multiple layers, Lyme Disease treatment is similar to peeling layers off an onion—or more accurately, peeling layers off a Lyme Disease colony. It takes time to remove each layer, and a full recovery is only possible after all layers of colonies have been removed. In theory, it may be possible to utilize a treatment that kills the entire colony at one time. However, there are a few serious obstacles that stand in the way of such an approach:

    a. First, such a treatment would likely be so toxic that it kills or causes severe damage to the patient him/herself. For example, extremely high temperatures (140° F and above) are known to degrade entire bacterial colonies, but obviously these temperatures would also kill a human being. Mildly increasing body temperature (i.e., to 100° F), while safe for the patient and somewhat helpful for killing bacteria, is not sufficient to eradicate entire colonies. Similarly, certain poisons or drugs at high doses may wipe out entire colonies but would also wipe out the patient.

b. Second, killing Lyme Disease bacteria results in herx reactions caused by circulating bacterial byproducts which lead to symptoms of immune system activation and inflammation. In moderation, these reactions are tolerable and even help the recovery process. In excess, they can be very dangerous or even fatal. If all the bacteria in the body were killed at one time, the resultant herx reaction may be so intense as to kill the patient.

3. Part of the reason that the Lyme Disease infection is able to persist chronically in the body is that conditions in the body are favorable to chronic infection. Toxicity, compromised immunity, obesity, poor diet, excessive stress, inadequate exercise, and other factors can lead to decreased ability for the body to ward off dangerous bacterial infections. "Bioterrain" is the word that describes the tissues throughout the body with respect to their affinity for accumulating toxins and harboring infections. Healthy bioterrain has a low level of toxicity, sufficient oxygen transport, healthy blood flow, and balanced immune activity. Lyme Disease bacteria will have a much more difficult time establishing infection in healthy bioterrain. In contrast, unhealthy bioterrain is characterized by low oxygen supply, deranged immune function, poor circulation, and the presence of dangerous, immunosuppressive toxins (such as mercury). Chronic bacterial infections thrive amid unhealthy bioterrain. To eliminate chronic Lyme Disease, unhealthy bioterrain must be converted to healthy bioterrain. This process does not happen overnight. It requires extensive and committed lifestyle changes and lots of time. Diet must be cleaned up, detoxification must be undertaken, an exercise program must be utilized, and various other

steps must take place. A speedy recovery from Lyme Disease is difficult (if not impossible) due to the slow process by which unhealthy bioterrain is converted to healthy bioterrain.

As you can see, there are some very profound reasons why the Lyme Disease recovery process is long. In the future, medical research may lead to a faster solution. History has taught that difficult challenges in treating disease can be obliterated as the result of a single breakthrough or discovery. Hopefully, such a discovery will occur in our lifetimes and render the Lyme Disease recovery process much shorter. Until this happens, the long recovery process is simply an unavoidable reality. This lengthy recovery process can be expected regardless of which anti-Lyme therapies you choose to use.

Instead of asking the pie-in-the-sky question of how we can shrink the recovery process from several years down to a couple weeks, it is more realistic for us to ask how we can optimize treatment planning and utilization to take as much time off the process as possible, and to make the process as convenient, comfortable, and affordable as possible. These are some of the goals of this book. The aim is not to replace the treatment guidelines set forth in my first book, but instead, to optimize and enhance them, with the ultimate goal of reducing the recovery time frame as much as possible and minimizing symptoms along the way. A friend and fellow research partner would always refer to the goal of shortening the recovery time as "shortening the runway."

It is important not to overlook the significance of time in healing chronic Lyme Disease. It takes the body a long time to develop chronic illness, and it will take a long time for the illness to be healed. Understanding and accepting the lengthy recovery process will prevent you from becoming discouraged. Additionally, because the recovery process is often not smooth but instead turbulent (much like a roller coaster ride), it is even more valuable to understand this at the outset. Seasonal symptom flareups are common (especially in spring and fall) and if these are not expected, they can be cause for doubt, discouragement, and undue stress.

Is there hope for someone with chronic Lyme Disease?

Yes. However, this can be a difficult question to answer for a couple reasons. First, it must be determined whether or not the person in question actually has chronic Lyme Disease. Second, the general health of the person in question must also be taken into account.

In many cases, Lyme Disease tests actually do more harm than good. Because these tests are often inaccurate, test results can point someone in the wrong direction. For example, many people who actually do have chronic Lyme Disease will get a negative test result. These people, if they do not seek alternate means of diagnosing the infection (such as a therapeutic probe of Lyme Disease treatment), may spend many years hopelessly searching for another diagnosis. Many of these people will never pick up this book because they do not believe they have Lyme Disease. Suffering will continue. These people, unfortunately, may never get well.

Conversely, there are instances where someone receives a positive Lyme Disease test result, yet does not actually have Lyme Disease. How is this possible? Such a person may have come in contact with the bacteria in the past, causing a positive test result (most Lyme tests have a difficult time differentiating between exposure to and infection with the bacteria), yet current symptoms may actually be caused by something other than Lyme Disease bacteria. Or, this person may have Lyme Disease bacteria in their body, but other problems may be causing the majority of their symptoms. We typically only focus on instances when someone is misdiagnosed with a condition that mimics an underlying case of Lyme Disease. However, the opposite can also happen: people are sometimes diagnosed with Lyme Disease when the real problem is something else. In these cases, recovery may be difficult due to inaccurate diagnoses.

So, the question of whether or not there is hope depends largely on an accurate diagnosis. It is critical that the treatments a person chooses are the correct treatments for their actual health problem. If properly diagnosed, there is hope. If improperly diagnosed (either with Lyme Disease or something else), there is not hope until an accurate diagnosis is found.

If we assume that a person is diagnosed accurately, then the next factor we must look at is the general state of health. Obviously, someone sick with Lyme Disease is in a poor state of health due to the bacterial infection. But that is not what we are talking about here. We are talking about other health factors such as:

- Obesity.

- Unhealthy habits such as smoking, excessive alcohol consumption, poor diet, etc.

- A compromised immune system due to the above unhealthy habits or other causes such as toxic exposure, old-age, other illnesses, etc.

- Inadequate or nonexistent exercise habits.

- Inadequate sleep.

- Unhealthy living environment, i.e., toxic materials in the home.

- Other diseases such as cancer, co-infections, genetic disorders, etc.

The human body itself is ultimately what provides the resources to defeat Lyme Disease. The immune system must engage to fight, and win, the battle. Yes, it is true that various antibacterial and supportive therapies are necessary to nudge the process along—thus the necessity and usefulness of this book. But the bottom line is that the treatments in this book are only useful to the extent that they support the primary healing process which is controlled by the immune system.

This is why it is so important to the healing process that the sick person support and strengthen their body during recovery. Anti-Lyme treatments will not do any good unless the body is prepared to step in and take over the fight. People who have had unhealthy habits throughout their entire life will have a much more difficult time beating Lyme Disease in comparison with those who have taken care of their bodies. People who have been victims of other circumstances beyond their control—cancer, genetic disorders, etc.—may also have a more difficult time defeating Lyme Disease. Unhealthy habits and other negative circumstances can be overcome, but doing so is challenging. People who are not willing to abandon bad habits and adopt a healthy lifestyle may have difficulty recovering.

As you can see, the question of whether or not there is hope for chronic Lyme sufferers is complicated. If someone actually does have chronic Lyme and not some other problem, and if this person takes care of their body and supports their immune system in the healing process, then there definitely is hope. However, if someone mistakenly believes they have Lyme Disease but actually has some other problem, and/or if someone's immune system is not capable of stepping up to fight the infection, then hope for recovery is limited.

The pill panacea

Modern medicine has an obsession with oral treatments, i.e., pills or liquids you swallow. Most popular medical treatments in both conventional and alternative paradigms involve swallowing pills or substances. Be it herbs, antibiotics, anti-inflammatory drugs, vitamins—the route of delivery is the mouth.

In many cases this is the logical way to heal the body—after all, as humans, we do receive nourishment from food and water by swallowing. Our digestive systems are ideal for distributing healing substances throughout the body via blood. Using the oral route of distribution for medical treatments is also very convenient and practical. This is obvious when one considers the many financial and lifestyle-related disadvantages of treatments delivered intravenously.

Treatments using the oral route of distribution are certainly valuable. Unfortunately, though, the money-driven modern medical paradigm has leveraged the ease and practicality of oral treatments into a pill panacea. In addition to the reasonable and health-focused advantages of pills, they are also easy to manufacture, sell, prescribe, and take. Pills are good business.

The pill panacea has rendered many other valuable, non-oral treatments unknown and obsolete. Examples of ignored non-oral treatments include saunas, exercise, and rife machines, to name a few. Remember, even alternative health care practitioners need to make a living and often sell not only their consultation services, but also various bottles of stuff. Alternative medicine magazines are jampacked with colorful, compelling advertisements for the latest supplement, herbal energy booster, antioxidant formula, etc. As is the case with rife machines, exercise, and saunas, many extremely beneficial, yet low-profit therapies remain secrets, inconspicuously tucked away from consumer consciousness.

While some oral treatments are highly beneficial, the simple fact is that they are not enough to eradicate a stubborn and insidious Lyme Disease infection. Even powerful pharmaceutical antibiotics often do not get the job done. The five core treatment protocols discussed in this book were chosen not based on their profitability, but instead, their effectiveness. Some of these therapies are very difficult to profit from so you will not find them in commercial medicine. Several of the therapies do not utilize the oral route. The advantage of reading this book is that you will gain a perspective untainted by profitability considerations. The only considerations given heed were those relating to effectiveness.

Part I:

The 5 Core
Treatment Protocols

Introduction to the five core treatment protocols

M any cases of early-stage Lyme Disease are resolved with standard, conventionally prescribed antibiotic therapy. Hence, the following 5 treatment protocols are intended for use only in cases of chronic Lyme Disease where previous antibiotic treatment has failed or provided unsatisfactory results. Pharmaceutical antibiotics as routinely prescribed by an LLMD are the first line of defense against Lyme Disease.

The following five breakthrough treatment protocols greatly differ from each other and represent cross-sections from several medical paradigms. Antibiotic therapy is based on the paradigm of using pharmaceutical technology to kill the bacteria. The Marshall Protocol relies on pharmaceutical antibiotics and also endeavors to create functional and hormonal changes in the body. The Salt / Vitamin C protocol is based on the paradigm of using adjusted quantities of natural nutrients to create an unfavorable environment for infections. Detoxification is based on the paradigm of reducing the toxic burden in a Lyme Disease sufferer's body. Rife machine therapy is based on the paradigm of electromedicine and coordinative resonance.

In writing this book, protocols of vastly differing ideology were chosen intentionally. Because of the hardiness and incredible survival ability of Lyme Disease bacteria, a multifaceted approach is necessary to beat the disease. In fact, Lyme Disease is such an ominous and difficult problem that recovery often *requires* the best of everything medicine has to offer: conventional and alternative, Eastern and Western, nutrition and exercise, rest and activity. You will probably find that use of one or two of these protocols is not enough—most people end up needing several or all of them over the course of their recovery process.

The simple fact is that Lyme Disease affects the body in numerous ways, and no single treatment can address the totality of the disease. Each breakthrough therapy chosen for this book focuses on a specific aspect of the Lyme Disease complex which other protocols are unable to address. In this way, while each therapy alone is merely beneficial, the sum of all of them amounts to a very powerful weapon for ousting the bacterial infection from the body. When integrated as part of a coordinated, organized protocol, these therapies are unrivaled in their ability to reverse chronic Lyme Disease. In Chapter 11, strategies for integrating these protocols will be discussed.

The 5 core protocols in Part I are intended to be the foundation of a Lyme Disease treatment program. The supportive supplements in Part II are not powerful enough to be used as core therapies, but instead, should be used in support of the core protocols.

You will notice that, throughout the book, rife machine therapy is frequently referenced. This is because, according to extensive research, rife machine therapy is the most important core treatment protocol. It provides continual bacterial load reduction and allows the other therapies to work synergistically with each other. Rife machine therapy should be used throughout the recovery process as the foundational treatment.

Chapter 1:
The Antibiotic
Rotation Protocol

Introduction to rational antibiotic use

T he Antibiotic Rotation Protocol describes a method by which antibiotics can be used effectively and safely. Before we examine how to use the protocol, let's begin with some background information.

You may have already begun to notice seemingly contradictory statements in my books (and elsewhere in the Lyme Disease community) about pharmaceutical antibiotics. Are they good or bad? Should they be avoided or used? Do you need breakthrough therapies *beyond* antibiotics or *including* antibiotics?

Are antibiotics your best friend or your worst enemy?

The answer is both. Pharmaceutical antibiotics can be your best friend *or* your worst enemy. This is true in the same sense that food can be both beneficial and harmful. Food is necessary to sustain your life but can also put it at risk. What determines whether food is good or bad for you is very simple: how much you eat and what you eat.

Antibiotics, in the much same way, can be either good or bad for treating Lyme Disease, depending on how much you use and which types you choose. Many common approaches to treating chronic Lyme Disease with antibiotics are analogous to eating a whole chocolate cake in one sitting instead of smaller portions of nutritious foods in several sittings. In other words, Lyme Disease doctors frequently choose the wrong type of antibiotic and use entirely too much of it. In this way, antibiotics become your worst enemy.

Antibiotics can, however, be your best friend if they are used rationally and carefully. This chapter discusses novel and creative ways to include appropriate antibiotics in a treatment protocol. Because successful antibiotic use depends on the type chosen and the amount taken, this chapter also includes a description of some of the best (and worst) antibiotics currently available, as well as a few simple tips for using them. But before we talk about the benefits of antibiotic therapy, let's look at some of the poor methodologies that often cause antibiotics to be your worst enemy.

Antibiotic treatment that employs poor methodology (i.e., that which administers wrong doses of the wrong type of antibiotic) is usually based on invalid or false assumptions. First we will examine these assumptions and then see how and why they lead to poor methodology in the treatment of Lyme Disease.

The first false assumption made by many Lyme Disease doctors is that conventional antibiotic therapy alone is the only hope for curing or controlling chronic Lyme Disease. Even if doctors recommend nutritional supplements, exercise, and rest, typically they still believe that pharmaceutical antibiotics are the only way back to health. Evidence of this assumption is the fact that standard treatment for chronic Lyme Disease prescribed by most LLMDs includes extensive, continuous, high-dose antibiotic therapy. The assumption on which such treatment is based is often false, and results frequently in limited benefit because chronic Lyme Disease is not always treated successfully with antibiotics alone. In some cases, it is treated successfully, however, in many cases, it is not.

Some people would say success occurs quite often; however, we must look at the definition of "success." In many cases, so called "success" is achieved only by using pharmaceutical antibiotics continuously and indefinitely, in toxically high doses, to maintain fragile improvement in symptoms. If antibiotic therapy is discontinued, a relapse often occurs, and the "success" ends. (It should be noted, also, that co-infections—specifically Babesia and Bartonella—can be a cause for continued sickness despite antibiotic therapy, as can other factors such as mercury poisoning, mold toxin exposure, and other co-factors.)

The problem is that antibiotics become increasingly toxic the longer they are used. If continued use of antibiotics is required to maintain improvement, toxic side effects can reach damaging and life-threatening levels. It is simply not practical to continue conventional antibiotic treatment indefinitely. This very typical treatment methodology is not truly successful—it is an adulterated form of symptom relief which is unsustainable and will eventually lead to a collapse of health. Extended antibiotic use brings only superficial and very vulnerable success, what some might call "hanging on by a thin thread."

The second false assumption is the belief that if antibiotics fail to provide satisfactory results, the best course of action is simply to use more antibiotics. If treatment fails, instead of exploring other treatment approaches, Lyme Disease doctors often will prescribe more antibiotics for a longer period of time. This is not a solution to the problem of antibiotic-refractory Lyme Disease. It is instead an amplification of the same futile approach that did not work in the first place. And, this approach leads to even more dangerous side effects. Doctors often do not recognize the limitations of antibiotics. In defense of Lyme Disease doctors, it should be noted that many of the alternative therapies discussed in this book are not FDA approved, so it may not even be an option for doctors to prescribe these therapies.

The third faulty assumption is that the Lyme Disease bacterium (Borrelia Burgdorferi) is adequately susceptible to pharmaceutical antibiotics. In actuality, Borrelia Burgdorferi exists in three different morphologic forms (and is capable of shifting from one form to another as the environment changes), each having different characteristics and vastly different vulner-abilities. Two of the bacterial forms are active and symptom-producing: the spirochete (a spiral shaped pathogen with an outer cell wall) and the cell-wall-deficient form (sometimes referred to as variant or L-form) with no cell wall. The third bacterial form is dormant and not symptom-producing: the cyst form, an irregular, compact ball with a dense outer capsule that makes it completely resistant and impenetrable to most envi-ronmental threats (including antibiotics). Spirochetes and cell-wall-deficient bacteria are somewhat susceptible to antibiotics. Cysts have very little susceptibility. None of the three forms are *adequately* susceptible. In fact, studies have shown that Lyme Disease bacteria can survive exposure to high concentrations of different types of antibiotics. Since antibiotics cause Lyme Disease bacteria to rapidly convert to the near-invincible cyst form, antibiotics can have a self-limiting effect.

Complicating the reality that Lyme Disease bacteria are not adequately susceptible to antibiotics is the fact that this bacteria often clumps together in densely packed colonies. Although the outer layers of the colonies are exposed to antibiotics circulating in the bloodstream, the deeper, inner layers are protected. So, not only can Lyme Disease bacteria survive expo-sure to antibiotics, a significant amount of the bacteria is never even faced with the threat due to the protective effects of the colonial structure.

The fourth false assumption is that a symptom-free state indicates that the bacterial load has been eradicated (or, at least, is under control). The truth quite often is that patients who achieve a symptom-free state by using antibiotics are in fact still harboring Lyme Disease bacteria. Antibiotic treatment sparks the conversion of Borrelia Burgdorferi from active spiro-chete or cell-wall-deficient forms to dormant cyst form as the bacteria go into survival mode to escape antibiotic activity. Symptoms have disap-peared not because the bacteria have been killed, but because they now exist in the inactive, asymptomatic, and highly resistant, cyst form.

This phenomenon is seen quite clearly in the experience of Lyme Dis-ease sufferers who, believing themselves cured, discontinue antibiotics only to experience a dramatic and complete relapse of symptoms. The relapse occurs because the antibiotic resistant and dormant cyst form of the bacteria reverts back into the active spirochete and cell-wall-deficient forms once antibiotics are discontinued. Relapses typically are not gradual—symptoms of a relapse do not begin mildly and slowly increase over time. Instead, relapses are often immediate and violent, with symptoms shifting overnight from nonexistent to debilitating. This quick transition between remission and relapse happens because remission was not attained by eradicating the bacteria. It was attained by the antibiotics having forced massive quantities of bacteria into dormancy. When these large numbers of dormant bacteria activate, symptoms are immediately present again. The absence of symptoms does not indicate the absence of bacteria. (It should be noted that an additional reason for immediate, violent relapses is the presence of co-infections).

Another reason that a symptom-free state does not always indicate that the bacteria are eradicated is the fact that antibiotics lead to symptom relief not just because of their antibacterial properties, but also their anti-inflammatory properties. In some cases, even when the bacterial infection is still present, antibiotics can reduce symptoms of inflammation so effectively that the disease may appear to have gone into remission.

All of the above faulty assumptions result in poor methodology when using antibiotics to treat Lyme Disease. Doctors who base therapy on these assumptions typically prescribe indefinite courses of antibiotics at dangerously high doses (even when it is clear that antibiotics are not working) because they simply do not know of any better option. If better, more effective treatment options were made known and became widely available, Lyme Disease doctors would undoubtedly stop using toxic doses of pharmaceutical antibiotics in extended courses—these doctors want the best for their patients and they really do believe that the therapy they prescribe is the best course of action in treating Lyme Disease. No sane doctor would use antibiotics for months on end unless they really believed the reward outweighed the potential risks.

As a consequence of basing clinical practices on invalid assumptions, chronic Lyme Disease treatment has gained the reputation of being extremely unpleasant and even dangerous as people fall victim to the unfortunate side effects of extended antibiotic use: raging Candida infections, loss of gallbladder function (due to IV Rocephin), elevated liver enzymes or liver damage, dangerously low white blood cell counts, and vision damage (after taking Plaquenil, an antibiotic commonly used to treat Lyme Disease). These are only a few of the side effects of long-term antibiotic therapy. There are many others. Sadly, even after undergoing extensive antibiotic treatment and enduring its adverse effects, many Lyme Disease sufferers still remain infected.

Of course, many people do get well by using long-term, high-dose antibiotic therapy. So, such therapy is not always considered poor methodology. However, as time goes on, an increasing number of Lyme sufferers are reporting that long-term, high-dose antibiotic therapy does not lead to a cure and may in fact have devastating side effects. If long-term, high-dose antibiotic therapy has yielded positive results for you, then you should feel encouraged! The goal is, of course, to get well; and if you are getting well, there is no need to change what you are doing. However, if you are one of the many people who were not cured with long-term, high-dose antibiotic therapy, then this chapter may be particularly helpful to you.

Fortunately, there are some great alternatives to extended, high-dose antibiotic therapy. Adjusting our assumptions and reevaluating Lyme Disease pathology opens the door to a whole new world of treatment options. Ironic as it may seem, the antibiotics that may have been your worst enemy under the circumstances described above are actually part of the solution. Amidst the fray of ghastly chronic Lyme Disease treatment practices, it is surprisingly true that, of all the tools in the Lyme Disease treatment toolbox, antibiotics are among the most helpful—if they are used rationally and moderately. One of the core discoveries upon which this book is based is that antibiotics are not ineffective, but instead are very powerful and potentially beneficial tools that, because of misuse, can end up being at best unproductive or at worst dangerous. If used excessively, antibiotics can be your worst enemy. If used rationally and moderately, they are your best friend.

Researchers and doctors who are creative and bother to think outside the box of conventional bacteriology (many Lyme Disease specialists included) pretty consistently come up with smarter and safer ways to apply the same old antibiotics. "Smarter and safer" refers, first of all, to the practice of choosing antibiotics with the best action against Lyme Disease bacteria. Smart therapy takes into account the characteristics of each form, ensuring that the antibiotics used do not cause conversion of the spirochete to either the difficult cell-wall-deficient form or the highly resistant cyst form. A proper treatment plan will find ways to make antibiotics effective without the prolonged use of dangerously high dosages. It will also determine how to minimize the negative impacts and side effects inevitable with any pharmaceutical antibiotic treatment. And, *most importantly*, smart, safe therapy means recognizing the weaknesses of antibiotics and interspersing other therapies throughout the treatment process which attack the bacteria from a different angle and give the body a rest from the effects of antibiotics.

There are dozens of Lyme Disease researchers and practitioners who have figured out how to use antibiotics properly, but, unfortunately, most of them are not yet in the mainstream spotlight, and most Lyme Disease patients and practitioners are not aware of their discoveries. One of the goals of this book is to help get the word out.

One such researcher is Trevor Marshall, Ph.D., whose Marshall Protocol (Chapter 2) is a result of breakthrough research in bacteriology that shows us how to use old antibiotics in new ways. The Marshall Protocol is so successful in leveraging benefits of pharmaceutical antibiotics that anyone considering antibiotic therapy should thoroughly investigate the protocol prior to commencing anti-Lyme treatment.

Another such researcher is Dr. James Schaller, an LLMD and prolific author with books published or in preparation on topics including Babesia, pediatric Lyme Disease, Bartonella, Artemisinin, and Lyme combined with indoor mold exposure. Dr. Schaller's wide traditional and progressive antibiotic options, his ability to treat Lyme biotoxins, and his new patent-pending tick-infection staining are a rare and powerful clinical mix. The later stain shows Babesia and Bartonella species in a profoundly vivid and clear manner that is stunning. Not only is Dr. Schaller advancing on Lyme Disease research, he is also on the cutting edge of patient-physician relationships—his approach is to develop an augmented, close relationship between patient and physician which allows for full knowledge of the patient's complex situation and the formulation of a highly individualized treatment plan. He has never treated two people exactly the same way, because he knows everyone's body, illness, emotions, and healing philosophy is always unique.

An additional example of innovative antibiotic use is the Salt / Vitamin C protocol discussed in Chapter 3. In this protocol, salt, not pharmaceutical antibiotics, is used to create an adverse environment for Lyme Disease bacteria in the body.

What you will find in this chapter are ways to use antibiotics as *one component* of a Lyme Disease treatment campaign, instead of *the whole* treatment campaign. In this way, antibiotics become powerful tools that are used sparingly and precisely and efficiently, instead of powerful tools that are used excessively out of desperation.

Remember, there are two variables which must be considered to ensure that antibiotics are our friend instead of our enemy: the type of antibiotic and how it is used. Let's first look at how antibiotics should be used, and then move on to examine specific antibiotic choices.

How to use the Antibiotic Rotation Protocol

Whenever we talk or think about antibiotics, we must recognize that no matter how effective an antibiotic is, the Lyme Disease bacteria will eventually become resistant to it. This is the driving principle of this chapter. The simple fact is that currently there is no single antibiotic available which is capable of complete action against Lyme Disease bacteria in its varying forms. If there were, Lyme Disease would be no more difficult to cure than strep throat. This is probably not an advanced concept for most Lyme Disease sufferers to understand—it is well known that antibiotic therapy often fails in the treatment of chronic Lyme Disease due to bacterial resistance.

This does not mean that antibiotics are useless, but instead that they can be extremely useful *before* bacterial resistance develops. It is after that point that they become ineffective, and it is here that many Lyme Disease doctors go wrong. They place a patient on an antibiotic, and, when they see that the patient is having productive herx reactions and is improving significantly, they assume that the antibiotic is magic pixie dust and should be used for 10 (or more) months straight. As bacterial resistance develops and the patient begins to go downhill, the doctor wonders what went wrong—the antibiotic worked so well in the beginning. What went wrong is simple: the Lyme Disease bacteria developed resistance, and the antibiotic no longer had any effect.

The following six principles comprise the Antibiotic Rotation Protocol. These principles acknowledge the constraints by which successful antibiotic therapy must be applied. The principles were also designed to match the unique traits of the elusive Lyme Disease bacteria with the antibiotic methodologies best suited to counter them. As such, they are the appropriate foundation of a rational, effective antibiotic treatment campaign.

Before looking at the following principles, I want to emphasize just how important these principles are. Antibiotics are a very powerful tool. However, the way in which they are commonly used to treat Lyme Disease does not come even close to taking full advantage of their effect. Simply taking a course of oral or IV antibiotics, regardless of how long the course is, pathetically under-utilizes the benefits of antibiotics. On the other hand, when antibiotics are used according to the following principles, they become much more safe and effective. The key is not just picking the right antibiotics, at the right dose, for the right amount of time. The key is optimizing antibiotic therapy with special consideration of other resources available and the characteristics of the bacterial infection itself. For such a purpose the following principles have been established. Note: this list is not exhaustive—your trusted physician may know of other valuable principles of antibiotic use.

PRINCIPLE # 1: EVERY ANTIBIOTIC HAS A SHORT TIME FRAME OF EFFECTIVENESS

The key to using antibiotics successfully is to recognize that they have limited benefit. This benefit is confined to the first few days or weeks that an antibiotic is used. After this time, bacterial resistance can develop, and the antibiotic is no longer productive. The period of time during which a given antibiotic will have strong antibacterial effect in chronic Lyme Disease is approximately 7-45 days.

Herx reactions (see Chapter 4 in *Lyme Disease and Rife Machines* for an explanation of the herx reaction) can be used as a gauge for evaluating the effectiveness of an antibiotic and determining when to discontinue its use. When an antibiotic is first started, it is necessary to ramp up the dose carefully in order to avoid severe or out-of-control herx reactions. However, after this process of gradually increasing dosage has been accomplished, and the target dose has been reached, the (controlled) herx reaction will continue for a while, reach a peak, and then diminish. When the herx reaction diminishes in intensity and eventually disappears completely, it can be concluded that the antibiotic is losing its antibacterial effect. The more intense the herx reaction, the more effective the antibiotic—lack of herx reactions indicates lack of bacterial die-off.

A given antibiotic should be promptly discontinued a few days or a week after herx reactions diminish. Not only does the antibiotic become less effective as bacterial resistance develops, but the probability of antibiotic-related side effects also increases dramatically the longer the antibiotic is used. In this way, the cost to benefit ratio of a particular antibiotic shifts dramatically into the negative zone the longer an antibiotic is used—as antibiotic use lengthens, effectiveness decreases, and side effects increase. What's more, after bacterial resistance develops, a given antibiotic can actually cause the Lyme Disease bacteria to proliferate as they undergo survival activities which ultimately lead to a more entrenched infection. As a general rule, each individual course of antibiotics should be limited in duration to about 7-45 days.

Some doctors may choose to use two or more classes of antibiotics simultaneously during a single course of antibiotic therapy. Known as combination therapy, this approach is valid and (as long as it is used according to the principles discussed here) may provide additional antibacterial action.

PRINCIPLE # 2: BREAKS MUST BE TAKEN BETWEEN COURSES OF ANTIBIOTICS

After an antibiotic loses effectiveness and is discontinued (as described above in principle #1), a break should be taken from all antibiotic therapy. Even if the antibiotic is non-pharmaceutical and does not have toxic side effects (such as mangosteen, Chapter 7), a break is still mandatory. The break can be relatively short (i.e., 1-4 weeks) or relatively long (i.e., 3-12 months) depending on individual factors which must be established by each Lyme Disease sufferer—some people do better with longer breaks and others with shorter breaks. As a general rule, the longer the break, the better. As recovery progresses, many people notice that they are able to take longer breaks without backsliding or relapsing.

At this point you may be wondering how it is possible to take breaks from antibiotic therapy. Won't the infection return? Won't a patient get sicker? The following principle answers these questions. In fact, the following principle is one of the core concepts of this book; the secret weapon of effective, safe antibiotic use.

PRINCIPLE # 3: RIFE MACHINE THERAPY IS USED AS THE PRIMARY ANTIBACTERIAL TREATMENT DURING BREAKS FROM ANTIBIOTICS

Rife machine therapy can be used during antibiotic breaks to maintain antibacterial coverage while giving the body a rest from the toxic effects of antibiotics. *Lyme Disease and Rife Machines* describes the schedule by which rife machine therapy should be applied. Because rife machine therapy is an extremely effective antibacterial tool, to which Lyme Disease bacteria cannot become resistant, its use will allow you to break from antibiotic therapy for as long as you desire. Many people find that they make the fastest progress when antibiotic use is kept at a minimum—for example, some people do best when they take antibiotics for a sum total of only two months (divided into shorter courses) per year. Other people progress faster when antibiotics are used more intensively—for example, five months (divided into shorter courses) per year. Either way, rife machine therapy makes it possible to restrict antibiotic use as desired while still maintaining antibacterial coverage.

The value of using rife machine therapy during antibiotic breaks goes even beyond allowing the body to rest from antibiotics. In fact, the very success of a Lyme Disease treatment campaign can quite literally depend on the use of rife machine therapy between courses of antibiotics. Rife machine therapy not only offers a respite from antibiotics but also attacks the infection from a different angle which causes significant bacterial load reduction. Switching back and forth between rife machine therapy and antibiotic treatment catches the infection off guard and blocks bacterial defense mechanisms which typically facilitate the pathogen's survival during anti-Lyme treatment. Additionally, rife machine therapy is most effective when antibiotics are not in use, so it is especially valuable to use it during antibiotic breaks (although it should still be used even during a course of antibiotics). A more detailed description of how this dynamic plays out is the primary focus of *Lyme Disease and Rife Machines*.

Alternating between the two therapies also allows rife machine therapy to be used more moderately. Although it is recommended that rife machine therapy be continued throughout the entire healing process *without* breaks (see *Lyme Disease and Rife Machines*), when antibiotics are in use, rife machine therapy is needed slightly less often. Even though there are no known side effects of rife machine therapy, common sense dictates that it (as any treatment) should still be used as moderately as possible.

Using rife machine therapy during antibiotic breaks permits both treatments to have maximum effectiveness with minimum side effects. Optimized antibacterial effectiveness is particularly crucial given the resistant and hardy nature of Lyme Disease bacteria. Side effect reduction is also welcome given the fact that anti-Lyme treatment must be continued for months or years to achieve complete success. Combining rife machine therapy and antibiotics in this way allows you to get the most out of the resources available to you. There are other methods by which antibiotic treatment and rife machine therapy can be used in conjunction with one another. However, at the time of this book's writing, the above described program optimizes the cost/benefit ratio of each therapy as much as possible.

PRINCIPLE # 4: A NEW AND DIFFERENT ANTIBIOTIC SHOULD BE USED FOR EACH ROUND OF TREATMENT

After completing a break from antibiotic therapy, another course of antibiotics can be undertaken. The next course should employ an entirely different antibiotic than the previous course because the infection will have already become resistant to the preceding antibiotic. The previous antibiotic may again be useful after a year or so.

When to begin the next course is a decision that must be made individually. Many people find that the right time to start another antibiotic occurs when they subjectively experience some degree of plateau in the progress they are making using rife machine therapy alone. If symptoms seem to be cropping up, it may be an indication that antibiotic use is appropriate. Antibiotics can be especially helpful in spring and fall, when symptom flareups are particularly common.

Pharmaceutical antibiotics are not the only ones that you can choose from for your courses of treatment. Non-pharmaceutical antibiotics (i.e., colloidal silver, herbal antibiotics, and even systemic enzyme therapy [Chapter 6]) may also be used as antibacterial therapy. The Salt / Vitamin C protocol described in Chapter 3 is considered to have antibacterial properties and can also be used as an antibiotic.

The decision as to which specific antibiotic to use for each round of treatment is more of an art than a science. Some people achieve optimal results when they alternate between pharmaceutical and non-pharmaceutical antibiotics. Others do better when they stick to using certain types of antibiotics and avoiding others. In still other cases, some will notice that they progress fastest when they use a certain type of antibiotic during a certain time of year. Do not be obsessive or over analytical in the choosing process. Instead, realize that trial and error will help you determine which pattern of antibiotic use works best for you. Be patient during the process of optimizing your antibiotic treatment schedules. Needless to say, the advice of a trusted physician can also provide guidance.

Because each course requires a different antibiotic, and because bacterial resistance will develop to every antibiotic, it is valuable to have as many antibiotics available as possible. As such, this book will not only describe common antibiotics but will also introduce you to less well-known (yet equally safe and effective) pharmaceutical and herbal antibiotics, where to get them, and how they compare to more common antibiotics. The goal is to expand your antibiotic arsenal as much as possible.

The above described process of taking breaks between courses of antibiotics, and using a different antibiotic each time, is known as "rotating antibiotics" or "antibiotic rotation therapy." Rotating antibiotics (with mandatory breaks in between), even when dosages are low, provides vastly increased antibacterial action in comparison with the antiquated method of using long courses and high doses of the same antibiotic. In fact, success of antibiotic therapy is less dependent on an antibiotic's dose and more dependent on the schedule by which antibiotic therapy is applied (as well as the use of rife machine therapy during breaks). Chapter 11 will help you see how the process of rotating antibiotics can be integrated into the big picture of a Lyme Disease treatment campaign.

PRINCIPLE # 5: VARIOUS ADJUNCTIVE THERAPIES CAN INCREASE THE EFFECTIVENESS OF ANTIBIOTICS

During your courses of antibiotic treatment, there are certain things you can do to render the antibiotics more effective. The most powerful way to augment the effectiveness of antibiotics (at the time this book was written) is the Marshall Protocol (Chapter 2). The Marshall Protocol capitalizes on certain weaknesses of Lyme Disease bacteria in order to help antibiotics work in a more powerful way. In fact, the Marshall Protocol is so proficient at this that antibiotics can be taken in relatively minuscule doses and still elicit extremely potent antibacterial effects.

Other therapies are also capable of augmenting the effectiveness of antibiotics. It is believed that systemic enzyme supplementation (Chapter 6) can help antibiotics work more effectively. Ginkgo biloba and other blood thinners may help antibiotics better reach bacterial colonies. Increased oxygenation (as is achieved, for example, by exercise or ozone therapy) is believed to potentiate antibiotic therapy. Increased body temperature has been proven by several scientific studies to greatly increase the susceptibility of bacteria to antibiotics. Other methods for augmenting the effectiveness of antibiotics not included in this book may also be useful.

It should be standard practice to utilize supportive therapies that increase antibiotic effectiveness.

PRINCIPLE # 6: ANTIBIOTIC USE MUST BE SPREAD OUT OVER A LONG PERIOD OF TIME

The beneficial practice of spreading out antibiotic use over a long period of time should not be confused with the harmful practice of using the same antibiotic at high doses for extended periods. Instead of lengthy courses of the same antibiotic, each individual course of antibiotic use can be kept short (determined by the herx reaction), with breaks taken between courses as described above. However, the total period of time during which these courses of rotating antibiotics are necessary can be quite long.

In other words, you should plan to continue short rounds of rotating antibiotic therapy for an extended period of time.

This principle is necessitated by the fact that the natural life cycle of Lyme Disease bacteria is measured in months and years, not days and weeks. Most bacterial infections, such as strep throat, have extremely short life cycles, measured in minutes or hours, and thus a short period of antibiotic use is effective. In contrast, Lyme Disease bacteria have a long life cycle which requires long-term antibiotic treatment. An antibiotic treatment campaign should be tailored in such a way that it is sustainable for the long haul. This includes the necessity of finding a practitioner who is willing to prescribe antibiotics for you on a rotational basis, according to the principles set forth here, for several months or years. It also includes procuring the financial resources necessary to sustain such a treatment campaign. Most important, it means taking breaks from antibiotics so that their side effects are kept to a minimum during the extended time frame.

Another contributing factor to the long treatment timeframe is the fact that Lyme Disease bacteria clump together in dense colonies, and outer layers of bacteria are eliminated before inner layers. Removing layers from a Lyme Disease colony is a similar concept to peeling layers off of an onion. The process of peeling layers off of Lyme Disease colonies is quite long, requiring months or years of patience and persistence. Research and experience have taught that layers are removed according to an independent and somewhat mysterious timetable. Significant progress in the recovery process seems to occur in spring and fall. This may have something to do with the lifecycle of the bacteria. One thing that is certain is that the process of peeling layers off Lyme Disease colonies cannot be accelerated by taking more antibiotics, or by using a rife machine more often. Patience must be practiced and the process must be allowed to unfold naturally. Here you can see why antibiotic therapy should be administered moderately: higher doses and longer courses of antibiotics do nothing to accelerate recovery but instead simply serve to increase side effects.

One Lyme Disease specialist articulately explained this process by stating that "treating Lyme Disease is a marathon, not a sprint." You should plan to use antibiotics moderately and intermittently over the course of months or years instead of intensely and continually over the course of days or weeks.

These principles of effective antibiotic use can be modified and tailored, with the help of your physician, to your own unique situation. The principles should be seen as general guidelines, not inflexible rules.

Now that we have looked at several principles by which antibiotics can be used rationally and moderately, according to the Antibiotic Rotation Protocol, let's evaluate the specific antibiotics available. We will start with pharmaceutical antibiotics and then move on to non-pharmaceutical (i.e., "natural") antibiotics.

Pharmaceutical antibiotics

Note: the below discussion of various types of antibiotics is not exhaustive in addressing their respective benefits, risks, and side effects. Always consult a physician before using any antibiotic. Also, thoroughly read the full prescribing information for any antibiotic you intend to take so you can identify potential side effects as well as the potential for dangerous or life threatening adverse reactions.

Pharmaceutical antibiotics are not all created equal. We tend to assume they are because they all look, taste, and appear to be approximately the same. They all come in little orange bottles from the pharmacy. The pills are all about the same size. You use them all the same way: by swallowing them a couple times a day. They all require a prescription and cost about the same.

Despite seeming similarities, antibiotics are very different from each other. Salt looks a lot like sugar, but of course we all know they are very different substances. Adopting a similar awareness about antibiotics is critical. Different antibiotics work by completely different methods of action and have completely different effects on bacteria. Lyme Disease bacteria are among the most advanced organisms in the world. These bacteria respond quite differently to variations in how you try to kill them.

This discussion will help explain differences in antibiotic classes and how these variations relate to treatment effectiveness. Because there are literally hundreds of different pharmaceutical antibiotics, this section cannot address all of them. Instead, the below discussion will highlight important classes of antibiotics in Lyme Disease treatment and will also identify the antibiotics to avoid. You can read or browse through this section or reference it when your physician tells you which antibiotic to take. Remember, because even the most effective antibiotics are best used according to the Antibiotic Rotation Protocol, with a *new* antibiotic for each course, it is very important to have as many antibiotics available for use as possible.

CELL WALL INHIBITORS

Cell wall inhibiting antibiotics are true to their name—they kill bacteria by preventing production of the bacteria's cell wall. Some bacteria can, however, live without a cell wall and are thus not killed by this class of antibiotic. Furthermore, the survival of some bacteria is actually facilitated and bolstered by cell wall inhibiting antibiotics. Borrelia Burgdorferi, the Lyme Disease pathogen, is one such bacterium.

Of the three known forms of Lyme Disease bacteria (spirochetes, cell-wall-deficient, and cyst form) spirochetes are the only type that have a cell wall and thus are the only form of Borrelia Burgdorferi susceptible to cell wall inhibiting antibiotics. This class of antibiotic has no effect on cell-wall-deficient or cyst forms of the bacteria.

Cell wall inhibiting antibiotics can break down spirochetes' cell walls. However, this does not necessarily kill them. Instead, cell wall inhibiting antibiotics force the spirochetes into survival mode where they rapidly convert to both cell-wall-deficient and cyst form. These forms are much more difficult to treat and are also responsible for causing Lyme Disease to become further entrenched and more serious. So, because cell wall inhibiting antibiotics cause spirochetes to convert into the two more dangerous forms, use of this type of antibiotic to treat Lyme Disease can lead to increased severity of symptoms and a protracted disease course. Trevor Marshall, Ph.D., inventor of the Marshall Protocol, hypothesizes that it may be possible to prevent many of the "incurable diseases" that are caused by cell-wall-deficient bacteria simply by avoiding cell wall inhibiting antibiotics.

Cell wall inhibiting antibiotics may lead to a temporary improvement in symptoms, but in the long run, symptoms will inevitably return and worsen significantly. This point cannot be emphasized enough. It is critical that Lyme Disease sufferers understand how dangerous and counterproductive cell wall inhibiting antibiotics can be. Many cases of debilitating, antibiotic refractory chronic Lyme Disease could have been avoided (or at least, rendered less severe) by avoiding treatment with cell wall inhibiting antibiotics.

CELL WALL INHIBITING ANTIBIOTICS CAN MAKE LYME DISEASE MUCH WORSE
These antibiotics should be avoided
or used very cautiously.

For these reasons, cell wall inhibiting antibiotics are *never* indicated in treating Lyme Disease. Rife machines can be used in the place of cell wall inhibiting antibiotics to kill spirochetes. The other antibiotics discussed below can also be used to attack the spirochete form, as well as the cell-wall-deficient and cyst forms.

For the sake of discussion, the only way I can conceive that cell wall inhibiting antibiotics could potentially be useful is if it were somehow beneficial to drive multitudes of spirochetes into cell-wall-deficient and cyst forms, and then to deal with the bacteria in those forms. If active spirochetes were causing more damage than the two other bacterial forms, then it could be argued that forcing conversion from spirochete to cell-wall-deficient and cyst forms via the use of cell wall inhibiting antibiotics would be beneficial. This may be the case in instances of out-of-control, acute Lyme Disease, and perhaps cell wall inhibiting antibiotics would have their place in such cases. However, in any case, use of these antibiotics should be approached cautiously. Once spirochetes convert to cell-wall-deficient forms, the damage has already been done. Many devastating and debilitating diseases—ranging from autoimmunity to severe mental disorders—are believed to be caused by cell-wall-deficient pathogens. The notion that only the spirochete form can cause these conditions is false; the other forms of Lyme Disease bacteria are also very dangerous. The decision to employ cell wall inhibiting antibiotics to attack spirochetes, knowing that this can trigger conversion into the cell-wall-deficient form, should not be taken lightly.

Additionally, it should be noted that in some cases of acute Lyme Disease, cell wall inhibiting antibiotics have been effective in permanently eradicating the infection. However, this scenario appears to be quite rare, and even more rare in cases of Lyme Disease which were not treated immediately following infection. Unfortunately, most cases are not treated immediately following infection.

In cases of Lyme Disease which have been previously treated with antibiotics, and in which the infection is not completely out of control, it would be much more difficult to justify use of cell wall inhibiting antibiotics. In these cases, because rife machine therapy is able to kill spirochetes *without* inducing their conversion to other bacterial forms, it seems only logical to conclude that rife machine therapy is a much better choice for attacking spirochetes than are cell wall inhibiting antibiotics.

There are some physicians and researchers who would disagree with this position regarding cell wall inhibiting antibiotics. Because so little is known about the Lyme Disease bacteria, my position is admittedly investigational and open for criticism and/or debate.

If you decide to use cell wall inhibiting antibiotics in your treatment program, proceed with caution. If this chapter does not talk you out of such a step, you will at least be able to proceed with full knowledge of the potential risks of these antibiotics, having been equipped with awareness of the issues and the debate surrounding their use.

In a few pages, you will see the Antibiotic Summary Chart, which is provided so that you can identify various types of antibiotics—including cell wall inhibiting antibiotics.

PROTEIN SYNTHESIS INHIBITORS

Protein synthesis inhibitors are a very useful class of antibiotic in treating Lyme Disease. Because both spirochetes and cell-wall-deficient bacteria require protein synthesis to survive, this type of antibiotic kills both of these bacterial forms. Protein synthesis inhibitors also prevent spirochetes from converting to the more dangerous cell-wall-deficient form, and, in turn, prevent cell-wall-deficient bacteria from converting to cysts. This class of antibiotic should be used as the core of a treatment program. There are many types of protein synthesis inhibitors. The below discussion will highlight some of the more useful and well studied of them.

Macrolides, lincosamides, and ketolides

The macrolide class of antibiotics consists mainly of erythromycin, clarithromycin, and azithromycin. Erythromycin is a first-generation macrolide and is generally not very useful in treating Lyme Disease. Clarithromycin and azithromycin are second-generation macrolides and are very useful. Clarithromycin is often sold under the brand name Biaxin, and azithromycin is sold as Zithromax. Azithromycin has a very long half-life which renders it extremely effective, but herx reactions can be intense because once a dose is administered, it takes up to two weeks before that dose leaves the body. For this reason, Lyme Disease sufferers must be cautious with azithromycin because once taken, there is no turning back. Both azithromycin and clarithromycin are prescription drugs commonly available in pharmacies. There are other macrolide antibiotics, including roxithromycin (available mainly in Europe), but they are either less effective or less available than azithromycin and clarithromycin.

Clindamycin, a lincosamide class antibiotic, is similar to macrolide antibiotics and equally as effective. Clindamycin is available with prescription from most pharmacies, typically sold under brand-name Cleocin. Clindamycin is a lesser-known antibiotic, but should be considered highly valuable because it has proven to be very effective in treating Lyme Disease.

A new class of antibiotics has recently been released: the ketolides. Because it is new, the only antibiotic in this class that has been developed thus far is telithromycin, sold as brand-name Ketek. Telithromycin is essentially a newer, more advanced macrolide. Telithromycin is an extremely effective antimicrobial agent, however, its side effects are more serious than those of previous macrolides, and include some significant cardiovascular effects. Additionally, because it is so new, it has not had a chance to prove its safety profile. One healthcare practitioner with whom I am in contact recently reported that this antibiotic has caused several of her patients to develop severe liver problems. For these reasons, use telithromycin with caution and before use, conduct additional research into the most recent warnings.

Tetracyclines

The most commonly used tetracycline antibiotics are tetracycline, doxycycline, and minocycline. Tetracycline itself is a first-generation tetracycline antibiotic and is the least useful in treating Lyme Disease. Doxycycline is much more effective. Minocycline is even more advanced and effective than doxycycline, having five times the killing power and five times the tissue penetration of doxycycline. Both doxycycline and minocycline are highly effective in treating Lyme Disease and are commonly available at pharmacies.

A little-known, yet very valuable member of the tetracycline class is demeclocycline, which is almost identical in chemical structure to minocycline. Demeclocycline is a valuable asset to Lyme Disease sufferers because it packs the same punch as minocycline and can be used after the bacterial infection has become resistant to minocycline. Demeclocycline is not commonly available but can be purchased with a prescription from The Falls Pharmacy in Snoqualmie, Washington, www.thefallspharmacy.com, (877) 392-7948. Demeclocycline is relatively expensive, but the price is easily justified because successfully treating Lyme Disease requires that a wide variety of antibiotics are used.

CYST-TARGETING DRUGS

Certain classes of antibiotics, while not designed with the intent to kill Lyme Disease cysts, have still been found to achieve this purpose. Hydroxychloroquine, typically sold under brand name Plaquenil, is an antimalarial drug which has proven to have anti-cyst activity. However, because Plaquenil can cause permanent vision damage, some researchers consider the risk/reward ratio of this drug to be undesirable. Therefore, if Plaquenil is used, pay close attention to possible vision changes. Frequent vision testing may be indicated—consult your doctor.

The 5-nitroimidazole class of antibiotics, typically used to kill parasitic infections, has also been shown to kill the Lyme Disease cyst—with fewer side effects than Plaquenil. For this reason, 5-nitromidizole antibiotics are an acceptable choice. The Lyme Disease infection can develop resistance to this class of antibiotics as it can to any others. Therefore, having a selection of different 5-nitromidazole antibiotics is beneficial. The oldest of this class of antibiotics is metronidazole, typically sold as brand-name Flagyl. Flagyl has a smaller molecule size than advanced generation 5-nitromidazoles so it has better tissue penetration, but it also has potential for the worst side effects. However, even with this risk in mind, Flagyl remains one of the most useful of the 5-nitroimidazoles.

Advanced generation 5-nitromidazoles include tinidazole, secnidazole, and ornidazole. These three antibiotics are very similar in chemical structure, but they have slightly different methods of action and thus each offers unique antibacterial activity against the Lyme Disease infection. These advanced generation 5-nitromidazoles have a larger molecule size and thus inferior tissue penetration in comparison with metronidazole, but their side effects are typically milder.

Prescription Flagyl is commonly available at pharmacies. Tinidazole was recently FDA approved and is readily available at most pharmacies.

Antibiotic Summary Chart

Antibiotic Class	Drug names in this class	Comments
Cell Wall Inhibitors	**Cephalosporins:** Aztreonam (Azactam® for injection) Cefaclor (Ceclor®), Cefadroxil (Duricef®), Cefamandole (Mandol®), Cefazolin (Ancef®, Kefzol®), Cefdinir (Omnicef®), Cefepime (Maxipime®), Cefixime (Suprax®), Cefoperazone (Cefobid®), Cefotaxime (Claforan®), Cefotetan (Cefotan®), Cefoxitin (Mefoxin®), Cefpodoxime (Vantin®), Cefprozil (Cefzil®), Ceftazidime (Ceptaz®, Fortaz®, Tazicef®, Tazidime®), Ceftibuten (Cedax®), Ceftizoxime (Cefizox®), Ceftriaxone (Rocephin®), Cefuroxime (Ceftin®, Kefurox®, Zinacef®), Cephalexin (Keflex®, Keftab®), Cephapirin (Cefadyl®), Cephradine (Anspor®, Velocef®), Imipenem and Cilastatin (Primaxin I.V.®), Loracarbef (Lorabid®), Meropenem (Merrem I.V.®) **Penicillins:** Amoxicillin (Amoxil®, Trimox®), Amoxicillin and Clavulanate (Augmentin®), Ampicillin (Principen®, Totacillin®), Ampicillin and Sulbactam (Unisyn®), Bacampicillin (Spectrobid®), Carbenicillin (Geocillin®), Cloxacillin (Cloxapen®), Dicloxacillin (Dynapen®, Dycill®), Mezlocillin (Mezlin®), Nafcillin (Unipen®), Oxacillin (Bactocill®), Penicillin G (Bicillin C-R®, Bicillin L-A®, Pfizerpen®), Penicillin V (Beepen-VK®, Veetids®), Piperacillin (Pipracil®), Piperacillin and Tazobactam (Zosyn®), Ticarcillin (Ticar®), Ticarcillin and Clavulanate (Timentin®)	**Worst Choice!**
Protein Synthesis Inhibitors	**Macrolides:** azithromycin (Zithromax®), clarithromycin (Biaxin®), dirithromycin (Dynabac®), roxythromycin (Rulid®) **Tetracyclines:** tetracycline, minocycline (Minocin®), doxycycline, demeclocycline **Lincosamides:** Clindamycin **Ketolides:** telithromycin (Ketek®)—caution: serious side effects	**Acceptable Choice**
Anti-protozoals and anti-malarials, (cyst-form drugs)	**5-nitroimidazoles:** tinidazole (Fasigyn®), metronidazole (Flagyl®), secnidazole, and ornidazole (Tiberal®) are three most used. Tinidazole, ornidazole, and secnidazole have the least side effects, but metronidazole has the smallest molecule size which might allow it to achieve higher tissue concentrations. (Plaquenil®).	**Acceptable Choice**

Secnidazole is very similar to tinidazole but is more difficult to locate. It can be purchased with a prescription from Apothe'Cure Pharmacy, Dallas, Texas, (972) 960-6601. Ornidazole is even more difficult to locate. It is available in Australia and New Zealand under brand-name Tiberal, manufactured by Roche. It can be ordered online from drugdelivery.ca, a Canadian online pharmacy.

Although metronidazole has a smaller molecule size and can be more effective, many practitioners prefer the advanced generation 5-nitroimidaozles because they typically involve fewer side effects. Individual circumstances should be considered.

The 5-nitromidazole class of antibiotics has been extensively studied by O. Brorson and S.H. Brorson, prominent Lyme Disease researchers who have published scientific studies in Norway and other countries. These researchers have established convincing evidence that this class of antibiotic is not only effective against the cyst form of Lyme Disease, but also the spirochete form, and perhaps even the cell-wall-deficient form. The Brorsons also report that they have observed situations in which the 5-nitromidazole antibiotics have led to clinical cures in chronic Lyme Disease. For these reasons, this class of antibiotics is among the most useful in treating Lyme Disease. The Brorsons' 5-nitromidazole of choice is tinidazole.

INTRAVENOUS ANTIBIOTICS

As discussed earlier in this chapter, treating Lyme Disease is a marathon, not a sprint. In other words, the most effective antibiotic therapy is that which is spread out over time in moderate doses, not that which is used at high doses for a short period of time. Because IV antibiotics are generally used in short courses at higher doses, they are not as desirable in the treatment of chronic Lyme Disease as are oral antibiotics. In addition, given the lengthy course of treatment necessary in chronic Lyme Disease, oral antibiotics are substantially more affordable, safe, convenient, flexible, and practical. Therefore, oral antibiotics should generally be preferred to IV antibiotics when treating chronic Lyme Disease.

Many Lyme Disease practitioners will disagree with this position because their philosophy is to hit the infection as hard as possible in a short period of time, and this is usually accomplished with IV antibiotics. It is true that certain people will recover by using that approach. In some cases, IV antibiotics do provide excellent results. However, the research relied on in writing this book points to the use of oral antibiotics instead of IV antibiotics.

Ultimately, all Lyme Disease sufferers must be empowered, do their own homework, do their own thinking, and come to their own conclusions. The truth is that chronic Lyme Disease treatment is a pioneering and experimental field, not a precise science. As such, there are gray areas that have yet to be completely understood. Instead of viewing this book as the final word in Lyme Disease treatment, view it as a platform from which you will be equipped to conduct your own research and make your own decisions. This goes for your conclusion about IV antibiotics as well.

It should be noted that there are certain cases in which IV antibiotic use is definitely preferred over oral antibiotic use. Discuss this issue with your physician. The advice of a trained physician who knows your unique situation should be considered superior to the information in this book. Hopefully your physician is open-minded enough to have an open discussion with you about these questions.

Non-pharmaceutical antibiotics

While typically less toxic, keep in mind that non-pharmaceutical antibiotics can have significant side effects and should be treated with respect. Non-pharmaceutical antibiotics should be used according to the same guidelines as pharmaceutical antibiotics, the guidelines set forth in the Antibiotic Rotation Protocol.

The methods of action of the following non-pharmaceutical antibiotics vary. Some of these antibiotics may act as cell wall inhibitors, in which case they should be used very cautiously, as previously noted. You may need to conduct additional research on the specific non-pharmaceutical antibiotic(s) you are considering using. The *PDR for Herbal Medicines*, a comprehensive 1,100 page reference book, provides excellent information on many antibacterial (and other) herbs, and can help you research / identify the methods of action of various herbal antibiotics.

COLLOIDAL SILVER (CS)

There are hundreds of websites and dozens of books about the groundbreaking and remarkable antibiotic capabilities of colloidal silver. CS possesses a broad-spectrum, powerful action against many microbes.

One of the dozens of books available is *Micro-Silver Bullet,* written in 1997 by Paul Farber, N.D., Ph.D., who himself had antibiotic refractory Lyme Disease and gained victory over it by using CS. The book is a very valuable resource for Lyme Disease sufferers. Other useful books include:

Colloidal Silver: Antibiotic Superhero
The Wonders of Colloidal Silver
Colloidal Silver: Making the Safest and
Most Powerful Medicine on Earth for the Price of Water
Colloidal Silver Today: The All-Natural, Wide-Spectrum Germ Killer
Colloidal Silver: The Hidden Truth

Two of the most accurate and informative websites are:
www.silvermedicine.org
www.silver-colloids.com

Online discussion forums include:
silverlist.org
health.groups.yahoo.com/group/colloidalsilver
health.groups.yahoo.com/group/colloidalsilver2

There is far too much important information about colloidal silver to include in this chapter. The important facts are that properly made colloidal silver may be the most effective non-pharmaceutical antibiotic available and is probably of more value than any pharmaceutical antibiotic in existence. Many companies sell CS, and it is also quite easy and affordable to make at home with an easily constructed, low voltage, colloidal silver generator. The quality of available CS varies greatly—additional information about what constitutes good and bad CS can be found through the above websites. Good CS is a powerful antibiotic, poorly made CS is worthless.

Of all the antibiotics discussed in this book, including pharmaceutical and non-pharmaceutical, colloidal silver has garnered the largest number of successful user reports. A detailed presentation of colloidal silver therapy and its benefits is beyond the scope of this book, but I would strongly encourage you to research CS thoroughly. If any antibiotic out there is capable of fighting Lyme Disease successfully, CS is probably it.

While colloidal silver is a profoundly powerful antibacterial, antiviral, and antifungal agent, you should be aware that silver toxicity is possible if you cross an unspecified threshold. Cases of irreversible skin discoloration have resulted from excessive use; this condition is known as argyria. Therapeutic use of colloidal silver should be approached cautiously.

T.O.A.-FREE CATS CLAW

Cats Claw (Uncaria tomentosa) is a powerful herb that has been long used to treat a broad variety of health problems. Although Cats Claw has proved somewhat helpful in the treatment of Lyme Disease, it has not been considered a breakthrough treatment.

Recently, however, a discovery was made about a specific form of Cats Claw herb, known as T.O.A.-free Cats Claw. This particular form is devoid of tetracyclic oxindole alkaloids (T.O.A.'s). Cats Claw lacking these T.O.A.'s is a completely different herb than common Cats Claw and has been found to possess amazingly effective antibiotic qualities as well as several other very important healing properties.

The most notable research about this T.O.A.-free Cats Claw was a controlled clinical study administered by Dr. Lee Cowden, M.D., a highly respected Fort Worth cardiologist. Dr. Cowden's research examined the effects of T.O.A.-free Cats Claw on 28 people who had confirmed Lyme Disease. The study was 10 weeks long and included diet, detoxification, and nutrition components. All 28 people were ill and disabled by Lyme Disease and flat-out broke from attempts to treat it. All of them had also failed conventional antibiotic therapy.

The results of Dr. Cowden's study were impressive. I talked with Dr. Cowden several times, and he explained to me that many of the study participants had shown improvement, some of it dramatic. Since this research was conducted, many Lyme Disease sufferers have used T.O.A.-

free Cats Claw with satisfying results. Because of these encouraging reports, the herb has earned its place as a useful Lyme Disease therapy.

Some researchers and proponents of T.O.A.-free Cats Claw have claimed (or alluded to the possibility) that it is the cure for Lyme Disease, if used long enough. Unfortunately, most available evidence does not support such impressive claims.

T.O.A.-free Cat's Claw does have direct antibiotic properties and is also an anti-inflammatory and immuno-modulator. The antibiotic component of the herb is attributable to the considerable quantities of quinovic acid glycosides found in the herb, which are natural precursors to pharmaceutical antibiotics known as Quinolones.

As an antibiotic, T.O.A.-free Cats Claw has antibacterial benefits, but it carries with it the same problems with decreasing efficacy that all antibiotics have. Three participants in the online Lyme-and-Rife discussion group conducted an unofficial, unscientific trial of the herb while undergoing treatment with rife machines. Their goal was to determine whether or not the herb eventually "stopped working," in much the same way that all antibiotics "stop working" due to developing bacterial resistance. The three found that the T.O.A-free Cat's Claw (brand name Samento®) had an initial beneficial impact, inducing herx reactions and improvement, but eventually it simply suppressed the Lyme Disease bacteria, leading to stagnated progress and even loss of previously made gains. While using Samento® the Lyme Disease patients noted that ultimately their herx reactions and the improvement achieved with rife machines was decreased. These three people concluded that T.O.A.-free Cat's Claw, as any antibiotic, can be beneficial for that short period of time before the bacteria develop resistance to the herb. After that point, using the herb becomes counterproductive. These conclusions should be included in any evaluation of the herb as therapy.

The two brands of T.O.A.-free Cats Claw commonly purchased by Lyme Disease sufferers are:

Nutramedix, product name "Samento®." Most Lyme Disease sufferers use the liquid Samento®.
www.nutramedix.com
1-800-730-3130

Nutricology, product name "Prima Uña de Gato"
www.nutricology.com
1-800-545-9960

Extensive additional information about T.O.A.-free Cats Claw can be found on the Lyme-and-rife online discussion forum. You can find help with dosing schedules and also read about the trials conducted by Dr. Cowden and the three Lyme Disease sufferers who used Samento® in conjunction with rife machine treatment.

Because Cats Claw is derived from the same substances that comprise the quinolone class of antibiotics, it shares similar side effects. Most notably, both the quinolone antibiotics and Cats Claw have been associated with tendon damage. This occurrence is quite rare, and new research shows that this side effect may be avoided if intracellular magnesium levels are brought back up to healthy levels (See Chapter 10). Nonetheless, proceed with caution when using Cats Claw.

OLIVE LEAF EXTRACT

Another natural supplement with antibacterial qualities is Olive leaf extract, a very powerful natural antibiotic, antiviral, antifungal, and antiprotozoal. It has broad spectrum activity against many microorganisms and is beneficial to the immune system. It can also be used against Candida infections.

The book *Olive Leaf Extract* By Dr. Morton Walker is an excellent source of information about this powerful herb.

The most trusted, highest quality brands of olive leaf extract are:

Ameriden
www.ameriden.com
888-405-3336

East Park Research
www.eastparkresearch.com
800-345-8367
(their Olive leaf extract product is called "d-lenolate")

TEASEL ROOT EXTRACT

Teasel Root extract has been found by some Lyme Disease sufferers to be an excellent natural antibiotic option which is effective against Borrelia Burgdorferi.

Teasel Root can be obtained from:
www.jeansgreens.com

An additional brand is SpiroNIL, available at various online stores.

SARSAPARILLA OFFICINALIS

Sarsaparilla, of the genus Smilax, is an herb that was once widely used as a Syphilis treatment. Because Lyme Disease and Syphilis are both spirochete infections, some Lyme Disease sufferers have used Sarsaparilla with good results (i.e., producing herx reactions and improvement).

Sarsaparilla Officinalis can be purchased from:
www.sourcenaturals.com
Product name "Smilax."

Several people have complained of irritated kidneys while using Sarsaparilla, and information available on the oral intake of Sarsaparilla associates it with kidney damage. Consult your physician before beginning this herb.

GRAPEFRUIT SEED EXTRACT
(not to be confused with grape seed extract)

Grapefruit seed extract is a powerful natural antibiotic that has produced herx reactions and improvement in Lyme Disease sufferers who use it. It is also commonly used for the prevention and treatment of Candida.

The brand of grapefruit seed extract most commonly purchased by Lyme Disease community members is:

www.nutriteam.com
Product name, "NutriBiotic Tablets"

LAURICIDIN®

Lauricidin® is a derivative of lauric acid, a component of coconuts. The antimicrobial properties of coconut oil have long been known. Lauricidin® harnesses these properties in a concentrated formula.

Lauricidin® has also been found to have broad-spectrum antimicrobial actions against a wide range of microorganisms.

Some researchers have also speculated that Lauricidin® has a helpful effect in removing the neurotoxin associated with Lyme Disease infection, through a soap-like or emulsifying action. This effect may result in breaking up infective Lyme Disease colonies.

Lauricidin is a very promising and useful antimicrobial that has been shown, through user reports, to have a strong effect against Lyme Disease.

More information and purchasing options can be found at: www.lauricidin.com.

Lauricidin is a frequent topic of discussion on the Lyme-and-rife online discussion forum.

MANGOSTEEN

Mangosteen fruit can be used as an effective non-pharmaceutical antibiotic. There is so much information available about mangosteen that a separate chapter in this book was justified. See Chapter 7 for more information.

SYSTEMIC ENZYME SUPPLEMENTATION

Systemic enzyme supplementation, as described in Chapter 6, can serve as a non-pharmaceutical antibiotic. In fact, it has proven to be highly effective and without side effects. Systemic enzyme supplementation offers many healing properties which benefit Lyme Disease sufferers.

STEPHEN BUHNER'S LYME PROTOCOL

In his book, *Healing Lyme* (available from www.amazon.com), Stephen Buhner describes an anti-Lyme protocol which uses various antibacterial herbs and supportive supplements. Many Lyme Disease sufferers have reportedly been helped by employing his protocol.

Chapter 2:
The Marshall Protocol

Preface and Disclaimer

The Marshall Protocol is a complicated therapy and one that continually evolves as a result of new research and information. Naturally, books are static and do not change. Therefore, in order to obtain the most recent information about this treatment, visit the official Marshall Protocol web site by pointing your browser to www.marshallprotocol.com.

This chapter is written by a layman, in layman's terms, and is intended only as an overview of the Marshall Protocol; it is neither an exhaustive explanation of nor instructions for using the program. Some of the information below is based on my own research of the treatment procedure, and my personal experience with it, and should not be interpreted as exhaustive or 100% accurate. I do not have formal training in understanding or applying Marshall Protocol principles; instead, I am simply an investigative journalist reporting what I have learned about the protocol. For precise, comprehensive, and official information about the protocol and how specifically to use it, visit the web site mentioned above.

This information has not been reviewed or approved by Trevor Marshall, Ph.D., the inventor of the protocol, and the statements made should not be construed as his statements. Also, much of the following information is experimental and investigational and should be viewed as such. The concepts presented below in relation to Vitamin D are still in the research phase, so they should not be interpreted as established, proven fact.

Introduction to the Marshall Protocol

The Marshall Protocol is perhaps the most significant breakthrough in Lyme Disease treatment since Doug MacLean discovered in the 1980s how to employ a homemade rife machine (see Chapter 5) to heal his own Lyme infection. The reason the Marshall Protocol is so significant is that it addresses an aspect of the Lyme Disease complex which no other treatment, protocol, supplement or herb can even come close to touching. The discoveries that led Trevor Marshall, Ph.D., to develop the Marshall Protocol have uncovered and exposed a critical part of the process which Borrelia Burgdorferi uses to establish and maintain infection in the host. The Marshall Protocol is the only known therapy which addresses this aspect of the bacterial survival process. If you take the Marshall Protocol out of the Lyme Disease treatment toolbox, there is no comparable tool to replace it.

The protocol builds on the work of Dr. Lida Mattman, one of the most influential medical scientists in modern history. With a master's degree in virology from the University of Kansas and a Ph.D. in immunology from Yale University, Lida Mattman has revolutionized the study of infectious disease and established the foundation for decades of progress in science and medicine. A 1998 nominee for the Nobel Prize in Medicine, Mattman found that a certain type of bacteria lacking a cell wall (known as cell-wall-deficient, variant, or L-form bacteria) are not only very common but are also the root cause of multiple health conditions that have baffled medical scientists for years. The presence of cell-wall-deficient pathogens in the human body is extremely difficult to detect and has thus been largely ignored by conventional medicine.

Dr. Mattman's studies have forced hundreds of physicians and researchers to accept the fact that this elusive and highly complicated class of bacteria is responsible for many previously-misunderstood ailments. Interestingly, Mattman's research findings bear a striking resemblance to the conclusions about microorganisms drawn by Dr. Royal Raymond Rife himself.

Although her breakthrough discoveries caused a light-speed acceleration in the field of bacteriology, no one has been able to figure out exactly what to do about the cell-wall-deficient bacteria identified by Dr. Mattman. We know they are there, and we know they cause many diseases considered untreatable or incurable by conventional medicine, but getting rid of them is a different story.

Fortunately, there is a handful of brilliant researchers who are currently studying these pathogens and are discovering ways to attack cell-wall-deficient bacteria, destroy them, and thereby heal incurable diseases. Trevor Marshall, Ph.D., is one such researcher. After failing to gain benefit from conventional treatment for his own affliction with sarcoidosis (a multi-system disorder characterized in affected organs by inflammatory lesions), Marshall was compelled to take a closer look at the pathogenesis of chronic disease. His research conclusions were very similar to those reached by Dr. Mattman: a surprisingly long list of chronic diseases are actually caused by cell-wall-deficient bacteria. Sarcoidosis and Lyme Disease, for example, share this root cause. If you are confused because you thought Lyme Disease was caused by spirochetes, not cell-wall-deficient bacteria, keep reading, we will answer that question.

Decades of studies by Dr. Marshall led him beyond the ability to merely identify cell-wall-deficient bacteria and their role in various disease processes. In developing the protocol which bears his name, he has created the means to actually counter their bacterial activity. The Marshall Protocol is a ground-breaking method of killing cell-wall-deficient bacteria in the human body and ultimately curing the previously untreatable diseases this pathogen causes. After Marshall employed his discoveries to treat sarcoidosis and heal himself, he went on to establish The Autoimmunity Research Foundation through which he collaborates with physicians and researchers around the world to help chronically ill people recover from various afflictions. Marshall has bridged the gap between simple awareness of the existence of cell-wall-deficient bacteria and knowledge of how to eradicate them.

Clarification of the root cause of Lyme Disease may be needed here. As mentioned earlier, the Lyme Disease pathogen, Borrelia Burgdorferi, exists in three distinct forms: spirochete, cyst, and cell-wall-deficient form. It is popularly (and erroneously) believed that the spirochete form of the disease is the only form—quite often, researchers and practitioners ignore the other two forms. This ignorance is the result of antiquated, inaccurate, and close-minded educational materials commonly presented at medical schools. In actuality, according to a burgeoning heap of published research, the spirochete form is in fact just a small part of the whole disease picture. Let's take a small detour to examine the three bacterial forms of Borrelia Burgdorferi.

Although not the totality of the disease, the spirochete form is highly dangerous and significant. It is responsible for the initial, rapid spread of the infection throughout the body and various organs due to its highly-mobile, drill-capable shape. The spirochete form is also responsible for many ongoing symptoms. It is, however, simply not the whole story.

The second form of Lyme Disease bacteria is the cyst form, which is also commonly ignored by mainstream practitioners and researchers. The cyst form is a symptomless, protective, survival-oriented form that is elusive, difficult to identify in laboratories, and nearly impossible to kill. Further discussion of the cyst form can be found elsewhere throughout this book and detailed discussion can be found in *Lyme Disease and Rife Machines*. Additionally, www.lymeinfo.net has an extensive collection of cyst form-related research and published studies.

The third form of Lyme Disease bacteria is the cell-wall-deficient form, which happens to be extremely dangerous, insidious, and also the target of the Marshall Protocol. Many of the most severe symptoms and organ dysfunctions associated with Lyme Disease occur as a result of the presence of cell-wall-deficient bacteria. Additionally, over time, the population of cell-wall-deficient bacteria tends to increase. This form can actually hide inside cells within the body to avoid detection. More amazingly, it can actually hide in immune system cells themselves. The cell-wall-deficient form must be addressed in order to heal, yet it is commonly overlooked, or worse, its existence is often completely denied, despite peer-verified research by the likes of such heavyweights as Yale graduate Lida Mattman.

Each of the three bacterial forms is capable of converting to the other forms under certain circumstances. Spirochetes convert to cell-wall-deficient and cyst forms as a survival tactic (cysts are much more treatment-resistant than spirochetes). Cysts convert to spirochetes occasionally—usually in spring and fall—as a proliferation tactic, to spread the disease to other tissues (spirochetes are more mobile and can more easily spread the infection than cysts). The cell-wall-deficient form is utilized for various reasons, including, of particular note, the ability of this form to survive numerous treatment approaches, including cell wall inhibiting antibiotics.

Different antibacterial approaches must be used for each of the three bacterial forms because each bacterial form has different weaknesses and vulnerabilities. Rife machines are highly proficient in killing spirochetes. Spirochetes can also be killed somewhat effectively with protein synthesis inhibiting antibiotics. Cysts respond to certain antibiotics (discussed in Chapter 1). Cysts can also be exposed and destroyed, with proper treatment, timing, and planning, by rife machine therapy. However, until the Marshall Protocol, there was not an effective treatment for cell-wall-deficient bacteria. There are several types of antibiotics (primarily protein synthesis inhibitors such as the tetracyclines and macrolides) which have activity against cell-wall-deficient bacteria, but these are minimally effective when used alone. The Marshall Protocol is the first therapy that has actually been able to comprehensively eradicate this form of the bacteria. This is why the Marshall Protocol is so important. Before the Marshall Protocol, there was simply no way to deal with the cell-wall-deficient form of Lyme Disease. Hence, before the Marshall Protocol, recovery was much more difficult to attain.

I first heard of the Marshall Protocol through Ron, a friend and fellow Lyme Disease sufferer who often participates in the Lyme-and-Rife online discussion group. Just as I had, Ron had benefited from rife machine therapy but still needed something to finish off the disease. Ron was tremendously successful with the Marshall Protocol. After due consideration I decided to try the protocol myself. Sure enough, results were forthcoming, and I couldn't help but notice that the Marshall Protocol seemed to provide improvement in areas where rife machine therapy lagged. The longer I researched, used myself as a guinea pig, and consulted with various patients and practitioners, the more obvious it became that the Marshall Protocol would play an important role in Lyme Disease recovery. As mentioned, it addresses an aspect of the Lyme Disease complex that, quite simply, no other treatment, supplement, or protocol can impact.

Those who use rife machines to fight Lyme Disease will be excited to find out that the Marshall Protocol appears to be compatible with rife machine therapy. More than compatible, actually. Each therapy compensates for weaknesses in the other. Because the method of action of the two therapies is entirely different, it is not redundant to use both during the course of a Lyme Disease treatment campaign. The therapies work together to accelerate the healing process.

The answer to many incurable, idiopathic diseases

The benefit provided by the Marshall Protocol does not stop with Lyme Disease. Thousands of actual patients with real medical conditions ranging from fibromyalgia and chronic fatigue syndrome to arthritis and obsessive-compulsive disorder have regained their health by using the Marshall Protocol. Their stories are very instructive. To communicate with thousands of Marshall Protocol users visit the discussion forum located at www.marshallprotocol.com.

The commonality which allows such differing illnesses to be treated successfully by the Marshall Protocol is their root cause: cell-wall-deficient bacteria. Visit www.marshallprotocol.com for a full list of conditions which may profit from the Marshall Protocol. Of course not all allegedly untreatable diseases are caused by cell-wall-deficient bacteria. Some such diseases may be caused by other pathogens or even problems like mercury poisoning and allergies. However, a large number of serious diseases are caused (or at least contributed to) by cell-wall-deficient bacteria and will respond accordingly to the Marshall Protocol.

Modern conventional medicine does not test for cell-wall-deficient bacteria during the process of diagnosing diseases. Hence, there is a wide range of symptom presentations having these bacteria as a root cause which end up being diagnosed with nonsense disease labels such as "fibromyalgia," "chronic fatigue syndrome," or "depression." These disease labels (and many others like them) are flawed because they provide only a description of symptoms but absolutely no useful information about the cause of the problem. Such diseases are those known in the conventional medical community as "idiopathic." The word means "without known cause" but is really just a fancy way to say "we have no idea what is wrong with you." Diagnosing muscle pains with the label "fibromyalgia" is like diagnosing a broken transmission in your car with the label "It Just Don't Work No More." Patients are told that there are no successful remedies for their diseases other than symptom-reducing, palliative treatments, because frankly, how could there be a successful remedy if no one knows what is causing the problem?

In many cases, the Marshall Protocol offers the only hope to people with idiopathic diseases, because the Marshall Protocol operates from a position of recognition and understanding of the actual problem, not just the symptoms.

While no one knows exactly how cell-wall-deficient bacteria infiltrate the body, or why some people are more susceptible to them than are others, open-minded scientists have long suspected their involvement in many health conditions deemed idiopathic. For example, consider autoimmunity, which is often alleged as the cause of diseases like those mentioned in the above paragraphs. Defined as an attack on the human body by its own immune system, autoimmunity itself has been hypothesized to be triggered by stealth pathogens (like cell-wall-deficient bacteria) which short circuit and confuse the immune system to the point of self-attack. It has been hypothesized that such stealth bacteria could hide away in host tissues, leading the immune system to mistake healthy, host tissues for the invading bacteria. The Marshall Protocol has helped to confirm this hypothesis; many people with autoimmune disorders have gained significant improvement, or even complete recovery, via the protocol. People with so-called "autoimmunity" are actually getting better when they are treated for stealth bacterial infections.

It may be difficult to understand and accept that cell-wall-deficient bacteria can cause diseases with so many diverse symptoms and presentations—from musculoskeletal disorders to mental disorders. The following three points help to explain why many diseases, commonly believed to be unrelated, can all be caused by cell-wall-deficient bacteria:

1. As a result of varying genetics, environmental factors, and other variables, illness will manifest differently in different individuals, leading to unrelated diagnoses despite analogous causes.

2. Many, possibly thousands, of different species of cell-wall-deficient bacteria exist, each having unique deleterious effects, leading to varied presentation of disease.

3. Cell-wall-deficient bacteria are capable of infecting every major organ and system in the body; the syndrome or disease label someone ends up with often depends on where a cell-wall-deficient bacterium establishes infection.

An analogy will further clarify how different diseases and different symptoms can have the same root cause: Allergies. Many people are allergic to pollen, yet allergic reactions vary greatly; some people get runny noses, others get asthma, some get red, itchy eyes. Some allergic reactions are only an uncomfortable nuisance, while others are life-threatening. In the same way, people react to infection by cell-wall-deficient bacteria differently—some moderately, some severely, typically all with symptoms that share some aspects in common but still vary wildly, as is the case with most idiopathic diseases. An interesting side note: many diseases which are caused by cell-wall-deficient bacteria result in part from allergic reactions to their bacterial toxins.

The bottom line is simply that many diverse diseases share the root cause of cell-wall-deficient bacteria. Because a multiplicity of conditions can be caused by cell-wall-deficient bacteria, the Marshall Protocol has applicability to many seemingly unrelated illnesses. If you or someone you know sufferers from an unmitigated disease, it is possible that it is caused by stealth bacteria unrecognized by conventional medicine. You have everything to gain and nothing to lose by exploring what the Marshall Protocol offers.

Now we will examine what the Marshall Protocol is and how it works. First we will look at the general principles and discoveries on which the protocol is based, and then we will look at the actual treatments and lifestyle recommendations that comprise the protocol.

Marshall Protocol principles

VITAMIN D DYSREGULATION

Also known as calciferol, Vitamin D was misnamed as a vitamin after its discovery in 1922. A vitamin is a type of organic substance that is required in the diet and essential to nutrition and metabolism. Vitamin D is unique because it is not required in the diet; instead, it is manufactured by the body via exposure to sunlight or artificial lights. Although we do consume Vitamin D in our diets, it is not technically a vitamin since it is not required in the diet.

For the purpose of explaining the Marshall Protocol, we are less concerned about the technical definition of Vitamin D and more concerned about how it affects chronic disease. Whether a true vitamin or not, Vitamin D plays a critical role in the pathogenesis of Lyme Disease and other illnesses involving infection with cell-wall-deficient bacteria. At the center of the Marshall Protocol is the breakthrough discovery that Vitamin D is not handled correctly in the bodies of people infected with cell-wall-deficient bacteria. Let's look at how this dysregulated handling of Vitamin D occurs.

As we mentioned, Vitamin D can enter the body in two ways: it is either synthesized in the skin after exposure to sunlight or artificial lights, or it is consumed in the diet. Once Vitamin D is inside the body, not all of it remains in static form. A small portion of Vitamin D is converted to a type of secosteroid known as 1,25 dihydroxyvitamin-D (abbreviated "1,25-D"). A hormone required for regular body function, 1,25-D is manufactured by the kidneys as a metabolite (or product) of Vitamin D. In healthy people, the body tightly regulates how much 1,25-D is made in the kidneys; although critical to health, too much 1,25-D can be very harmful. If present in excessive quantities, 1,25-D can be immunosuppressive and cause a plethora of physical and psychological symptoms.

In people infected with cell-wall-deficient bacteria, the production of 1,25-D can spiral out of control and rapidly reach damaging levels. This happens because, as an evolved survival mechanism, cell-wall-deficient bacteria are capable of catalyzing the process by which Vitamin D is converted to 1,25-D. Instead of a slow, controlled conversion which occurs only in the kidneys, 1,25-D production becomes uncontrolled, occurring throughout the body inside cells infected with cell-wall-deficient bacteria. Specifically, immune system cells harboring cell-wall-deficient bacteria can turn into tiny, unrestrained factories producing excessive amounts of 1,25-D. Bacteria catalyze the 1,25-D conversion process intentionally to cause immune system suppression and create a more favorable living environment in the body.

The result of catalyzed 1,25-D production is a subclinical yet devastating immunosuppression syndrome that allows Lyme Disease (and other types of cell-wall-deficient) bacteria to persist chronically in the body. When present in appropriately controlled quantities, 1,25-D is a critical nutrient and is important to health, as we have said. However, when present in excessive quantities, 1,25-D is immunosuppressive and inhibits the immune system from fighting infections. This process is one of the core survival mechanisms of Borrelia Burgdorferi. The excessive levels of 1,25-D often present in people harboring chronic infections leads to a greatly inhibited host defense system. By accelerating conversion of Vitamin D to 1,25-D, these tiny bacteria are basically able to neutralize the human immune system.

Additionally, as we have alluded to, elevated levels of 1,25-D itself (even without infections on board) can cause a plethora of disease symptoms. So, an elevated level of 1,25-D has a two-fold impact: it suppresses the immune system and also creates numerous other symptoms of malaise. This is why it is so important to address elevated 1,25-D levels when treating Lyme Disease.

The aforementioned principles are at the core of the Marshall Protocol. One of the primary objectives of the Marshall Protocol is to reduce the excessive levels of 1,25-D in the body. Since 1,25-D is a metabolite of (or product of) Vitamin D, the process of reducing 1,25-D levels in the body requires that a person suffering from infection with cell-wall-deficient bacteria decrease their consumption of Vitamin D foods and supplements, and also reduce their exposure to sunlight and bright lights. Both of these actions are primary components of the Marshall Protocol that will be examined in a few pages. By curtailing the amount of Vitamin D that enters the body, 1,25-D production is also reduced, bringing the immune system back into balance. While Vitamin D consumption (and exposure to sunlight and other artificial lights) may be neutral or even beneficial to healthy people, it can be poison to people infected with cell-wall-deficient bacteria because of this pathogenic process.

In addition to Dr. Marshall, Dr. James Schaller has also found that 1,25-D is involved in other inflammatory processes. Specifically, 1,25-D levels have been found to be higher in inflamed, damaged, and arthritic joints in comparison with healthy joints. This observation further confirms the principles on which the Marshall Protocol is based.

Spotlight on Vitamin D
Is Vitamin D a Health Restorer or Destroyer?

In recent times, Vitamin D has been highly touted by modern researchers and healthcare practitioners across the world as a beneficial nutrient for both healing disease and health maintenance. Studies show that it reduces symptoms of numerous chronic afflictions and that it contributes to health and vitality. In reality, however, the subject of whether or not Vitamin D is a beneficial nutrient to consume is actually quite controversial.

Controversy arises because there is more than meets the eye when it comes to Vitamin D. In some instances, its intake can actually be toxic and counterproductive to healing, even while it can trigger perceived symptom improvement. There is a very large cross section of sick people who can actually be harmed by the nutrient, despite the fact that it initially makes them feel better.

What separates people who benefit from Vitamin D from people who do not? The presence of pathogenic cell-wall-deficient bacteria in the body. Infection by cell-wall-deficient bacteria contributes to excessive production and disturbed handling of one of the metabolites of Vitamin D, known as 1,25-D. While often leading quickly to symptom improvement, excessive levels of 1,25-D ultimately slow healing and prolong illness.

How does excess 1,25-D lead to symptom improvement? Since 1,25-D is a similar substance to steroid anti-inflammatory drugs, it can have a similar effect as those drugs. Consider what happens when Lyme Disease is treated with steroidal anti-inflammatory drugs: immediate improvement in symptoms is experienced as the inflammatory response of the immune system (the primary cause of symptoms) is reduced. Yet, behind the scenes, steroids actually cause the Lyme Disease infection to worsen, considerably. With the immune system shut down and inflammation eliminated, the bacterial infection is free to proliferate and spread. Joseph Burrascano, M.D., one of the nation's leading Lyme doctors, has repeatedly said that steroids can cause severe aggravation of Lyme Disease—leading, in some cases, to permanent damage—despite the fact that steroid drugs make you feel better.

Steroid anti-inflammatory drugs typically result in dramatic symptom reduction in Lyme sufferers—but at an unacceptable cost. Similarly, people suffering from infection with cell-wall-deficient bacteria may feel better when supplementing Vitamin D (which is a precursor to 1,25-D), *(continued)*

Now that you have some background in the nuances of Vitamin D, we'll turn our attention back to the role Vitamin D plays in the Marshall Protocol. In the Marshall Protocol, the goal is to reduce excessive 1,25-D levels (which are almost always present in Lyme Disease sufferers). This is *(continued)* or when exposed to sunlight or bright lights, but in reality these things worsen their disease. Like steroid drugs, excess levels of 1,25-D can make you feel better but actually be bad for you.

This counterintuitive principle can lead patients, physicians, and researchers to mistakenly conclude that Vitamin D is beneficial in the treatment of chronic infections and other diseases such as multiple sclerosis and fibromyalgia (which may actually be caused by chronic infections). In the same way that doctors sometimes erroneously prescribe steroid drugs to the detriment of their Lyme patients, some Lyme sufferers may intentionally increase their Vitamin D consumption and exposure to sunlight only to their own detriment.

It is easy to conclude that feeling better indicates true healing. After all, in most sicknesses (such as colds and flu) improvement in symptoms does indicate healing. In actuality, however, Vitamin D—which is a precursor to 1,25-D—can be a poison to Lyme sufferers. Instead of eradicating the infection, it masks symptoms and provides a false sense of relief.

The situation gets even more confusing because the opposite scenario can occur: Vitamin D avoidance can feel *bad* but actually be *good* for you. When the Marshall Protocol is used to reduce Vitamin D consumption and thus 1,25-D synthesis, the immune system is freed up to function properly. As a result, inflammation and herx reactions occur as the body engages in the battle with the bacterial infection. This phenomenon is often experienced subjectively as an increase in symptoms, so it can be erroneously identified as an exacerbation of the disease. Although symptoms are increasing, healing is in fact occurring.

In my first book, *Lyme Disease and Rife Machines,* it was noted that though herx reactions are extremely unpleasant and feel like backsliding, they are a necessary part of the healing process. The same is true of Vitamin D avoidance. Vitamin D reduction leads ultimately to true and permanent healing even though it can feel like backsliding.

The Marshall Protocol is based on an entirely new paradigm, unaccepted by and directly opposed to much traditional medical thinking. We are in the midst of the birth pains of an entirely new way to think about Vitamin D and its relationship to infectious disease. For many people, the breakthrough discoveries of Trevor Marshall, Ph.D., mean restored health and an end to the chronic infections caused by cell-wall-deficient bacteria. The challenge at this point in time is providing accurate information and education about this new paradigm, not only to patients but also to health care practitioners and researchers. You are encouraged to frequently check the official Marshall Protocol web site (www.marshallprotocol.com) to stay up to date with the latest information.

accomplished by intentionally avoiding exposure to sunlight and bright lights and by decreasing consumption of Vitamin D-containing foods and supplements. We will further discuss these topics in a later section of this chapter. First, though, before moving on, I am sure some of my readers will be scratching their heads and wondering if they should actually consider Vitamin D reduction as a valid Lyme Disease therapy. Let's take a small detour with some additional discussion of that issue.

It is natural to be skeptical that intentional reduction of Vitamin D in the body could be healthy. Vitamin D supplements line the walls of your favorite health food store. Vitamin D may be a part of your daily supplement routine. New research is available almost daily detailing the benefits of Vitamin D. However, you need to shift the platform from which you view Vitamin D. Any good thing can become a bad thing under certain circumstances. Water, for example, is essential to sustaining life, but it can also cause death. No one would tell a drowning person not to worry because water is our friend. Vitamin D is no different. People infected with cell-wall-deficient bacteria will find that Vitamin D can and does become toxic. The effects of elevated levels of the Vitamin D metabolite known as 1,25-D are, quite frankly, responsible in part for the word "chronic" in "chronic Lyme Disease."

There is no one-size-fits-all formula for Vitamin D. Some health conditions may benefit from its supplementation, while others are harmed. Consider, for example, the analogous nutrient, iron. Too much iron makes you very sick (my father has this condition, called hemochromatosis, and has to give blood every couple weeks to lower his iron levels). Conversely, we all know that too little iron leads to anemia. In the case of iron it would be misguided to argue about whether iron is good or bad. The *right* amount is good, and the *wrong* amount is bad. The same is true of Vitamin D—in some cases it may be too low, and, in other cases, too high.

If you need objective verification that your 1,25-D levels are in fact abnormal, several laboratory tests are available. These tests look at levels of 1,25 dihydroxyvitamin-D, 25 hydroxyvitamin-D and angiotensin-converting enzyme. The codes for these tests are LabCorp #081091, #081950, and #010116, respectively. A physician trained in applying the Marshall Protocol can help you understand, order, and interpret these tests. You can get a referral to such a physician and learn more about these tests at www.marshallprotocol.com.

If you do not have access to a Marshall Protocol-trained physician, the tests are still worth doing because they can help you convince your current physician that your Vitamin D levels are indeed problematic and that the medications and lifestyle modifications advocated by the Marshall Protocol are indicated. Test results are also helpful for patients themselves to see, as they can objectively identify Vitamin D dysregulation and establish that the protocol may be helpful. Seeing objective test results can dispel doubt in the protocol and establish a scientific basis for its use.

In the case of Lyme Disease, laboratory tests, while helpful, are not a necessary prerequisite to proceeding with the protocol. The tests can be quite expensive and are often not covered by health insurance. I personally never had Vitamin D tests done. The results of these tests are not always a perfect indicator of the treatment's potential usefulness and should not in any case be relied on too heavily. In lieu of or in addition to the tests, a therapeutic trial of the protocol can potentially determine whether or not a specific patient will find benefit.

Because the goal of reducing Vitamin D in the body is so unusual, many of you may be wondering why you should even consider it at all. After learning the basic principles of this protocol, I was asking the same question. However, after using the protocol, the answer became clear: I used the protocol because it works. It provided enormous, sustained improvement even after many other therapies failed. This improvement did not occur overnight, and there were some counterintuitive experiences along the way. We have already seen some of the counterintuitive principles involved in the Marshall Protocol, but lets take a closer look to ensure that these important concepts are fully covered.

As we have said in the *Spotlight on Vitamin D* SideBox, people infected with cell-wall-deficient bacteria may actually feel better with higher levels of Vitamin D on board, but this leads ultimately to increased severity of their disease. As Vitamin D is converted into 1,25-D by cell-wall-deficient bacteria, immune system activities (inflammation) are diminished. This results in a symptom-reducing effect. The superficial improvement experienced may even lead Lyme patients to seek out Vitamin D sources. The appropriate course of action, in actuality, is to reduce levels of Vitamin D in the body.

When Vitamin D levels are lowered to the point that bacteria are no longer able to stimulate production of 1,25-D, the immune system can again begin to perform properly. Herx reactions will accompany the reviving immune system as it begins to attack the infection and kill bacteria. If you have read *Lyme Disease and Rife Machines*, recall that herx reactions are a necessary, albeit uncomfortable, part of the recovery process. Be aware that it is easy to misinterpret what is actually going on. Herx reactions that occur as Vitamin D levels are lowered may seem like worsening of the disease. These herx-related symptoms may even be misinterpreted as Vitamin D deficiency. In reality, such symptoms are not indications of disease worsening, nor are they signs of Vitamin D deficiency, but instead, they are indications of true healing.

In the short term it is easy to conclude that the Marshall Protocol's Vitamin D reduction is harmful—it seems to increase symptoms. It is also natural to conclude that Vitamin D supplementation is beneficial—symptoms are alleviated. Because of this confusion and the counterintuitive nature of Vitamin D's effects in someone infected with cell-wall-deficient Lyme bacteria, it is important to study thoroughly and understand fully the Marshall Protocol. Vitamin D avoidance can be confidently relied on only if you feel comfortable in your understanding of its mechanism of action.

Please remember that the information in this chapter about Vitamin D is experimental and investigational. There may be negative side effects to Vitamin D reduction. Consult your physician.

AMPLIFIED EFFECT OF ANTIBIOTICS

The second foundational principle on which the Marshall Protocol is based is intimately connected with restoration of proper Vitamin D regulation: upon restoring healthy 1,25-D levels, not only is the immune system revived, but another related, and very significant, benefit is seen. Also at the core of the Marshall Protocol is the breakthrough discovery that standard pharmaceutical antibiotics have greatly enhanced effect when Vitamin D levels are properly balanced. This was first discovered by Dr. Marshall in relation to treating his own case of sarcoidosis.

In the past, sarcoidosis patients have received only minimal benefit from antibiotic therapy. But Dr. Marshall discovered that, upon reduction of 1,25-D levels, sarcoidosis patients can actually be cured with antibiotic therapy. Eventually, dozens of people with other chronic illnesses (including Lyme Disease) discovered the same to be true: having given up on antibiotic therapy due to disappointing results, they found relief and even remission when taking antibiotics after reducing 1,25-D levels. These discoveries launched the Marshall Protocol: a program that eradicates cell-wall-deficient bacteria by utilizing a coordinated schedule of particular antibiotics in combination with various methods of Vitamin D control.

When Vitamin D levels are appropriately reduced (which leads to decreased production of 1,25-D), antibiotics not only work better, they can become hyper-effective. So effective, in fact, that only a minuscule dose is needed to elicit powerful antibacterial action. This outcome is seen even in patients who have previously failed to respond to high-dose antibiotic therapy. For example, someone who previously experienced only mild benefits when taking 300mg/day of minocycline will experience dramatic benefits during use of the Marshall Protocol even though doses as low as 10mg/day may be used. Incredible, isn't it?

The amplified effect of antibiotics has a twofold benefit. First, it means that antibiotics will actually start to work for people who had not previously responded to them; and second, it means that antibiotic side effects are kept to a minimum during use of the protocol because doses can be kept low. This is great news! The Marshall Protocol solves two of the primary problems facing Lyme Disease sufferers: the marginal effectiveness of antibiotics and the toxic side effects associated with their use. Of course, increased effectiveness of antibiotics also means that herx reactions can be much more severe, thus, special care and caution is necessary.

Marshall Protocol components

Now that we have seen the principles that govern the protocol, let's examine the practical steps that comprise its use: lowering 1,25-D levels in the body and subsequent antibiotic dosing to eliminate the cell-wall-deficient bacteria.

CORRECTING VITAMIN D LEVELS

The Marshall Protocol establishes three primary means of lowering (correcting) 1,25-D levels: reducing exposure to sunlight and bright lights, avoiding Vitamin D containing foods, and taking Benicar, a special drug which both weakens cell-wall-deficient bacteria and lowers 1,25-D levels.

Reducing exposure to sunlight and artificial bright lights

While using the Marshall Protocol it is very helpful to protect both the skin and eyes from exposure to sunlight and bright lights. This action is beneficial because, when skin and eyes are exposed to sunlight and bright lights, Vitamin D is produced, which leads to 1,25-D synthesis by the bacteria. Avoidance is accomplished by wearing clothing which covers as much of the body as possible when outside (even on cloudy days) and when indoors if significant light sources are present (such as bright over-head lights, halogen, fluorescent lighting, etc.). This means long-sleeved shirts and long pants at all times, with the face and neck protected by a sun hat when outdoors. Eyes should also be carefully protected with special sunglasses that block not just harmful UV rays but also other types of light. When indoors the eyes must be protected from bright computer screens and televisions, either by avoiding them, viewing them through sunglasses, or decreasing contrast and brightness settings. To learn more about which types of sunglasses are appropriate, visit www.marshallprotocol.com.

Sun sensitivity often develops after the protocol is started (if it was not already present), which can include worsened symptoms of disease after exposure of the skin and eyes to sunlight (and/or bright, artificial lights). Some Lyme Disease sufferers may have had no prior symptoms of sensitivity to the sun or other bright lights before beginning the Marshall Protocol, so it may appear that the protocol is harming them if sensitivity begins to develop. This is another aspect of the Marshall Protocol that may seem counterintuitive. You may be thinking, *"I do not have sun sensitivity issues before the Marshall Protocol, but after I get started on it, I will develop sun sensitivity? This is absurd—how can a protocol that causes me to become unduly sensitive to the sun possibly be beneficial?"*

These questions and concerns are reasonable, but they are easily addressed once you understand how the Marshall Protocol works. Prior to using the Marshall Protocol, if your 1,25-D levels were high and out of control, sun exposure would not have made much of a difference in the levels or in how you feel. However, after you intentionally lower 1,25-D levels and the healing process begins, exposure to the sun or bright lights will cause 1,25-D levels to creep back up, thus halting progress and increasing symptoms. Although protecting yourself from the sun and bright lights may be difficult at first, it will eventually become natural as you simply feel better while complying.

To better understand how the process works, consider this example: someone with poor vision may not even be aware of the problem until getting glasses or corrective contacts. Although they may have never noticed a problem with their vision before, after it is corrected, the contrast makes the prior deficiency obvious. And if this person then tries to stop using corrective lenses, it will be even more obvious that their vision is less than sufficient. The realization will only come after having experienced corrected vision. In the same way, you will recognize the effects of high 1,25-D levels only *after* those levels are corrected and stabilized. At that point you will experience tremendous healing and improvement, and avoiding sunlight and bright light will no longer be a chore because you can clearly see the benefit to be gained.

If this concept still does not make sense to you, you can read about my personal experiences with the protocol at the end of this chapter. In that narration, you will gain a better understanding.

Many people on the Marshall Protocol joke that they are "cave dwellers." The lifestyle restrictions involved in the Marshall Protocol are significant and may cause some to go off the protocol prematurely. However, people who are very sick often experience such a change for the better while on the protocol that the lifestyle restrictions will seem a small price to pay. Those who embark on and succeed with the Marshall Protocol are usually desperate and have such a strong desire to get their lives back that they will gladly do what the protocol prescribes if it means relief from symptoms and the beginning of healing. Complying with the lifestyle restrictions of the Marshall Protocol is somewhat difficult, but the rewards can be overwhelmingly joyful.

The importance of avoiding sunlight and bright lights does decrease over time, fortunately, as cell-wall-deficient bacteria are eliminated from the body. The point in the Marshall Protocol when avoidance of sunlight becomes less important is approximately 18 months into the program. Although difficult and inconvenient, compliance during these 18 months is more than worth it because it helps you get your life back.

Specific guidelines for this aspect of the protocol can be found at www.marshallprotocol.com. At the time of this book's publication, a great deal of new information has become available regarding the issue of sun and light sensitivity/exposure. Please visit the website for the latest.

Avoiding Vitamin D sources in food and supplements

The next component of the protocol involves avoiding various high Vitamin D foods, including eggs, foods with egg products (such as mayonnaise and ranch dressing), all seafood and fish, seaweed and kelp. Many other products also have unacceptably high Vitamin D content. In order to reduce production of 1,25-D, not only must you prevent the Vitamin D synthesis that occurs after exposure of your skin to sunlight and bright lights, you also must prevent Vitamin D from entering your body via your diet.

The first and most obvious step to avoiding ingestion of Vitamin D is checking labels. Many cereals, processed foods, snacks, drinks, etc., contain added Vitamin D. Most milk is fortified with Vitamin D (although a careful search at your local grocery or natural foods store will most likely turn up a brand of milk that does not contain additional amounts). Many supplements also contain Vitamin D, and these must be avoided.

Many people feel noticeably worse when they accidentally consume Vitamin D (in the same way that inadvertent sun exposure will cause problems). This result serves as added motivation for avoidance. If noticeable negative effects are not felt immediately, they may still occur a few days after consumption of the Vitamin D and therefore not be consciously attributed to the offending food. The same goes for sunlight exposure: a symptom flareup several days after accidental sun exposure may not be obviously attributable to the offending episode.

Vitamin D becomes less of an issue over time. Just as the necessity of avoiding sun becomes less of a concern, the need to avoid Vitamin D containing foods will diminish.

Benicar lowers Vitamin D levels and weakens the bacteria

Benicar (olmesartan medoxomil, Sankyo Pharma Inc.), a drug conventionally used to lower high blood pressure, is called for in the Marshall Protocol because it acts to further regulate Vitamin D levels, weaken cell-wall-deficient bacteria, decrease nonproductive inflammation, and allow the antibiotics (which you'll learn about in the next section) to help the immune system kill the cell-wall-deficient bacteria. Avoidance of sun and diet sources of Vitamin D is not enough. The additional action of Benicar is necessary.

The blood pressure lowering effect of Benicar (the effect for which the drug was originally intended) is irrelevant to the Marshall Protocol—it is simply a side effect. The real value of Benicar is that, as an off label use, Dr. Marshall discovered that it serves to control the level of 1,25-D in the body and weaken the cell-wall-deficient bacteria. In treating diseases which are caused by cell-wall-deficient bacteria, use of a blood pressure lowering drug is simply a necessary evil that must be endured in order to realize the healing benefit of the Marshall Protocol. In other words, in the cost/benefit ratio of components of the Marshall Protocol, the benefit of using Benicar is healing from a disease conventionally believed to be incurable, at the cost of using a pharmaceutical drug that you would not otherwise take.

Fortunately, communications with the FDA have indicated that Benicar is among the safest of drugs currently available. Benicar-related effects noticed by people with chronic infections are typically herx reactions indicative of healing, not adverse side effects.

This is the part of the protocol that many people have the hardest time understanding. At this point you may be tempted to discount the treatment and say, *"This is ridiculous, I am supposed to take a blood pressure medication to lower Vitamin D levels in order to treat Lyme Disease?"* Despite the strangeness of it, the Marshall Protocol is arguably the most effective way to eliminate pathogenic cell-wall-deficient bacteria from the body. Although the program seems somewhat extreme, the simple fact is that it works. The most convincing evidence that the protocol is based on valid science is seen in the reports from hundreds of chronically ill people who have used the protocol with excellent results. In researching and determining whether or not you should use the Marshall Protocol, be sure to talk with other Marshall Protocol users. Their stories will help you gain confidence in the validity of the protocol's methodology, or help you decide that the protocol just isn't for you.

The concerns of those who already have low blood pressure or do not feel comfortable using a blood pressure lowering drug are valid. Fortunately, Benicar is one of the weakest blood pressure-lowering drugs on the market and has already been replaced by drugs more effective for this purpose. Benicar's blood pressure lowering effects are mild. Because chronic infection itself often leads to low blood pressure, many people reading this book will be concerned about taking a medication which might lower it further. But although a very minor blood pressure drop may be seen initially, chronically ill people with low blood pressure often notice that their blood pressure actually increases or stabilizes on the Marshall Protocol as a result of bacterial load reduction. Quite often, blood pressure actually normalizes as a result of the Marshall Protocol. This statement is based not only on the research substantiating the Marshall Protocol, but also on the reports of people using it. Although some people choose to purchase and use a blood pressure monitoring device, or have their blood pressure monitored by their physician, most patients quickly abandon these practices after it becomes obvious that blood pressure variations are insignificant.

A prescription is required to obtain Benicar, so you'll need either to find a Marshall Protocol-friendly physician or produce documentation explaining the treatment to your existing physician in order to familiarize him/her with the protocol so he/she can supervise your use of it. Referrals to Marshall Protocol-friendly physicians can be attained by visiting the Marshall Protocol website at www.marshallprotocol.com. Instructions detailing exactly how to use Benicar can also be found on that website.

ANTIBIOTICS

The next component of the Marshall Protocol (which also requires a physician's prescription) involves the use of specially selected antibiotics on a preplanned, precise dosing schedule in conjunction with Vitamin D avoidance and Benicar use.

In my first book, and elsewhere in this book, I explained how use of certain antibiotics (namely, cell wall inhibitors) in Lyme Disease can be extremely detrimental to the healing process because these drugs induce spirochete bacteria to convert to highly resistant cyst and cell-wall-deficient forms. I also explained that other types of antibiotics (namely, protein synthesis inhibitors) are less likely to cause bacterial conversion and are of great value to the healing process. These principles have not changed. However, since *Lyme Disease and Rife Machines* was published, evidence has been building which indicates that the most effective use of protein synthesis inhibiting antibiotics is achieved when they are administered as part of the Marshall Protocol, not when they are used alone. In fact, the Marshall Protocol so greatly increases the effectiveness of antibiotics that, in light of current knowledge, it is hard to justify antibiotic use outside of its parameters.

It is encouraging to me that both Trevor Marshall and I arrived at similar conclusions about antibiotic classifications even though our areas of research and experience are very different. We both agree that protein synthesis inhibiting antibiotics are the most beneficial, and we also agree that cell wall inhibiting antibiotics can be potentially harmful. This is one more indication to me that we are on the right track.

The most important concept to understand in relation to the antibiotic component of the Marshall Protocol is how differently the body, and the cell-wall-deficient bacteria inside the body, will respond to antibiotics when they are used as part of the Marshall Protocol. Because elevated 1,25-D levels in people with chronic infections cause immunosuppression, antibiotic therapy becomes much more powerful and effective when 1,25-D levels are lowered, as a result of enhanced immune function. In addition, Benicar itself weakens the cell-wall-deficient bacteria. This one-two punch of enhanced immune function and weakened bacteria renders antibiotics an entirely different treatment than when used without regard to the Marshall Protocol.

As we have said, the amplified effect of antibiotic therapy that occurs with the Marshall Protocol is so powerful that antibiotics are used in much smaller doses and taken much less frequently than is typical in non-Marshall Protocol antibiotic regimens. Yet herx reactions are often much more intense than when antibiotics are used in higher doses as part of other treatment plans. The reactions can be so intense that antibiotic doses must be gradually ramped up from initial, *very* small amounts. Even if a Marshall Protocol user has previously taken the same antibiotics indicated in the protocol without experiencing significant effect, the application of Marshall Protocol principles will most certainly augment antibiotic activity and lead to amplified herx reactions. This greatly amplified effect of antibiotics is just another reason the Marshall Protocol is so valuable. It simply gets to the root of the matter and gets the job done right.

Any level of improvement previously experienced as a result of using antibiotics will be greatly amplified on the Marshall Protocol. The antibiotics which never worked before have new, incredibly powerful effects, despite their greatly reduced doses. Because such small doses are required on the protocol, many side effects commonly experienced with higher doses of antibiotics are avoided. Candida, immune system suppression, disturbed digestion, and other such problems happen less frequently.

Of utmost importance in the Marshall Protocol is the selection of the specific antibiotic classes to be used. There is a tendency for people to believe erroneously that all antibiotics are similar in function and result. In reality, and especially in relation to the treatment of cell-wall-deficient bacteria, different classes of antibiotics will have totally different effects, even to the point of making or breaking the success of the treatment protocol. In fact, the problem of cell-wall-deficient bacteria in the first place is likely a result of overuse of the wrong antibiotics: cell-wall-deficient bacteria are often caused by forced conversion from other bacterial forms as a result of using cell wall inhibiting antibiotics.

This book will not present the specific antibiotics used in the Marshall Protocol. See www.marshallprotocol.com for further discussion on the topic of antibiotic selection.

My experience with and commentary on the modified Marshall Protocol

Now that you have been introduced to the Marshall Protocol, I would like to share my personal experience with it.

Many protocols have predetermined, rigid guidelines. In reality, despite these guidelines, everyone is different and certain people will need variations of a given protocol. Such was the case with myself. After using / experimenting with the Marshall Protocol for over three years, I came to discover that what worked best for me was slightly different than the standard protocol. In this section I will share the variations that worked for me, and why I believe these variations were beneficial. However, I must disclose that the information below is my experience and opinion only, and should not be mistaken for the official Marshall Protocol developed by Dr. Marshall. For this reason, I am referring to my experiences in this section as the "modified Marshall Protocol." Please realize that this section includes only the experiences of one person.

Before looking at how I personally modified the protocol, I would like to share some related background information.

The story begins in fall of 2002, when my Lyme Disease symptoms first began to get out of control. Looking back, I now believe that I had been infected with Lyme Disease for my whole life—but the disease did not take over and become unmanageable until fall of 2002. (Note that this occurred in fall, not another season, which verifies the conclusions drawn in *Lyme Disease and Rife Machines* about the significance of spring and fall in Lyme Disease bacterial activities.) Shortly after the infection worsened in those autumn months, I started to notice a strange reaction to the sun. Each time my skin was exposed to the sun for more than a few minutes, I could feel something changing in my body—changing for the worse. Then, after I got out of the sun, whatever had changed did not completely go away. It was as if whatever was happening in the sun was causing some type of permanent changes in my body. Each subsequent time I would get sun exposure, I noticed the same thing would happen, over and over, leading to a sustained worsening of symptoms. Because it was still early in my illness, I had absolutely no idea what was happening, and I did not know if it was important or not. Now I know that it was very important.

Eventually, I reached a point when these reactions no longer occurred and sun exposure did not have any effect. At the time, I believed that this meant I was healing—whatever ugly disease process had caused the sun sensitivity had most certainly resolved, I thought to myself. After all, the reactions had stopped, right? The only problem was that the worsened symptoms that resulted from the sun reactions did not go away. The reactions themselves stopped happening, but it felt as if permanent damage had been done.

It would be two more years before I even heard about the Marshall Protocol. When I began reading about the Marshall Protocol and what it said about sun exposure, I was intrigued and immediately interested because of my strange experience with the sun in 2002. Although various aspects of the Marshall Protocol seemed outlandish to me, I did not write the protocol off because it was the only protocol I had ever seen that potentially explained my experiences with the sun.

Amazingly, when I first began to use the Marshall Protocol, it actually felt as if I were reversing the damage done during those sun exposure episodes in the fall of 2002. As I followed the Marshall Protocol guidelines of avoiding sun exposure and Vitamin D consumption, using Benicar, and taking Marshall Protocol antibiotics, I literally felt the same reactions as I did in 2002, except this time, I was experiencing reduction in aggregate symptoms instead of an increase in symptoms. Needless to say, this experience immediately convinced me that this protocol was significant and dealt with an aspect of the Lyme Disease complex that to date, no other protocol has successfully addressed. Later during my use of the protocol, this conclusion would only be strengthened as I experienced continual progress and healing.

Hindsight is 20/20. Looking back, I now know that when the reactions I had to the sun in late 2002 diminished, it was not a sign that I was getting better. It was instead a sign that I had reached an unhealthy equilibrium in which Vitamin D levels in my body had greatly increased, aiding the bacterial infection in its survival and proliferation. Although the reactions had stopped, my symptoms were greatly worsened—and remained greatly worsened all the way up until I first started using the Marshall Protocol. I did not return to feeling relatively well until the Marshall Protocol helped me reverse those reactions and return to a healthy equilibrium. It is important to note that my experiences were very counterintuitive. When my initial reactions of 2002 went away, it actually meant I was worse. When the reactions returned as a result of using the Marshall Protocol, it meant I was getting better.

I believe I was lucky that my initial experience with the sun in 2002 was so acute and dramatic, and, therefore, memorable. I was also lucky that I noticed, upon beginning the Marshall Protocol, that the resultant reactions were somehow related to my earlier experiences with the sun. I'm sure that many people undergo the same processes that I did but do not experience them as vividly. It would be much harder for these people to evaluate their response to the Marshall Protocol (or any protocol for that matter). People who cannot interpret their responses to the Marshall Protocol might conclude that the reactions are harmful, instead of concluding that they are an indication of the reversal of previous damage done. After all, the Marshall Protocol is somewhat unusual, and without personal experiential evidence like my own, it might be hard to rationalize use of the protocol.

Experiencing acute, intense, perceptible changes and reactions during the course of my chronic illness was not limited to my experiences with the sun and the Marshall Protocol. For some reason, most of what has happened to me during my struggle with Lyme Disease has been this way. I have been very aware of my body and usually I am able to tell quite clearly what is taking place. I believe this acute perception is one of the factors that have allowed me to write the books that I have written. Having a unique ability to perceive reactions that most Lyme sufferers do not notice has given me a 6th sense with regard to interpreting and evaluating various treatments. Since modern medical science leaves much to be desired in the area of Lyme Disease understanding, my 6th sense is a special, invaluable resource. Of course, the subjective experiences of one person are not sufficient to draw scientific conclusions from. However, they sure do help!

There is one more experience I would like to share before moving on to the ways in which I modified the standard Marshall Protocol. When I first began taking Benicar, the reaction I had was so strong and alarming that I wrote it off as a horrible side effect of the drug itself and not a herx reaction. The reaction lasted for almost a week after just one tiny dose of

Benicar. It was so severe that I stopped using the protocol and did not revisit it again for a long time. Many other Lyme Disease sufferers have had similar experiences. Such experiences are responsible for the reputation the protocol has earned as a very extreme, potentially dangerous protocol. However, although it may be natural for the people who experience strong reactions to conclude that those reactions are horrific side effects, I later learned (via research, future experiences of my own, and communicating with other Lyme Disease sufferers) that said reactions are not side effects but instead, genuine herx reactions resulting from attacking and challenging the Lyme Disease infection. The disease itself, in response to the treatment, produces the monstrous reactions as the disease fights to win the battle and persist in the body. It is no secret that chronic Lyme Disease is an entrenched, stubborn, strong infection. It is also no secret that there are very few ways to actually remove the infection. When you begin to make progress in uprooting the bacterial colonies, a full-scale war is the result. And believe me, war is what you feel. The reactions are a result of forcing the body to move from a sick equilibrium to a healthy equilibrium. This is most certainly not a comfortable process. However, comfortable or not, you cannot blame the protocol for these reactions, you can only blame the disease.

One of the convincing factors that prompted me to conclude that reactions to the Marshall Protocol are herx reactions and not side effects is the fact that people who are not chronically infected with cell-wall-deficient bacteria do not experience horrific reactions to Benicar. Remember, Benicar is nothing more than a commonly used drug for lowering blood pressure. Sure, Benicar does have some documented side effects. No pharmaceutical drug is without side effects. However, the documented side effects for Benicar are nothing even close to what people harboring cell-wall-deficient bacteria experience. Some of the documented side effects for Benicar include back pain, bronchitis, creatine phosphokinase increase, diarrhea, headache, hyperglycemia, influenza-like symptoms, rhinitis and sinusitis. Yet, what I experienced when I first started taking Benicar was an undeniable and extreme flareup in my Lyme Disease symptoms (or symptoms similar to my Lyme Disease symptoms). Although severe, these reactions were not drug side effects.

My personal experience is another factor which supports my conclusion that Marshall Protocol reactions are not side effects but instead herx reactions: as I progressed on the protocol, despite continuing to use Benicar, the reactions diminished and so did my overall disease symptoms. My state of health and well-being increased dramatically the longer I used the protocol. Theoretically, if what I was experiencing was drug side effects, they should not have dissipated over time but instead intensified. Yet, the opposite is what occurred. Presently, as I write this, I am able to take the full Marshall Protocol dose of Benicar with close to zero reaction. And, I credit a large portion of my recovery to the Marshall Protocol. If Marshall Protocol reactions were somehow harmful, then how do you explain these occurrences?

With all that said, it is important to note that even though Marshall Protocol reactions are indeed genuine herx reactions, it is still possible that these reactions can be dangerous or even life-threatening. The fact that the reactions are productive and result from the disease, and not drug side effects, does not provide free license to let these reactions get out of control, and does not mean that these reactions are categorically safe. In fact, herx reactions as a result of the Marshall Protocol or any other Lyme Disease treatment can be very dangerous and frightening, and should be respected. Herx reactions can be as or more dangerous than side effects of pharmaceutical drugs. Important steps must be taken to control and minimize these reactions during use of the Marshall Protocol. This book will not describe what these steps are. You can learn about how to safely control Marshall Protocol reactions at www.marshallprotocol.com. **It is absolutely critical to have a solid understanding of how to control Marshall Protocol reactions before you use the protocol!**

Now I will share the modifications to the protocol that I personally found to be beneficial. Remember, these modifications have not been evaluated or approved by Dr. Marshall or other official researchers of the protocol. They are simply my experiences. These modifications, while beneficial to me, may be harmful to others. So as you read on, please keep in mind that this information is experimental.

The first modification to the protocol I eventually found beneficial was using it in a pulsed manner. "Pulsing" a therapy simply means using it for a time, then taking some time off, then using it for a time again, then taking some time off, and so on. There are several reasons why I pulsed the protocol. Some of the reasons are related to my subjective experience of the protocol and other reasons are related to philosophical conclusions I arrived at with regard to the protocol. Here are the reasons I pulsed the protocol:

1. Because Benicar is a drug, I desired to give my body a rest from its use. Additionally, the Marshall Protocol calls for using a relatively high dose of Benicar. This further solidified my decision to take breaks from the protocol. I did experience what I believe were a few mild side effects of Benicar including some heartburn and indigestion. Breaks from the protocol were one solution to this problem.

2. Being on the Marshall Protocol was quite intense, even after the initial reactions dissipated. I found my quality of life was unacceptably compromised if I used the protocol continuously. Many Marshall Protocol users have commented that this diminished quality of life is justified and should simply be tolerated. However, in my case it was not. If I were forced to use the protocol either continuously or not at all, I would have chosen not at all. Therefore, using the protocol in a pulsed fashion, in my opinion, was more beneficial for me than not using it at all. Results may have been slower than they could have been, but nevertheless, results were still forthcoming.

3. In general, I believe that most, if not all, Lyme Disease treatments have the highest level of benefit and lowest toxic impact when they are used in a pulsing manner. You will notice this theme throughout my books with regard to lots of different types of therapies. I hold this position both because of philosophical conclusions and my subjective experiences during the recovery process. In short, pulsing various Lyme Disease treatments ensures that the bacterial infection never has time to adapt to the treatment, and that the infection is always caught off guard. It also reduces side effects and

gives the body time to figure out what to do on its own during breaks from therapy.

4. My health insurance did not cover Benicar or the antibiotics used in the Marshall Protocol. Ideally, my financial state should not have any influence on how I built my treatment campaign. In reality, however, finances are just as real as Lyme Disease bacteria. The protocol was more affordable when breaks were taken.

5. Because the Marshall Protocol utilizes pharmaceutical antibiotics, I believe it can potentially interfere with the progress of rife machine therapy (see *Lyme Disease and Rife Machines* for more information on this topic). I still believe that rife machine therapy is the foundational treatment upon which the recovery process is built. Therefore, any treatment that compromises the success of a rife treatment campaign is unacceptable. Using the Marshall Protocol in a pulsed manner ensures that rife machine therapy is not hindered.

I found that the best time to use the Marshall Protocol was typically during the winter, between the months of September and April. This does not mean I used the protocol continuously during this time frame, but instead, this was the time frame in which pulsed applications of the protocol were most beneficial for me. During the summer months of April to September, my symptoms were generally at a minimum, and I did not feel the need to use the protocol. This summer symptom reprieve is consistent with what Doug MacLean, inventor of the first rife machine used to fight Lyme Disease, also experienced. Some would argue for continuing to use the protocol during the summer months despite the symptom reprieve. And, maybe my recovery would have progressed faster had I done that. For that matter, maybe my recovery would have progressed faster had I not made any modifications to the Marshall Protocol at all. However, the fact remains that based on my philosophical conclusions and subjective experiences, these modifications to the protocol were justified.

I also found that using the Marshall Protocol during spring and fall helped mitigate the inevitable spring/fall flareups. Particularly, I found

Benicar use to be valuable during these times. In fact, sometimes I would use only Benicar and not take antibiotics at all. As I progressed through the recovery process, I found more and more that Benicar was the ingredient that helped the most, and that the antibiotics were not as important. This observation was not categorically true, especially in the beginning. At first, I noticed that the antibiotic component of the protocol was critical. So, clearly, things changed as time went on. The antibiotics eventually lost most of their effect, but Benicar did not.

Avoiding sun exposure and Vitamin D consumption was another component of the protocol that did not lose its beneficial effect. This component continued to be helpful throughout my entire healing process. In fact, as a very important note to my readers, I should mention that even during breaks from the protocol, I still followed the recommendations of staying out of the sun (or wearing long sleeves, a sun hat, and sunglasses when in the sun) and avoiding food sources of Vitamin D. For me, taking time off from the protocol meant that I was not using Benicar and antibiotics. Continuing to avoid sun and Vitamin D foods was very natural for me to do even while on breaks from Benicar and antibiotics because if I failed to do this, symptoms would quickly return. My body quite clearly communicated to me that sun avoidance and Vitamin D food avoidance was the proper course of action. Returning symptoms upon sun exposure would feel very similar to the initial harmful reactions I experienced in fall 2002. This was a blatant indication that continual avoidance of sun exposure was critical. In my opinion, staying out of the sun and avoiding Vitamin D foods even while taking breaks from Benicar and antibiotics is what prevented me from losing the gains I had made.

Sure, the lifestyle restrictions involved in avoiding Vitamin D foods and especially avoiding the sun are significant, especially considering that I continued to comply with these restrictions even during my breaks from the protocol. The lifestyle restrictions were even more cumbersome for me, as a person who thrives in the outdoors and loves to hike, mountain bike, and just plain be outside. However, having been so sick and so miserable with chronic Lyme Disease, complying with these restrictions was something I was willing to do. I did not just comply with these restrictions due to philosophical or theoretical information. I complied because the protocol was helping to give me my life back—and I felt this in a very real way. Symptoms kept diminishing and my overall quality of life kept increasing. If I failed to stay out of the sun and avoid Vitamin D containing foods, I would backslide. Truthfully, real symptom improvement is just about the only thing that could actually convince someone to comply with such inconvenient lifestyle restrictions. Not to mention the silliness of wearing long pants and shirts in the heat of summer, and the associated, inevitable funny looks and questions.

Thankfully, I was still able to participate in many of the outdoor activities I loved simply by wearing long sleeves, long pants, a sun hat, and sunglasses while partaking in them. Fortunately, I live high in the mountains, and there were only a few weeks of the summer during which the temperatures were high enough to make it very uncomfortable to participate in outdoor activities with the excessive clothing I had to wear.

Many people disagree with the Marshall Protocol premise that sun avoidance is beneficial. Quite a few respected sources on health and physiology actually conclude the opposite of what the Marshall Protocol states. Most healthcare practitioners and researchers say that Vitamin D is healthy and beneficial to healing chronic disease. Numerous studies have shown that Vitamin D aids in healing. It has been documented that some forms of chronic disease actually result from Vitamin D *deficiency*.

I cannot, nor will I try to, argue with the evidence that Vitamin D is beneficial for various health problems. I know very well that intentionally avoiding both Vitamin D and sun exposure for long periods of time seems to be contrary to established wisdom. However, I also cannot argue with what I experienced. Use of the Marshall Protocol greatly accelerated my healing in many ways. I believe that my body knows what it needs. The long-term, sustained, unrelenting symptom improvement I got from using the Marshall Protocol was far more than I gained with most of the other Lyme Disease treatments I used. I do not claim to fully understand the mechanism by which it is possible for something as beneficial as Vitamin D to be so detrimental to people with Lyme Disease. I'm not sure anyone completely understands this, although Dr. Marshall probably has the best grasp of the science. Did the caveman understand the physiological reasons why drinking water is life-sustaining? No. But of course, the caveman still drank water and lived. All I can do is share what I have experienced and let you come to your own conclusion.

Trial and error vs. laboratory testing

There seems to be two groups of Lyme sufferers: one group that benefits greatly from the Marshall Protocol and may even require it to get well, and another group that sees minimal or no benefit from the protocol. At the time this book was written, it is not known exactly why some people fall into one category while other people fall into the other category. It seems likely that, quite simply, those whose cases of Lyme Disease involve the physiological problems which the Marshall Protocol addresses will require the protocol, and those whose cases of Lyme Disease do not involve those physiological problems may not need the protocol.

The best (and possibly only) method of finding out which group you fall into is simply to try the protocol. Instead of over-researching, over-analyzing, and over-questioning the protocol, the better course of action is to just take it for a test drive and see what happens. Benefit from the protocol can be identified and measured by symptom improvement and the accompanying productive herx reactions. It is important to remember that the Marshall Protocol typically causes dramatic herx reactions—these reactions are not an indication that the protocol isn't working; instead, quite often, they are an indication that the protocol *is* working.

If the protocol works for you, then keep using it. If it does not help you, then discontinue it. It really is that simple. This trial-and-error philosophy appears throughout my books as a result of the fact that I do not have a high degree of confidence in the reliability of the majority of Lyme-related tests and diagnostic procedures. Instead of fancy tests, I think it is a better option to simply use a therapeutic trial of a given treatment (whether that treatment is rife machine therapy, the Marshall Protocol, or something else) to determine whether or not it has applicability in a specific individual's case of Lyme Disease. Lyme Disease and its associated physiological effects are just too complicated and poorly understood by modern medicine to assume that current testing procedures can accurately identify the disease or even the appropriate treatment protocols for the disease.

Rife machines vs. the Marshall Protocol

Many people have asked me whether I believe the Marshall Protocol can replace rife machine therapy or whether rife machine therapy can replace the Marshall Protocol. Ideally, we should use as few treatments as possible. If only one of these treatments is necessary, there would be no need to use both. However, after studying, using, reading about, and analyzing the two treatments, the conclusion I reach is that each treatment targets an aspect of the Lyme Disease complex that the other treatment misses. In this way, as far as I know, neither treatment is superfluous, and when used together, the two treatments have synergistic value.

A final word

Although relatively new, the Marshall Protocol is among the most promising of Lyme Disease therapies. Its potential should be thoroughly investigated by all Lyme Disease sufferers. Even though the concepts on which the protocol is based are seemingly counterintuitive and can take a while to get used to, the therapy has an unrivaled ability to eradicate cell-wall-deficient bacteria and elicit permanent clinical improvement in many sufferers of Lyme Disease and other allegedly incurable illnesses which share cell-wall-deficient bacteria as their root cause.

This chapter has not provided sufficient information to enable someone to begin using the Marshall Protocol as part of a Lyme Disease treatment program. Instead, the chapter is intended only as an introduction. The Marshall Protocol must be employed very carefully, according to a specific, step-by-step process. For detailed instructions and comprehensive information about the full protocol, including an internet discussion group with over 3,000 members, visit www.marshallprotocol.com.

Chapter 3:
The Salt / Vitamin C
Protocol

A new discovery

As early as 2002, reports began appearing on the internet and in Lyme Disease support groups indicating that intake of salt and Vitamin C may have potential benefit in the treatment of Lyme Disease and its co-infections.

The first hint was found on a web site (www.lymephotos.com) authored by several Lyme Disease sufferers who reported that they had achieved remission from their symptoms by using an oral salt and Vitamin C treatment. The website was fairly obscure and not well-known in the Lyme community, and even where it was known many questioned the protocol and the veracity of the website. Some Lyme sufferers tried the protocol, but (according to one researcher) a full two-thirds discontinued it when unexpectedly pronounced herx reactions (microbial die-off symptoms) were encountered.

When I published my first book in January of 2005, user reports were still sparse and scientific research on the protocol even harder to come by. There was enough information for Lyme patients to know that the Salt / Vitamin C protocol appeared promising, but not enough information to draw any conclusions. So the therapy earned a passing mention in my first book, but nothing more.

Interest in the protocol broadens

Just several weeks after my first book was published, another intriguing mention of the protocol appeared, this time in print. The January, 2005 issue of *Townsend Letter for Doctors and Patients*, a monthly alternative medicine periodical, included a story entitled "Lyme Disease, Potential Plague of the 21st Century." The article was written by several well-respected researchers, including Professor Robert Bradford of the Bradford Research Institute, and contained not only coverage of the oral Salt / Vitamin C protocol but also the first working hypothesis I had seen describing how and why the protocol works.

It was around this time that interest in this newly emerging protocol began to grow.

A fellow researcher and friend of mine who had applied an extensive array of treatments to his own Lyme Disease infection, including traveling to other countries for cutting-edge treatments not available in the United States, began to research the protocol intensively. A wide-ranging investigation of relevant studies and abstracts as well as direct collaboration with a Lyme Disease research laboratory convinced him of the scientific validity behind the protocol as described at www.lymephotos.com. Additionally, an apparent synergy was identified with regard to using salt and Vitamin C together that was not found with use of each item individually. Discussions with individuals with biological, microbiological, and medical science backgrounds provided further confirmation that the treatment can be a valuable addition to the Lyme Disease treatment toolbox.

As a result of his research and growing confidence in the protocol, my friend applied the protocol to himself and with its use became free of Lyme Disease symptoms. A Yahoo! online discussion group focusing on the Salt / Vitamin C protocol was established shortly thereafter. As this group grew in numbers, user data began to accumulate rapidly which indicated that the protocol was indeed helping many Lyme Disease sufferers. Today, the group has grown to more than one thousand members, many of whom have publicly reported that the Salt / Vitamin C protocol is the most effective treatment they have used for Lyme Disease. A number of these folks have reported that their Lyme symptoms have gone into remission. Those achieving these encouraging results represent all age groups, both male and female, as well as various durations of infection (from a few years to decades). You may follow a link to this discussion group and join by visiting: www.lymebook.com/resources.

One user report of particular interest detailed the experience of a single Lyme Disease sufferer who had been using rife machine therapy for approximately 18 months. Having improved greatly, even to the point of being able to walk on her own again without a walker, she began to relapse and felt that rife machine therapy was no longer working. At the time, evidence seemed to indicate that the type of machine she was using was not sufficient to provide sustained improvement, and many fellow Lyme Disease sufferers recommended a machine upgrade. There was also evidence to indicate that her machine may have been broken. However, this particular Lyme sufferer decided to try the Salt / Vitamin C protocol.

She began to improve rapidly and regained her progress, even reaching a level of health which her rife machine had not provided. Although it is likely that a more efficient rife machine would have provided the same results, it was the oral Salt / Vitamin C protocol that got her back on track.

In experiences similar to this, many other rife machine users have reported that rife machine therapy restores their health to about 90% of pre-Lyme levels but that the last 10% is more difficult to achieve. The oral Salt / Vitamin C protocol, in addition to the other therapies discussed in this book, appears to have a synergistic effect with rife treatment, possibly serving as the missing link needed for achieving the last 10%. In this way, the protocol should not be thought of as a replacement for rife technology, but, instead, a supportive treatment.

User reports such as these, which were at first subtle and easy to miss but became more substantial over time, led to inclusion of the oral Salt / Vitamin C protocol as one of the top 10 Lyme Disease treatments discussed in this book. Although the protocol is still in its infancy, it warrants investigation by every Lyme Disease sufferer.

One of the most exciting aspects of the protocol is that it appears to provide clinical benefit against not only Borrelia Burgdorferi itself but also numerous co-infections. The researchers who developed the protocol believe that Lyme Disease involves many complicated infective organisms, including even microfilarial worms which live symbiotically with bacteria and protect them from the activity of antibiotics. Because all microorganisms rely on a delicate sodium balance to survive, and because this protocol fundamentally changes that balance, the researchers conclude that many different types of microorganisms associated with Lyme Disease may be targeted.

The first explanation of why it works

At this point in time, most of the information establishing the effectiveness of the oral Salt / Vitamin C protocol comes from anecdotal user reports. However, the article in *Townsend Letter for Doctors and Patients* provides the beginnings of a scientific basis upon which further studies may be conducted. The authors of the article hypothesize that salt helps kill microorganisms in two ways.

First, salt enhances the activity of elastase, an enzyme which contributes to white blood cell function and immunity. During acute inflammatory responses, elastase is released by white blood cells called neutrophils. The released substance generates fibers in surrounding tissues that may facilitate phagocytosis (the break down and destruction of pathogens) by trapping bacteria and focusing enzyme activity on their elimination. The *Townsend Letter* states that "through oral salt (12 g per day), combined with large doses of Vitamin C, the indirect killing ability of elastase is dramatically increased."

Second, increasing sodium concentration surrounding microorganisms like Borrelia Burgdorferi leads to bacterial death as sodium ions enter the spirochete form of the bacterium. To be precise, "an increased intracellular sodium concentration, combined with a decreased potassium concentration, leads to spirochete death." Specific cause of death is by activity of an antimicrobial peptide in neutrophils known as LL-37.

What about the Vitamin C component of the protocol? Research indicates that Vitamin C, when used with salt, greatly accelerates the healing process by stimulating and restoring the immune system as well as detoxifying the body.

One distinct advantage of the oral Salt / Vitamin C protocol is its simplicity: it can be used at home, without a prescription, at a very low cost. It can also be combined safely with most other Lyme Disease treatment protocols. To date, there are no known adverse side effects of the protocol; however, some researchers have expressed concern over potential negative impact on the kidneys. A few Lyme Disease sufferers have reported kidney pain while using the protocol. It is unknown whether this pain is a side effect of the protocol (undesirable) or a herx reaction occurring as a result of bacterial die-off (desirable). Based on medical and veterinary abstracts it has been found that the kidneys are primary targets of the Lyme Disease pathogen and its co-infections, so it is possible that reactions experienced in the kidneys may simply be bacterial die-off. Evidence supporting this conclusion includes the fact that, to date, laboratory tests conducted on protocol users who experience kidney pain have shown no kidney problems. Many such individuals have had their doctors carefully test liver and kidney function and have received favorable results. Additionally, the kidney pain is typically reported to be transitory and, according to some reports, eventually fades during the protocol process.

Reports have also shown that approximately 5% of Salt / Vitamin C protocol users may experience blood pressure and water retention problems. The protocol should only be used under the careful supervision of a licensed physician. Remember, this therapy is experimental.

How is the protocol used?

According to lymephotos.com, the treatment involves the oral intake of 8-16 grams of salt and 8-16 grams of Vitamin C per day. The dose of each component should be started at much lower levels and increased gradually according to personal die-off (herx) reaction tolerance. Diarrhea and other detoxification reactions may occur as pathogens are killed and eliminated from the body. More information is available on the lymephotos.com website. The exact description of what is known as the "scale-up method" of dosing can be found at the Yahoo! discussion group mentioned earlier.

The type of salt used is of critical importance. Only pharmaceutical-grade salt tablets (the kind used to make saline solution) or natural salts such as unprocessed sea-derived or Himalayan salts are acceptable. A good brand is Real Salt, www.realsalt.com. Standard, store-bought table salt was found to be adverse and toxic, made harmful due to extreme heating in production as well as the addition of aluminum hydroxide, silica aluminate (aluminum has been implicated in Alzheimer's Disease), sodium ferrocyanide, tri-calcium phosphate, stearic acid, and other substances. The aluminum additives leave a bitter taste so manufacturers add dextrose, a refined sugar, which has been found in studies to disrupt the body's equilibrium.

Most types of Vitamin C are acceptable; however, buffered Vitamin C (for example, Ester-C) is more easily tolerated in the high doses called for by the protocol. The buffered form of Vitamin C allows for avoidance of excess acidity caused by use of Vitamin C in its common ascorbic acid form.

Because both salt and Vitamin C are water-soluble, lots of water should be consumed throughout the day in order to maintain hydration and to circulate the salt and Vitamin C throughout the body and flush them from the system.

We have described here only the basics of this new, important Lyme Disease therapy. At www.lymebook.com/resources, you can find links to more detailed and advanced information. One available resources is an instructional E-Book which explains exactly how to use the Salt / Vitamin C protocol. At the time of this book's writing, the fee to download the E-Book was $29.95. The cost includes access to information about the protocol and how it was developed, available research on it, methods of action of both salt and Vitamin C, how to use the "scale up" dosing schedule, and the materials needed for the treatment and where to get them. The book also looks at the protocol's safety and describes appropriate information to present to doctors. To learn more, visit www.lymebook.com/resources.

Chapter 4: Detoxification

A toxic world

E liminating waste is just as important as eating. Stop eating for awhile and you are dead. Stop exhaling, urinating, and having bowel movements, and you are dead even faster. The human body is equipped with many tools and metabolic processes that are designed to prepare excess or harmful substances for elimination from the body—a process called detoxification. A healthy body in perfect condition, surrounded by a perfectly clean environment, does not need help to remove wastes. However, there are many aspects of life in the 21st century which can cause us to accumulate more wastes than we can remove. If not properly eliminated, waste products accumulate in the body and become toxic. There are two primary reasons why this can happen:

1. In the manufacturing process of the products we use every day (food, automobiles, homes, clothing, dental and medical products, personal care products, etc.), industrialized society has found it most efficient and profitable to use synthetic substances and chemicals which our bodies do not have the native ability to detoxify. Products and food that contain these toxic substances are all around us, so entrenched in our lifestyle that they are impossible to avoid regardless of how health-conscious we are.

2. Typically we do not take sufficiently good care of our bodies to keep detoxification processes at optimal functionality. Diet, exercise habits, and amount of rest we get are all culprits in suboptimal detoxification. And, in conjunction with point number one, industrialized products, foods, and chemicals further weaken and stress the detoxification organs of the body.

As a result of these factors, the body's detoxification processes do not happen perfectly, and dangerous toxins can easily outpace the body's ability to eliminate them. A toxin is basically any substance that causes harm to our bodies and undermines our health, and there are as many resultant health afflictions as there are different types of toxins. Autoimmune disorders, chronic infections, degenerative conditions, cancer, high cholesterol, high blood pressure, and many other illnesses are often caused or worsened by an accumulation of toxic substances. For gaining further understanding, a great book on the subject is *Detoxify or Die*, by Sherry Rogers, M.D.

Toxins can accumulate in the bodies of all of us, young and old, healthy and sick, black and white, rich and poor. Unfortunately, if you have Lyme Disease, you have even more to worry about. Like everyone else, you live in a society which exposes you to dozens of synthetic toxins in your clothing, food, environment, vehicle, job, home—and just about everywhere else. But your Lyme Disease infection produces additional and very potent toxins which wreak havoc on every major system in the body. These toxins are produced continuously, twenty-four seven, by the bacteria which cause Lyme Disease. Not only are you faced with the same toxic exposure as anyone else who lives in the industrialized world, you are also forced to deal with these added bacterial toxins. To make matters worse, Lyme Disease sufferers typically use high doses of synthetic drugs (such as antibiotics). These drugs can accumulate in tissues and reach toxic levels, which add to the already toxic condition and the need for detoxification.

Additionally, the inflammation and physiological stress created by a chronic infection such as Lyme Disease puts an incredible burden on all of your internal organs, including detoxification organs like the liver and kidneys. Industrialized toxins, Lyme Disease toxins, build up of synthetic drugs, and stress from a chronic illness all mean that most Lyme Disease sufferers have a much higher concentration of accumulated toxic substances in their body than do other people.

Toxins are classified as either water-soluble or fat-soluble. The primary difference between the two is that the fat-soluble type is most often associated with long-term, debilitating, chronic illness, while water-soluble toxins are usually associated with rapid-onset, acute, short-term illness. Our focus in this chapter will be on fat-soluble toxins, so detoxification processes and therapies for water-soluble toxins will not be covered. For example, because the kidneys primarily eliminate water-soluble toxins, a discussion of the kidneys is not included.

Lyme Disease toxins and most of the toxins produced by industrialized manufacturing are fat-soluble, so named because they accumulate in the body's fat stores. Fat-soluble toxins pose a danger to our bodies for three reasons. First, even in very thin people, there is enough fat in the body to store a colossal amount of fat soluble toxins. Second, because the brain is comprised mostly of fatty tissue, these toxins can end up saturating the brain. And third, removal of this type of toxin is extremely difficult.

When the body's detoxification mechanisms become overloaded with fat-soluble toxins, the body intentionally stores them in body fat. If toxins are allowed to remain in circulation, they pose a threat to critical body systems. When detoxification pathways are maxed out, storage of fat-soluble toxins in body fat is really the body's only option. It is a better solution than allowing them to remain in the circulatory system where they cause the most immediate damage.

Whether or not detoxification pathways become overwhelmed (leading to toxin storage) depends on several factors. These include the innate genetic strength and constitution of a person's detoxification organs, the quantity and type of toxins to which that person is exposed, and other factors like stress, healthy (or unhealthy) diet, rest, and lifestyle habits. Harboring a Lyme Disease infection adds to the toxic burden, making it even less likely that the body will be able to handle all the toxins it encounters.

So what is the problem with storing toxins in our fat? If these toxins are safely out of the way, maybe we shouldn't have to worry about them, right? Wrong. Unfortunately, although the body does everything it can to get these excess toxins quarantined off, storing fat-soluble toxins in tissues throughout the body is not an adequate solution to the problem of our toxic world.

First, although less harmful when stored, these toxins still exert ill effects on the body. Second, when in storage, the toxins occasionally break loose from the fatty tissues in which they reside and enter circulation, resulting in symptoms of sickness/poisoning and weakening of important body functions. Third, if a person does not change whatever circumstances and conditions have led to increasing toxicity in the first place, there will come a point when even the storage sites have reached maximum capacity, and new toxins will begin to accumulate in the bloodstream and in the brain, which is itself composed primarily of fatty tissue.

When putting toxins in storage, the body will initially place them in fatty tissues other than the brain. However, as these other storage compartments fill up, the brain becomes an inevitable reservoir in which fat-soluble toxins begin to accumulate. Additionally, because the body is not 100% proficient in handling toxins in the first place, some end up in the brain regardless of the body's efforts against this.

Many of the world's most devastating illnesses are caused by fat-soluble toxins which accumulate in the brain. Many psychiatric illnesses are caused or exacerbated by toxins stored in the brain. These include schizophrenia, depression, memory loss, bipolar disorder, Alzheimer's disease, obsessive-compulsive disorder, and the like. Physical disorders such as multiple sclerosis, Parkinson's disease, and dementia are also caused or contributed to by toxins in the brain. The brain becomes a toxin trap.

Examples of fat-soluble toxins include heavy metals (mercury, lead, arsenic, etc.), pesticides commonly found in foods, plastics and other synthetic substances used to produce modern products, and of course, Lyme Disease toxins produced as bacterial waste. Each toxin has a different set of deleterious effects on the body. As an individual becomes affected with any of these poisons, detoxification pathways and organs will be weakened and stressed, and additional toxins are even more likely to accumulate. In this way, the toxic burden can be a downward spiral.

Additionally, chronic infections like Lyme Disease can thrive more easily in a toxic environment because toxins weaken and disable the immune system. Toxic pockets can form in various parts of the body, eventually becoming breeding grounds for infectious micro-organisms. Because chronic infections themselves produce toxins, infections and toxins feed off each other synergistically: the more toxic a person becomes, the more likely it is that chronic infections will take hold; and the more chronic infections on board, the more likely that toxins will begin to accumulate.

This relationship between infections and toxins has been documented throughout recent medical history by some of the most brilliant thinkers in science and medicine. Numerous health experts have hypothesized that all human disease is a result of either or both toxins and infections. While I would not go as far as to say that *all* disease results from these two factors, it seems likely that a great majority does. It is no accident that you are reading about toxins in a book about infections.

The scope of this chapter is not broad enough to encompass a detailed description of every fat-soluble toxin and its associated health effect. Instead, this chapter will give a short description of the fat-soluble Lyme Disease toxin and will then describe various detoxification protocols which help the body remove it. Fortunately, the detoxification therapies which are most effective for Lyme Disease toxins also happen to be useful for most other fat-soluble toxins. In this way, a detoxification protocol used as part of a Lyme Disease treatment campaign will have the bonus effect of ridding your body of toxins you may have picked up years before you acquired Lyme Disease.

Detoxification therapies not presented in this chapter (including those which address the accumulation of water-soluble toxins) such as colon cleanses, fasting, certain herbal remedies, and others, may also have value in the treatment of chronic Lyme Disease—this chapter is not the final word.

The Lyme Disease toxin

As a part of its normal life cycle, and as a strategy to weaken its host, Lyme Disease bacteria continuously secrete a very potent fat-soluble toxin which wreaks havoc on the human body. Additionally, when Lyme Disease bacteria are killed with antibacterial treatments, an intense rush of these toxins will flood the body—this flood of toxins is partially responsible for the famed herx reaction that occurs during recovery from Lyme Disease. Because the Lyme Disease toxin's negative effects are primarily exerted on the brain, the toxin is considered to be a neurotoxin. But this toxin's effects are not limited to just the brain; it also affects all other organs and body systems.

Believe it or not, the vast majority of Lyme Disease symptoms are not caused by the physical presence of Lyme bacteria in the body, but instead by the toxins which those bacteria produce. It is quite amazing that a single toxin can adversely affect so many body functions and systems. For example, according to Dietrich Klinghardt, M.D., Ph.D., James Schaller, M.D., and other Lyme Disease researchers, Lyme Disease toxins can be:

1. Carcinogenic.

2. Responsible for decreasing hormone output and disrupting hypothalamus, adrenal, and thyroid function, leading to a cascade of symptoms.

3. A primary cause of explosive inflammation in the brain and even in DNA.

4. A cause of lethargy, fatigue, muscle soreness, and fibromyalgia-like symptoms.

5. Responsible for Lyme-related psychological, emotional and neuro-logical symptoms such as depression, obsessive-compulsive disorder, rages, schizophrenia, brain fog, memory loss, a profound decrease in reasoning abilities and insight, panic attacks, agitation, confusion, personality changes, mania, seizures, strokes etc. In fact, Lyme toxins can cause nearly any psychiatric or neurological disorder.

6. A cause of eating disorders and appetite suppression, even anorexia.

7. Immunosuppressive.

8. Responsible for weakening the body's detoxification ability such that other toxins accumulate.

9. A disruption to the process of cellular energy production.

10. Damaging to vision and eye function, leading to blindness, blurred vision, eye pain, night blindness, etc.

11. A cause of a variety of other symptoms and health conditions.

It is important to understand that the Lyme Disease toxin is more than just a bacterial byproduct; it is a highly evolved survival-promoting substance that is intentionally produced and secreted by the bacteria to undermine numerous hormonal and functional processes in the body. An in-depth and enlightening description of other damage caused by Lyme Disease toxins can be found on page 134 of *Lyme Disease and Rife Machines*, as written by Marc Fett, a Lyme Disease expert and contributor to my books.

One of the most devastating aspects of poisoning with Lyme Disease neurotoxins is that Lyme Disease bacteria *continuously* secrete these toxins. Additionally, they are produced *inside* the body. Because Lyme Disease bacteria often infect the brain, these toxins are immediately present in the last place you want them—the brain—so neurotoxins disturb brain function *constantly*. This is in contrast to toxins which are transmitted from the external environment, such as those found in food, the elimination of which the body has many opportunities to accomplish through its detoxification pathways before the brain is affected.

Because these factors render the effects of Lyme Disease neurotoxins unremitting and severe, detoxification therapies are critical to symptom reduction throughout the healing process. In fact, proper detoxification can result in faster symptom reduction than any other type of Lyme Disease therapy. When the toxins are removed from the body, you feel a lot better, right away. While it can take weeks, months, or years to see improvement from antibacterial therapies, it often only requires a couple days to see improvement from detoxification.

Detoxification itself will not cure Lyme Disease because it does not provide antibacterial action to eliminate the infection. However, because detoxification greatly reduces symptoms and lifts the toxic burden from all internal organs, it should be part of a core Lyme Disease treatment protocol.

All detoxification therapies require that toxins circulate in the bloodstream before finally being removed from the body. The bloodstream is simply the only intermediate pathway between areas where fat-soluble toxins are stored and the organs which eliminate them. Lithium supplementation as discussed in Chapter 8 can protect the brain from toxins until they are eliminated during a detoxification protocol.

Now let's move on to explore the two organs that are primarily responsible for ridding the body of fat-soluble toxins: the liver and the skin. We will also investigate proper detoxification therapies associated with each organ.

The liver as a detoxification organ

The liver is one of the most incredible and hard-working organs in the body. It has many functions so critical to life that if any of them should stop for even a few days, we would die.

First we will take a broad look at the liver and how it functions. Then we will examine several therapies which support the liver in its detoxification processes.

THE LIVER DETOXIFICATION PATHWAY

One of the liver's key functions is detoxification. For our purposes of understanding detoxification, the liver acts as a filter which grabs fat-soluble toxins out of the bloodstream and processes them for elimination. After these toxins are captured, they are combined with bile, a fluid produced in the liver to aid in digestion. The manufacture and secretion of bile are the liver's primary tools for removing fat-soluble toxins from our bodies—bile acts as the vehicle which transports toxins out of the body. Bile is responsible for both digestion and detoxification processes.

Via the gallbladder, the liver secretes the toxin-saturated bile into the upper region of the small intestines where it is responsible for digesting fats. As digestion occurs, bile makes its way down the digestive tract through the small intestine and into the large intestine. Most of the bile is absorbed in the large intestine and routed back to the liver for reuse. Some of the bile, however, along with the toxins contained in it, is eventually eliminated from the body via the stool. Bowel movements are brown in color because of their bile content. After a quantity of fat-soluble toxins have been removed in this way, and the liver detoxification pathway is clear, the body will pull additional toxins out of storage in fatty tissues and place them in the bloodstream to be grabbed and processed by the liver.

This process repeats continually throughout your life and removes many fat-soluble toxins from your body. Unfortunately though, as is evidenced by the fact that many people do suffer the effects of poisoning by fat-soluble toxins, the process is not perfect. There are several reasons why toxins may not be eliminated properly.

To begin with, toxins are pulled from deeper tissues to be processed by the liver at the same rate bile is produced—and no faster. New bile is produced only when existing bile is eliminated from the body. This would not be a problem if bile were readily eliminated in the stool. However, a portion of bile—as much as 90%—is actually absorbed in the large intestine and brought back to the liver. This circular motion in which bile travels is known as enterohepatic circulation. Absorbed bile is recycled for future fat digestion. So, only about 10% of the bile moving through the digestive tract is actually eliminated from the body via the stool.

Bile recycling, which allows the body to conserve resources, causes slowed toxin removal in two ways. First, a significant portion of the toxins contained in bile is absorbed along with the bile in the large intestine. The circular motion in which bile moves also creates a circular motion in which toxins move—keeping them in the body longer. Second, bile absorption means that less bile production is necessary. Remember—toxins are pulled from deeper storage sites only at the speed at which new bile is produced. Thus, the rate at which toxins are pulled from their fatty storage sites is slowed, sometimes even stagnant, simply because bile production is slow due to bile absorption and recycling.

In addition to the absorption of bile in the large intestine, other factors can slow the process of bile, and thus toxin, elimination. Toxin removal through bile is dependent on good, healthy bile flow. In many cases, sick people do not have good bile flow because of blockages like gallstones which impair bile production and excretion, poor diet that does not include foods which create and stimulate bile production, and weak digestive organs. The very presence of Lyme Disease bacteria in the liver can create inflammation and weaken the liver. Even so simple a condition as constipation can contribute to decreased toxin removal by slowing the transit time during which bile is moved through and out of the body.

These imperfections in the liver's detoxification process can cause the rate of toxin accumulation to exceed the rate of bile production and thus waste removal. If this happens, toxins will build up in the body faster than they are eliminated. Nine out of ten Lyme Disease sufferers experience a net accumulation of toxins instead of a net elimination of them. One way to think of this process is to imagine a bathtub full of water. The bottleneck which prevents water from leaving the bathtub is the drain. If the drain is closed or clogged, and someone is continuously pouring water into the tub, the tub will fill up instead of empty.

The liver detoxification therapies presented on the following pages are designed to overcome such obstacles. Their goal is to support the liver and accelerate the process by which bile is able to remove fat-soluble toxins from the body.

The only other vehicle aside from bile that can effectively eliminate fat-soluble toxins from the body is sweating. This is the mechanism by which the skin acts as a detoxification organ. Sweating is an extremely important detoxification therapy and will be discussed later in the chapter.

LIVER DETOXIFICATION THERAPIES

The cleansing laxative

I learned about this procedure from Elmer Cranton, M.D., a highly accomplished alternative medicine physician, now retired, who founded Mount Rainier Clinic in Yelm, Washington (www.drcranton.com). Dr. Cranton's work has led to breakthroughs in EDTA chelation therapy, Candida elimination, hormone replacement therapy, hyperbaric oxygen chamber treatment, and nutritional supplementation. Dr. Cranton developed his own line of nutritional supplements which I believe are among the highest quality in the world. He has written several excellent, influential books on topics ranging from bypassing bypass surgery to anti-aging.

Cleansing laxatives are accomplished by drinking a mixture of water and 10 grams of powdered Vitamin C. When water is mixed with a high quantity of Vitamin C, the resultant solution contains too much Vitamin C for the body to absorb. So, when the solution is swallowed, it simply passes through the digestive tract (taking everything on the way with it) and produces diarrhea within several hours.

This laxative rapidly increases digestive transit time and facilitates detoxification in several ways. First, it resolves any constipation and increases the rate at which bile moves through the digestive tract. Second, it causes more bile to be eliminated in the stool because transit time is too rapid for bile absorption. Third, it allows for absorption of a portion of the Vitamin

C, which has its own beneficial nutritional and detoxification properties. The laxative can also help reduce symptoms of intense herx reactions.

When a cleansing laxative is used and a large amount of bile is expelled from the body, the liver immediately begins to manufacture more bile. As this occurs, the liver pulls toxic substances from fatty body tissues to attach to the bile. Thus, the cleansing laxative accelerates the rate at which toxins are removed from deeper tissues. Although many over-the-counter and prescription laxatives can accomplish the same thing, this mixture of Vitamin C and water happens to be nontoxic, side effect free, and provides an infusion of Vitamin C.

Cleansing laxatives are not appropriate for long-term use because they may cause discomfort, emergency trips to the bathroom, dehydration, inhibited food absorption, and even dependency. They should generally be used very sparingly and work well for an occasional case of constipation.

Some people use enemas to accomplish roughly the same goal as the cleansing laxative. Various substances are sometimes used in enema solutions to elicit certain effects. For example, some people put coffee in enema solutions—this is believed to stimulate the liver to release toxins which are then eliminated from the body with the coffee solution. Many Lyme Disease sufferers have found rapid and significant relief from enemas, especially coffee enemas. However, there are certain disadvantages. Enemas can be inconvenient, require set-up time, and most important, create potential for injury. Although enemas are a valid detoxification therapy, the cleansing laxative provides a safer, more moderate alternative. It should certainly be noted, though, that numerous Lyme Disease sufferers consider coffee enemas to be life savers.

The cleansing laxative is cheap and can be done without help from a physician. Powdered Vitamin C is available at most health food stores. Ten grams of powdered Vitamin C should be mixed into 16 ounces of purified water until completely dissolved. The solution should be consumed relatively quickly.

The Hulda Clark liver cleanse

Hulda Clark, who holds a doctoral degree in physiology, was one of the first researchers to discover that a vast majority of health conditions can be caused by infections or toxins or a combination of both. Her 1995 book, *The Cure for All Diseases*, has sold thousands of copies throughout the world and has become one of the most important sources of information on the subject of eliminating hidden infections and chronic toxicity.

Clark stays active in the alternative health community by educating the public through appearances, lectures, and publications. She often appears as a keynote speaker at the large and well-known alternative health conventions held across the country. Of note is her frequent attendance at the Rife International Health Conference (www.rifeconference.com) which typically takes place in Seattle, Washington, during the fall.

One of the detoxification treatments which Hulda Clark pioneered is the liver cleanse (also sometimes referred to as the "liver flush"). This cleanse uses all-natural, over-the-counter ingredients to accomplish several purposes. First, it causes the liver and gallbladder to release bile rapidly. Second, it quickly escorts this bile from the body (instead of allowing it to be absorbed). Third, it makes this process as safe, comfortable, and efficient as possible. Some people believe that this cleanse can also eliminate gallstones.

Many patients and researchers have concluded that the liver cleanse can improve or cure numerous seemingly unrelated health problems, from musculoskeletal pain to multiple sclerosis to acne. Although evidence supporting these claims is mixed, there are literally thousands of accounts from sick people who have used the liver flush to rid themselves of dozens of health problems. Many report much improved health and attribute this improvement to the liver cleanse. The logic supporting claims that this therapy can resolve so many different health problems is simply that a congested liver and impeded bile flow can have a profound negative effect on the entire body—on each and every organ. For additional information and user reports, visit www.curezone.com.

Convincing support for the use of this treatment is the fact that variations of it have been recommended for decades by dozens of healthcare practitioners of many disciplines. Although Hulda Clark's book is one of the most well-known sources of information on the procedure, numerous other books have described similar treatments. Some researchers believe that the liver cleanse has been used for hundreds if not thousands of years by many different tribes and cultures throughout the world. Today, leaflets and loosely stapled handouts describing the liver cleanse can be found in the waiting rooms of hundreds of the nation's best alternative medicine physicians. This liver therapy is one of the most well-known and frequently used alternative health procedures in modern times.

Think of the cleanse as being similar to an oil change for your car. Bile elimination is accelerated by the procedure, the liver is required to manufacture new bile, and in the process, fat-soluble toxins are removed from storage to be processed for elimination. As a result of this rapid toxin removal, many people report feeling much improved after the procedure— better than they have in years. They report such benefits as clearer vision, better sleep, a more positive attitude, new energy, and a feeling of being younger. Often, this rejuvenated feeling is short-lived. However, additional cleanses can move one toward a more permanent state of better health. As toxins are removed from the liver and the body, the above improvements may become permanent, or at least longer lasting.

Below we will describe one of the most popular versions of the liver cleanse, adapted and compiled from several different books and sources. Other versions of the therapy can be found at www.curezone.com. Completing the cleanse takes about a day. It should be done on a day when responsibilities and activities can be kept to a minimum. Also, the day after should be reserved as a day of rest.

Precautions: before using this treatment, you should thoroughly research it in sources which contain more extensive information than does this book. A good place to start is www.curezone.com in the cleansing section. Rare incidences of severe pain and discomfort have been reported. In a patient with gallstones, the Hulda Clark cleanse could be dangerous as it may cause a gallstone to become lodged in the common bile duct (an extremely rare occurrence). This treatment should be used only under the consent and supervision of a licensed physician.

Necessary ingredients:

½ cup extra-virgin olive oil
4 tablespoons epsom salt
1 grapefruit and 1 lemon
3 cups water

Procedure:

<u>**Morning and afternoon up to 2:00 p.m.:**</u> Eat a no-fat breakfast and lunch such as oatmeal, fruit, baked potato, or cooked vegetables. This causes bile pressure to build up in the liver and gallbladder. Do not eat or drink anything after 2:00 p.m.

<u>**6:00 p.m.:**</u> Mix one tablespoon of epsom salt into an 8 oz. glass of water and drink. This solution can taste absolutely awful, so have something nearby, such as a piece of candy, to place in your mouth after you finish drinking. Do not swallow the candy but instead spit it out after it has served its purpose of eliminating the taste of the epsom salt solution. A grape, raisin, or other pleasant tasting food will also work (just remember not to swallow it).

<u>**8:00 p.m.:**</u> Repeat exactly the 6:00 p.m. step above.

<u>**10:00 p.m.:**</u> Mix ½ cup extra-virgin olive oil with juice from a freshly squeezed grapefruit and lemon. After mixed, your olive oil / grapefruit / lemon juice solution should be at least 1 cup. Because you need to mix this solution thoroughly, it is easiest to make the solution in a jar which you can tightly seal and shake. After it is well mixed, drink the solution and go <u>immediately</u> to bed.

Next Morning: When you wake up (no earlier than 6:00 a.m.), repeat exactly the 6:00 p.m. step from last night. Expect diarrhea throughout the morning—remain close to a bathroom.

2 Hours After Waking: Again repeat exactly the 6:00 p.m. step from last night. Two hours after this final epsom salt drink, you may begin to eat again. Your first meal should be very light, and as the day progresses you should return to normal eating. By dinnertime you will be able to consume a regular meal.

This therapy should be done no more often than every two weeks. There are important aspects of the cleanse which are not discussed in this book. See www.curezone.com for more information. Caution: consult a physician before using this liver cleanse.

The Shoemaker Neurotoxin Elimination Protocol

The Shoemaker Neurotoxin Elimination Protocol (SNEP) was developed by Ritchie Shoemaker, M.D., a practicing physician in Pocomoke City, MD. Dr. Shoemaker received his medical degree from Duke University and has published four books and numerous articles in various scientific research journals. Detailed information about the SNEP can be found on Dr. Shoemaker's web site: www.chronicneurotoxins.com.

The SNEP is based on the theory that many chronically ill people are sick because they have been exposed to toxins which their body cannot eliminate. Dr. Shoemaker concludes that this toxic condition is often a result of infections which produce biotoxins as a part of their microbial life cycle. Lyme Disease, according to Shoemaker, is an example of one such infection. The accumulation of Lyme Disease toxins in the body can cause chronic illness.

Shoemaker also suggests that many other chronic conditions may be caused by a similar phenomenon. Some of the conditions which may involve biotoxin poisoning include depression, chronic fatigue syndrome, fibromyalgia, irritable bowel syndrome, multiple sclerosis, and sick-building syndrome. Even Bell's palsy, learning disabilities, endometriosis, sensory-neural deafness, poor vision, and chronic soft tissue injury may be caused by biotoxin poisoning.

The diagnosis of biotoxin poisoning is made, according to Dr. James Schaller, by determining a patient's history of exposure to Lyme Disease bacteria, indoor mold toxins, and/or the presence of physical exam findings such as rashes, slowed cognition, and painful joints, to name a few. Additionally, using what Dr. Shoemaker refers to as the Visual Contrast Sensitivity Test (VCS) helps confirm the diagnosis. According to his research, people with biotoxin poisoning sometimes have certain subtle vision problems which can be picked up by the test. If the VCS test is positive, possible biotoxin poisoning is diagnosed and the SNEP is indicated. Because people with confirmed Lyme Disease are already known to be affected by bacterial biotoxins, the VCS is optional when using the procedure to treat Lyme Disease.

The SNEP is similar to the Hulda Clark liver cleanse in that its purpose is to remove more bile from the body than would occur in the natural digestion process. The SNEP induces the body to speed up production of bile. As this occurs, the liver pulls toxins from their storage sites in fatty tissue to be deposited in the newly synthesized bile. This process is similar to our example of removing the plug in a full bathtub to allow the water to drain out.

What separates the SNEP from the Hulda Clark liver cleanse is the means by which bile is eliminated. As part of the SNEP, cholestyramine (a pharmaceutical drug which is FDA approved for lowering cholesterol) is taken orally. Cholestyramine combines with bile to form an insoluble compound which is not absorbed as it passes through the digestive tract. Thus, bile and the toxins it carries with it are eliminated through the stool instead of being absorbed in the large intestine. Because cholesterol is a major component of bile, cholestyramine reduces cholesterol by continuously removing bile from the body. The cholesterol-lowering effects of cholestyramine are merely a side effect of the SNEP. In terms of detoxification, the primary effect is the elimination of bile and consequent acceler-ated detoxification of fat-soluble toxins.

Various brands of cholestyramine are available. Some contain sugar and other additives. Others are more desirable because they do not have unwanted sweeteners or preservatives. Cholestyramine can be obtained at most common pharmacies with a prescription. It is typically taken on an empty stomach 1-4 times per day depending on the version of the protocol used and patient tolerance. Patients with sensitivity to cholestyramine can be given stomach-soothing agents which eventually allow for full, effective therapeutic doses to be used. One example of a soothing medicine is high quality Aloe Vera gel at 1 tablespoon twice daily taken at a different time of day than cholestyramine. The SNEP can be administered by any physician or nurse practitioner with drug prescribing privileges. Detailed information about the protocol can be found at www.chronicneurotoxins.com.

Many Lyme Disease sufferers have experienced great improvement us-ing the SNEP. Some Lyme Disease sufferers have noticed no significant benefit. Others still have found that the protocol made them worse. Worsening while on the protocol probably results from the fact that this detoxification process causes neurotoxins to be stirred up and moved into circulation before they are eliminated. This can be a very uncomfortable process, and some people stop the protocol before they reach the point when enough toxins have been removed so that improvement is felt. Dr. Shoemaker recommends several interventions to make the detoxification process more tolerable. More information is available at
www.chronicneurotoxins.com.

In my opinion, the SNEP is not a cure for Lyme Disease because it does not directly attack and kill the bacterial infection. As long as the bacterial infection is present, biotoxins will be produced. Additionally, long-term use of cholestyramine has several disadvantages, not the least of which is the cholesterol lowering effect. Many Lyme Disease sufferers already have low cholesterol and this may disqualify them from using cho-lestyramine long-term. In some cases, cholesterol may be so low that even short-term use of cholestyramine could be dangerous.

Aside from its cholesterol lowering abilities, cholestyramine has other side effects. Because the drug does not get absorbed systemically, these side effects are mostly mild. However, some can be significant. The most frequent side effect associated with cholestyramine is constipation. Additional side effects include abdominal discomfort and/or pain, flatulence, nausea, vomiting, diarrhea, eructation (belching), anorexia, steatorrhea (oily, bulky stools caused by excess fat), and rash and irritation of the skin, tongue, and perianal area. More severe and far less common side effects include bleeding tendencies due to hypoprothrombinemia (vitamin K deficiency), vitamins A (one case of night blindness reported) and D deficiencies, and osteoporosis. Hypercholeremic acidosis (high blood acidity) has occurred in children, and rare reports of intestinal obstruction, including two deaths, were reported in pediatric patients. Occasional calcified material has been observed in the biliary tree, including calcifications of the gallbladder, in patients to whom cholestyramine has been given. As with any drug, careful consideration of cost-to-benefit ratio is necessary.

The SNEP has been quite helpful to some Lyme Disease sufferers and should be considered a valuable tool in the Lyme Disease treatment toolbox. Because cholestyramine requires a prescription, a physician's supervision is needed to use this protocol. See www.chronicneurotoxins.com for more information.

One final note: according to research by Dr. Shoemaker, repeated by Dr. James Schaller (who wrote the Foreword for this book), patients that have a type of genetically determined cell surface pattern, known as either 15-6-51 or 16-5-51, will never remove Lyme's biotoxins without use of cholestyramine. So, in these people, cholestyramine use may be more than just optional; it may be mandatory. The code for the test that looks for these genetic factors is LabCorp test #012542. The name of the test is the HLA DRB, DBQ Disease Evaluation. Quest Laboratory also offers a similar test, but only offers 40% of the data available in the LabCorp version. For more information, Dr. Schaller recommends reading the book *Mold Warriors*, by Ritchie Shoemaker.

Diet, nutrition, and supplementation

The above described protocols for liver detoxification can be very useful in treating Lyme Disease. However, one of the most beneficial and least risky actions you can take to bolster liver health is improving your diet and consuming nutrients which support the liver. These topics are beyond the scope of this book. However, several excellent books are available, the most notable of which is *The Liver-Cleansing Diet*, by Sandra Cabot. One of the most helpful liver supplements, milk thistle, will be discussed later in this chapter, as will mineral supplementation. It is recommended that, as part of your Lyme Disease research, you seek additional materials relating to liver health.

In general, most of the habits which you know to be healthy will benefit the liver. If you are attempting to recover from Lyme Disease, you should do everything you can to eat right and exercise moderately. The health of your liver quite literally depends on it.

Next we will turn our attention to the body's second primary mechanism for eliminating fat-soluble toxins: the skin. The skin detoxification mechanism will be described, as will several therapies which support it.

The skin as a detoxification organ

The skin is the largest organ in the body. It covers more than 20 square feet in an average adult and accounts for as much as 15% of our total body weight, more than any single internal organ. The average square inch of skin contains about 20 blood vessels, 60,000 melanocytes (which produce pigment), more than a thousand nerve endings, and 650 sweat glands. The skin has multiple functions, not the least of which is simply to hold your body together and prevent entrance of foreign objects and pathogens into the bloodstream and tissues. Often referred to as our third lung, the skin acts as an interface between our internal and the external environments as it regulates exchange processes like absorption and elimination. Skin is a semipermeable barrier through which your body can not only absorb substances but can also release them.

First we will examine the skin as a detoxification pathway, and then we will look at individual therapies that aid the skin in detoxifying the body.

THE SKIN DETOXIFICATION PATHWAY

Sweating is one of the primary functions of the skin. It accomplishes both temperature regulation (cooling) and toxin removal. Your sweat is made up many different components. These include water (up to 99%), and substances like salt and other electrolytes, sugar, metabolic wastes like ammonia and urea, metals and heavy metals, and drug metabolites. Because our sweat can be as revealing as urine, sweat analysis is becoming an ever more common clinical procedure for detecting a multitude of substances in the body. For example, a recent innovation in the science of drug testing is the "sweat patch," a device which offers an accurate and non-invasive way to monitor drug use and abuse.

Sweat in humans is produced by two types of glands. The eccrine sweat glands are present over the entire surface of our bodies and are especially concentrated on the palms of our hands, soles of the feet, and the forehead. They produce sweat composed mostly of water and salts. Apocrine sweat glands are predominant in the armpits and genital area. Apocrine sweat contains protein and fatty materials and is the source of the sweat odor which is caused by bacterial breakdown of organic compounds.

When sweat glands are stimulated to increase production, they secrete a substance (sweat) which is synthesized from the fluid which fills the spaces between our body's cells (the interstitial spaces). This fluid comes from blood plasma leaked into the tissues by capillaries. Any circulating toxins present in the blood system are carried into the interstitial spaces along with the plasma. In this way toxins make their way into sweat, which is a filtrate of the plasma. Heat stress and exertional activities speed up the circulation of blood and thus accelerate the release of fluid into the interstitial spaces. This in turn prompts sweat glands to produce more toxin-laden sweat.

Most people living in modern times do not sweat very much. Lack of adequate exercise, the prevalence of climate control technology at home and in the workplace, and the non-physical nature of most jobs contribute to minimal sweating. Unfortunately, decreased sweating means decreased toxin removal.

Nenah Sylver, Ph.D., in her book *The Holistic Handbook of Sauna Therapy*, cites several published scientific studies which illustrate the ability of the body to detoxify via sweat production. For example, from her book we know that nickel, mercury, and cadmium are eliminated more effectively through sweat than through urine. Also, people with known chemical exposure who have symptoms of peripheral neuropathy and/or multiple sclerosis can obtain between 90 and 99% reduction of symptoms through the skin detoxification pathway.

Although skin detoxification is beneficial to anyone living in industrialized society, there are several reasons why it is specifically helpful to Lyme Disease sufferers. As we have seen, those with Lyme Disease accumulate a greater quantity of toxins than do healthy people. Sweating can help eliminate these toxins. The advantages of efficient skin detoxification for Lyme Disease sufferers do not, however, stop there. Unlike most healthy people, Lyme Disease patients have burdened livers and kidneys due to the stress incurred by the inflammation and toxic burden created by a chronic infection. As a result, Lyme Disease patients often have very weak livers and kidneys. Because the liver and kidneys are the primary detoxification organs of the body, detoxification is often stagnant. This can lead to overwhelming symptoms of poisoning by the Lyme Disease neurotoxin.

Detoxifying through the skin (via sweat) lifts the burden from the liver and kidneys because it completely bypasses them. Sweat production allows toxins circulating in the blood to be excreted directly through the skin, removing the necessity for the liver and kidneys to process, store, and eliminate toxins. The vast surface area of the skin allows quick, efficient detoxification without placing a burden on other detoxification organs.

The detoxification abilities of the skin through sweating are limitless. Even a completely healthy set of liver and kidneys cannot process more than a small amount of toxins in a given period of time. In contrast, there is virtually no limit to the amount of toxic material that can pass through the skin. In this way, sweating can greatly accelerate toxin elimination, even in people with healthy detoxification systems. Sweating is the "shortcut" to detoxification. The following therapies are intended to facilitate the skin's detoxification processes.

SKIN DETOXIFICATION THERAPIES

Sauna therapy

Note: The information in this entire sauna section is based in large part on information from Nenah Sylver's excellent book, *The Holistic Handbook of Sauna Therapy*. This book, in my opinion, is the most accurate, complete and useful book currently in print on the topic of sauna treatment.

Sauna therapy is one way to integrate sweating into a modern lifestyle. People have been using saunas and sweat therapy to detoxify for thousands of years. In comparison to other methods of skin detoxification, sauna therapy is the most affordable, effective, and established method. By increasing both circulation and lipid (fat) metabolism, the heat generated by a sauna causes the release into general circulation of a wide range of toxins stored in fatty body tissue. This process has been well documented in medical studies. Sauna therapy is so effective that the U.S. government recommends it for detoxification of dozens of poisons.

In addition to accelerating detoxification, saunas provide numerous other benefits due to increased body temperature. From Nenah Sylver (as well as Lawrence Wilson, M.D., author of *Sauna Therapy*, another valuable sauna book), we know that saunas have the following benefits:

1. Immune system stimulation and activation

2. Direct antibacterial action

3. Balancing of the autonomic nervous system

4. Improving oxygenation

5. Relieving internal congestion

6. Relaxing muscles and enhancing flexibility of tendons and ligaments

7. Alkalizing the body

8. Increasing circulation

9. Resolving edema

10. Normalizing enzymatic activity

11. Relieving pain

12. Increasing energy and clearing the mind

13. Normalizing body temperature

Below, we will examine specific types of sauna therapy, and then we will look at another type of detoxification treatment involving the skin: the Epsom salt bath.

→ What is a sauna?

A sauna is an enclosure in which you sit or stand and in which temperature is raised to cause sweating. You can use a sauna at a health club or spa or build or purchase your own. Cost of purchasing or building a sauna ranges from $50-$5000. Owning a sauna makes treatments much more convenient.

Many people believe that different types of saunas are all about the same. In actuality, there are some important differences among styles of saunas. Less important is the shape and size, and more important is the type of heating element and the material used for construction. There are also other variations, including whether or not ozone or steam is used inside the sauna. First we will examine different heat sources and then take a look at building materials and other variations in sauna therapy.

→ Traditional saunas

Traditional saunas are heated by a wood-burning or gas stove, hot rocks, or an electric coil or other electric heating element. The traditional sauna is basically a room with a heater. The heater often has a few rocks on top, onto which you can throw water to create steam in the sauna. In modern times, traditional saunas mainly use radiant electric heat as opposed to the sun, fire, or hot sand which were popular heating mechanisms before electricity became technologically feasible.

Traditional saunas have been used for centuries, but in modern times they gained popularity about 60 years ago when L. Ron Hubbard pioneered their use for drug and alcohol detoxification. Hubbard also developed a program which uses the traditional sauna for detoxification of other toxic chemicals. More than 500,000 people have used his program with success.

Traditional saunas heat only the surface of the body, mainly through convection (the transfer of heat from hot air to the body). Because the heating effect is generated from warm air in the sauna, traditional saunas operate at high temperatures between 150-210°F. Healthy people can use these saunas daily; however, the high temperature renders the sauna dangerous for people with certain types of health problems and cardiovascular weakness. Since this type of sauna primarily heats the body through convection, the effect is similar being outside on a hot day. In this way, traditional saunas utilize a very natural form of heat to induce sweating, and many people consider them to be the safest and most reliable method of sauna therapy.

→ Far infrared radiation saunas (FIR saunas)

Infrared radiation, a type of electromagnetic energy, was discovered in 1800 by Sir Frederick William Herschel, a German musician and astronomer who was well-known in his time.

Infrared radiation is emitted from numerous sources: the sun, animals and plants, fire, sand, a warm sidewalk—actually, all objects emit some amount of infrared energy. "Far" infrared energy occupies a narrow section of the infrared radiation spectrum. Infrared radiation is invisible to the human eye because it exists on the electromagnetic spectrum just beneath the frequencies of visible light. Interestingly, some animals can actually see infrared energy. A rattlesnake, for instance, can identify warm-blooded prey in the black of night. Humans have learned to detect infrared energy by using machines such as night goggles and IR cameras.

FIR saunas were introduced about 30 years ago and are heated by metallic or ceramic elements which emit far infrared radiation. They heat the body through radiant energy, and unlike the convection method of heating used in traditional saunas, radiant energy does not require the air in the sauna to actually be hot. Similar to the sun, radiant energy causes heating by transferring energy into physical objects—even though the sun is millions of miles away, it can still heat the earth via radiant energy.

FIR saunas operate with a much lower ambient air temperature than traditional saunas (110-140°F in comparison to 150-210°F). Additionally, because FIR saunas emit radiant heat, the body is warmed from the inside as well as on the surface—radiant energy penetrates the body up to about 1.5 inches. Some researchers believe that a lower ambient temperature and ability to heat the body from the inside out cause FIR saunas to be both more comfortable and more effective than traditional saunas. Also, FIR sauna heating elements are more efficient than those in traditional saunas, so energy used and cost of operation is lower with the FIR sauna.

Many Lyme Disease sufferers have received great benefit from FIR saunas. The FIR sauna is considered part of a core treatment protocol by some of the most well respected Lyme literate healthcare practitioners in the world. However, readers should be aware that some researchers do not feel comfortable with FIR saunas and consider them to be potentially dangerous. While these researchers are definitely in the minority, it is important to note that controversy does exist. Those who desire to avoid FIR saunas can use a traditional sauna instead.

→ Moisture and steam in the sauna

Steam and moisture in the air can be achieved when taking a sauna by spraying or throwing water on rocks which are heated by the sauna's heating element. Because the rocks are hot, this water will make a sizzling noise and quickly evaporate, increasing moisture content in the air. Some cultures throughout the world consider steam in a sauna to be mandatory and will even conduct sacred ceremonies around the process of throwing water on hot rocks. Other cultures and schools of thought in sauna therapy prefer dryness and lack of moisture. Neither approach is right nor wrong, and in the end, whether or not steam is used in a sauna is largely determined by personal preference. Still, advantages and disadvantages to each method can be listed.

Advantages to steam:

1. Steam in the sauna produces negative ions which have numerous health benefits. Positively charged ions in the air are known to cause fatigue and restlessness, partly because they can attract carbon dioxide and other harmful substances. Negative ions, on the other hand, lead to healing. Negative ions are created by plants during photosynthesis, by fire, and by moving water. Negative ions are common around waterfalls, the ocean, and other sources of moving water. This explains why people often feel rejuvenated and relaxed near such bodies of water. The healing effect of negative ions has been well studied. NASA even uses negative ion generators to help astronauts recover after spaceflight. Some hospitals in Europe use negative ion generators in hospital rooms.

2. Moisture in the sauna has a lubricating effect on the mucous membranes and the respiratory passageway. This can prevent dust and other debris from reaching the lungs.

3. Steam can raise the temperature in the sauna.

Disadvantages to steam:

1. Because steam can significantly increase the temperature inside the sauna, it can be difficult to tolerate for many people.

2. Sweating and toxin removal can be significantly lessened when steam is used. The body produces sweat to cool down. If the air already has higher moisture content, less sweat is needed. Studies have shown that sweating and toxin elimination in a steam sauna can be as low as half that achieved in a dry sauna.

3. If purified water is not used to produce the steam, steam saunas can result in vaporization and absorption through the skin of toxic chemicals found in tap water such as chlorine, fluorides, and possibly other volatile organic chemicals.

4. Too much moisture in the air can be uncomfortable and cause difficulty breathing.

A person can experiment with dry saunas and saunas with a higher moisture content to determine which option is preferred.

→ Ozone saunas

Ozone gas, which is discussed thoroughly in *Lyme Disease and Rife Machines*, not only has incredible detoxification properties but also is antibacterial and has other healing effects on the body. These effects include oxygenation, cancer prevention, and increased circulation. Ozone also creates a feeling of greatly increased energy. In fact, ozone is one of the most powerful healing substances known to man. Although ozone can be introduced into the body in numerous ways (including drinking ozonated water, ear and rectal insufflation, and inhaling ozone which has been bubbled through olive oil) the most effective method of ozone treatment is its use in the sauna.

Ozone gas is created in an ozone generator and introduced into the sauna's environment via a tube which is connected to the sauna. Ozone can only be used in a sauna cabinet that allows the patient's head to protrude from the cabinet because pure ozone is harmful to breathe. The sweating induced by a sauna is necessary for ozone to be absorbed through the skin because sweating opens the pores and allows ozone to enter.

An ozone sauna is one of the most potent healing methods in existence. Not only are the already-discussed benefits of heat and sweating realized, but also the effects of ozone are harnessed in the most powerful way possible. For this reason, ozone saunas can elicit dramatic effect in the treatment of many diseases (not just Lyme Disease). Ozone saunas have been shown to be particularly beneficial for treating cancer.

The ozone sauna has a shotgun effect in healing—it does not target just one or two health problems in the body, but instead, it has profound healing effect on the majority of problems which can occur in the body. While this powerful effect is obviously useful, it can be dangerous as well. The sicker the person, the more intense the healing reaction. Healing reactions can be so intense as to require weeks for recovery, especially in treatment of advanced cases of Lyme Disease. Because of the powerful action of ozone saunas, they must be used carefully and in moderation, especially in cases of more serious illness.

Mercury toxicity (which will be discussed later in this chapter) is one condition which is greatly impacted by ozone saunas, leading to massive amounts of mercury being detached from tissues and dumped into the bloodstream. Although some mercury is excreted through sweat during the ozone sauna, much of it is redistributed and attached to other tissues. This can be very dangerous. Although some researchers view ozone as an ideal treatment for mercury poisoning, it is not a good therapy for people severely poisoned with mercury because the small amount of mercury actually eliminated from the body does not justify the large-scale mercury redistribution that is possible. As you will read in a few pages, there is a safer way to accomplish mercury detoxification. People who are severely mercury toxic should probably avoid ozone saunas. In some cases, people with severe mercury toxicity may need to avoid all types of saunas.

One type of healing reaction which occurs in most people who use an ozone sauna is a red, itchy rash that appears all over the body. Although not actually dangerous, the rash's intense itch can be very uncomfortable, even debilitating. If ozone saunas are temporarily discontinued, the rash will dissipate. Ozone sauna veterans claim that the post-sauna rash will no longer appear after a number of saunas have been taken and the body is sufficiently detoxified. In any case, if you intend to use an ozone sauna, it is necessary to be forewarned about the rash because it can be quite intense!

→ **Sauna building materials**

There are a variety of materials used for building saunas, but this brief discussion will address only the advantages and disadvantages of the two most common materials: wood and plastic.

Wood is a common material used to build sauna enclosures and is suitable if it is natural and has not been treated with chemicals. Wood must be thoroughly dried before it is used as a construction material because wood with higher moisture content will eventually warp and crack due to the repeated heating and cooling that takes place in the sauna.

One of the disadvantages of wood is that its porous nature can allow absorption of the dirt and toxins produced in sweat, leading to a smelly, unsanitary sauna after several months or years of use. The naturally aromatic properties of wood can also cause reactions in chemically sensitive people. Additionally, many types of wood have been pretreated by their manufacturers with chemicals which render wood ill-suited for people with chemical sensitivities.

Plastic, fiberglass, and other synthetic materials are also used to construct sauna cabinets. Intrinsic advantages to these materials include ease of cleaning, lack of a propensity to absorb toxins and other chemicals, imperviousness to water, and durability. The main disadvantage is that synthetic materials can outgas (release toxic gasses) for weeks, months, or years after they are built. However, most sauna users find that outgassing odors diminish beyond perceptibility after only several weeks of use.

Fiberglass, a material similar to plastic, is often the material of choice for construction of saunas in which ozone gas is used. This is because fiberglass is one of only five known substances which do not break down in the presence of pure ozone. Anyone intending to use ozone in a sauna must first verify that their sauna is constructed out of a material that will not be corroded by ozone. Because of the advantages listed above, and because Lyme Disease sufferers often find ozone to be quite beneficial, fiberglass saunas are recommended over wood.

The epsom salt bath

The skin functions the same way as a two-way road. Not only can the body eliminate toxins through the skin, it can also absorb substances via the skin. For example, many medications are administered cutaneously (through the skin). These include nicotine patches, birth control patches, insulin patches for diabetics, etc. The fact that the skin is the largest organ in the body with an enormous amount of surface area allows it to absorb significant amounts of various substances with which it comes in contact. This property of the skin can be both a positive and a negative attribute, depending on the type of substance in question.

The absorptive properties of skin have the potential to cause harm to the body because we often absorb toxins and undesirable substances through our skin. People take care to drink filtered water, yet take showers in tap water containing chlorine and other harmful chemicals. Many common skin products contain synthetic chemicals and other toxins. We are aware that birth control patches cause medication to enter the body—why are we not also aware that moisturizing lotion, chemicals in shower water, and bug repellent can enter the body as well?

Skin detoxification depends almost exclusively on the release of toxins in sweat, but the body's ability to absorb substances through the skin can also be employed in the service of detoxification and healing. One such example is the simple addition of Epsom salt (a form of magnesium) to a hot bath.

Epsom salt has many positive effects in the Lyme Disease healing process. Among these are alkalinization of body tissues and blood, restoration of healthy magnesium levels, and neutralization of Lyme Disease neurotoxins. As we've seen, Lyme Disease neurotoxins are one of the primary causes of Lyme Disease symptoms, and thus their pacification and elimination can result in tremendous benefit and symptom reduction. An Epsom salt bath has a profound symptom-reducing effect.

Epsom salt may be taken orally, but this is uncomfortable and impractical because it is a strong laxative and, frankly, tastes awful. Administering it in a hot bath allows for efficient absorption into the system, and, as a bonus, enhances detoxification via sweat at the same time (a hot bath, similar to a sauna, causes sweating). In comparison to other types of therapies, an Epsom salt bath has several advantages:

1. Affordability (enough Epsom salt for use in one bath costs less than a dollar).

2. It can be done in the privacy of your own home on your own schedule.

3. Increased core body temperature.

4. Relaxation and stress reduction.

5. The benefits of this wonderful do-it-at-home therapy are gained by balancing and restoring equilibrium in the body, not superficially suppressing symptoms.

This single therapy alone can make the Lyme Disease recovery process much more bearable. It is especially helpful during herx reactions. People often find that after a hot bath with Epsom salt, they feel refreshed, rejuvenated, relaxed, optimistic, and ready for the day. Muscle soreness, fatigue, lethargy, depression, and other symptoms are washed away. These positive results are temporary, but they are still worthwhile because, for a very small investment of time and money, a high degree of palliation is achieved.

The only way to permanently eliminate neurotoxin poisoning is to eradicate the infection that causes it. Epsom salt baths do not do this. For the purpose of actually eradicating the infection, entirely different therapies are available—such as the Marshall Protocol, antibiotics (herbal and pharmaceutical), and rife machine therapy. In addition, according to Dr. James Schaller, it is also important to address indoor mold toxins as well as co-infections such as Babesia and Bartonella which are both profoundly unappreciated, incapacitating, deadly infections.

Other healing substances can be administered through the skin during a hot bath, such as apple cider vinegar (long known for its alkalizing and healing qualities). A significant amount of hydrogen peroxide can be absorbed through the skin by spraying it onto the body in a spray bottle after a hot shower and then rinsing it off.

Additional detoxification therapies

Now that we have examined both the liver and skin detoxification pathways, and also looked at therapies which support those functions, let's move on to examine other helpful detoxification modalities.

DETOXIFICATION SUPPLEMENTS

One of the effective approaches to detoxification is supplementation with herbs, vitamins, and other substances which are taken to accomplish one of two goals: they either directly pacify and neutralize toxins, or they support and strengthen the detoxification organs that pacify and neutralize toxins. The supplementation approach to detoxification is a very gentle approach because, unlike liver cleanses for example, it does not involve forcing immediate changes in liver or bile function.

There are dozens of herbs, nutrients, and minerals which accomplish the goals listed above. However, the purpose of this book is not only to introduce you to effective treatments but also to encourage use of a Lyme Disease treatment protocol which is simple, affordable, practical, and convenient. This means avoiding long lists of "helpful supplements." Many books and web sites offer an overwhelming number of supplements which you just can't live without for this or that reason. All too often, these must-have supplements are just overpriced food source nutrients which, in most cases, are provided in ample amounts in a balanced diet. Furthermore, American consumerism and marketing hysteria in the arena of alternative medicine have led the public to believe that hundreds of expensive supplements lining the walls of health food stores are mandatory for recovering from illness. The truth is that only a small percentage of available supplements actually help reverse chronic disease.

Because a Lyme Disease protocol involves many different aspects (not just detoxification), a treatment program can become overwhelming and costly if you feel that you need to take 100 pills a day. So, to help you keep your treatment regimen as simple as possible, we will present only two detoxification supplements. As you progress on your healing journey you will inevitably encounter other beneficial supplements that may be worth a try. Just remember to keep it simple: more is not always better.

Milk thistle (silymarin)

The first supplement we will look at is milk thistle, also known as silymarin. The "king" of liver supplements, milk thistle is extremely effective, affordable, well studied, and is associated with numerous benefits in the detoxification process. This single supplement alone is capable of providing a great deal of liver support because it protects the liver from toxins, increases bile production and flow, and regenerates weak or dying liver cells. In addition, milk thistle has been shown to increase intracellular glutathione levels and modulate the immune system.

The seeds, fruit, and leaves of the milk thistle plant have been used since Roman times as a liver tonic. Milk thistle is native to Europe and is believed to have originated in the Mediterranean region. In the United States, it is grown in California and on the East Coast. It is a tall plant with large, prickly leaves and has a reddish purple flower. Milk thistle has so many amazing liver-related benefits that it would take dozens of pages to present each individual study evidencing this herb's value. According to

Pub Med., the U.S. government's database of published scientific studies, there have been over 894 scientific studies on the effects of milk thistle. To view some of the studies, visit Pub Med online at www.ncbi.nlm.nih.gov/entrez and search for milk thistle.

Perhaps the most convincing evidence in favor of using milk thistle for liver support comes from the U.S. government itself—an entity which typically looks down on herbal and alternative treatments. The United States AHRQ (Agency for Health Care Research and Quality), which exists to "improve the quality, safety, efficiency, and effectiveness of health care for all Americans," under a program entitled Evidence-Based Practice Program, reviewed the available scientific literature on milk thistle to determine its efficacy.

AHRQ describes the plant as "a member of the aster or daisy family that has been used by ancient physicians and herbalists to treat a range of liver and gallbladder diseases and to protect the liver against a variety of poisons." The report states that milk thistle is believed to be "hepatoprotective (protective of the liver) through the following mechanisms of action: antioxidant activity, toxin blockade at the membrane level, enhanced protein synthesis, antifibriotic activity, and possible anti-inflammatory or immunomodulating effects."

The *PDR for Herbal Supplements*, edited by Jeoerg Gruenwald, Ph.D., Christof Jaenicke, M.D., and Thomas Brendler, explains that milk thistle has the following beneficial effects:

1. Hepatoprotective activity which includes preventing toxins from entering liver cells, bolstering the outer membrane of liver cells, decreasing production of superoxide anion radicals and nitric oxide, inhibiting leukotriene formation, and increasing glutathione production.

2. Increased regenerative ability of the liver resulting from stimulation of RNA polymerase 1 (this effect is so profound that milk thistle is used as a remedy against death-cap mushroom poisoning).

3. Anti-inflammatory qualities through inhibition of leukotriene production.

4. Preventing kidney damage after exposure to certain toxins.

5. Reduction of secretion of intracellular prostate-specific antigen (PSA) and inhibition of cell growth in hormone-refractory prostate cancer.

6. Increased rate of recovery in liver disease induced by alcohol abuse.

According to the Research Triangle Institute, a nonprofit research and technology corporation, "milk thistle has unappreciated therapeutic benefit in cancer since it is known more widely as a protectant from environmental and pharmaceutical liver toxicants." Other sources cite milk thistle as an effective treatment for depression and a way to increase bile production and flow.

Because of these benefits, milk thistle is an excellent supplement to add to your Lyme Disease treatment protocol. Milk thistle supplements are generally available at most health food stores. Proper dosing and administration is fairly simple and can generally be done according to instructions on the bottle.

Milk thistle may be contraindicated in certain situations, so consult your physician before use.

Alkalizing minerals

Many, possibly all, diseases and their symptoms are associated with an acidic body pH. Health and vitality, in contrast, occur with an alkaline body pH. Because diseases can both be caused by acidic pH and also create and worsen acidic pH, a downward spiral can precipitate. According to Stephen Heuer, a health consultant in Scottsdale, Arizona, body acidity can be responsible for a wide range of diseases, even cancer. Acidity can decrease oxygen levels, reduce cellular energy, reduce the body's ability to absorb nutrients, and create mineral deficiency. These problems can cascade into dysfunction of nearly every organ in the body.

Bringing acidic body pH back to alkaline can be very challenging. Yet doing so is one of the fastest ways to stop symptoms NOW, especially in the case of Lyme Disease. Although the presence of a bacterial infection is the root cause of Lyme Disease, the majority of ongoing symptoms are actually caused by circulating Lyme Disease toxins. Because alkalizing nutrients neutralize Lyme Disease toxins, alkalizing the body simply makes you feel better quickly. In Lyme Disease, acidic pH can be the cause of numerous symptoms (especially during herx reactions), including extreme sugar cravings, fatigue, lethargy, depression, poor digestion, and a plethora of other symptoms. When alkalizing treatments are used, these symptoms often disappear instantly.

There are several tests you can do to determine your body pH, the easiest of which is the use of pH test strips to measure the pH of your saliva or urine upon waking in the morning. The test results should show a pH within the range of 6.4 to 7.0. If pH is below 6.4, this indicates the body is in a state of physiological acidity.

The strip tests are very inexpensive and can be useful to have as an objective measurement of a disease process which is often elusive and subjective. Additionally, because increased acidity occurs after effective antibacterial treatment as a result of bacterial die-off and toxin release, pH tests can be used to prove objectively the effectiveness of certain types of Lyme Disease treatments. One Lyme Disease sufferer who participates in the Lyme-and-Rife internet discussion group has reported that his pH becomes consistently, significantly more acidic 24 hours after a rife machine treatment. Inexpensive pH test strips can be purchased from most health food stores.

Although helpful, interesting, and inexpensive, pH testing is not absolutely necessary to find out whether you are suffering from an acidic body pH—if you feel sick and tired and have Lyme Disease, your body is likely acidic.

Before further discussion of using alkalizing minerals to treat Lyme Disease, an important caveat is necessary: Restoring alkaline pH in the body requires much more than just supplementation—it involves making permanent changes to your diet and lifestyle. People with Lyme Disease must continually struggle to attain an alkaline pH because their efforts are tirelessly thwarted by ongoing bacterial toxin production. The book *Alkalize or Die* by Theodore Baroody offers excellent tips on diet and other modifications to achieve alkalinization. It is important to note that, while the supplementation discussed below can help, the primary means of restoring alkaline pH in the body is through lifestyle and diet changes. Supplementation cannot substitute for this. Unfortunately, many popular foods (such as red meat, soda pops, and fast food) greatly contribute to an acidic body pH. In contrast, healing foods such as fruits and vegetables greatly contribute to an alkaline body pH.

Although not a replacement for comprehensive diet and lifestyle modifications, mineral supplementation is a simple action you can take to encourage alkalinization in the body and achieve relatively immediate symptom-reduction. In addition to its alkalizing effect, mineral supplementation strengthens the immune system, helps crowd out unwanted heavy metals, improves mental function, aids digestion, and has numerous other benefits. Mineral supplementation is also important when undergoing sauna therapy (as discussed earlier in this chapter) because it replaces minerals lost during sweating.

The most important mineral to supplement in Lyme Disease is magnesium, as discussed in Chapter 10. Molybdenum is also very helpful because it has been found by Lyme Disease sufferers to specifically address symptoms of Lyme Disease neurotoxin circulation, especially during herx reactions. Zinc can be beneficial because it prevents copper toxicity and boosts the immune system. A multi-mineral product is also important.

Magnesium and zinc are easy to find at health food stores. Molybdenum can be a little more difficult to locate but is readily available at many online supplement stores. A wide range of multi-mineral brands and formulations is available. One product that has greatly helped many Lyme

Disease sufferers is "ConcenTrace Trace Mineral Drops," manufactured by Trace Minerals Research, www.traceminerals.com. Mineral supplementation is affordable, non-toxic, and offers excellent detoxification properties.

MERCURY DETOXIFICATION

Although the liver grabs toxins out of circulation from the blood and processes them for elimination, some toxins can become so tightly bound to tissues throughout the body that they never even enter circulation. In addition, some toxins can have such a severely damaging effect on the liver that when they are in the bloodstream, the liver is unable to process them for elimination. In serious cases, these toxins can accumulate in and suffocate the liver, leading to liver damage or even death.

An example of this type of stubborn toxin is the heavy metal mercury. Although mercury is a fat-soluble toxin similar to the toxin produced by Lyme Disease bacteria, special therapies and procedures are necessary to deal with mercury poisoning because of the metal's dangerous and problematic characteristics. For this reason, and because mercury poisoning can seriously complicate Lyme Disease treatment, a special section on mercury and its detoxification is included here.

Mercury is one of the most harmful toxins on the planet and is a catalyst to infection. It is directly immunosuppressive. Although conventional medicine has yet to acknowledge its full potential for harm, mercury is one of the most common, dangerous toxins to accumulate in the body. Mercury poisoning is a BIG problem, not a small one. Once mercury is in the body it is difficult to remove because it binds very strongly to human tissues.

All people (sick or healthy) are exposed to this toxin. Some exposure occurs naturally because mercury is a part of our environment, some occurs through direct contact with mercury products (such as mercury amalgam dental fillings or thimerosal-containing vaccinations), and some occurs via inadvertent contact with mercury-contaminated locations or objects. Even someone careful to avoid such products and contaminated areas will find that mercury is present everywhere in the environment: in the air, water, food, all around us.

So, mercury toxicity is not always a question of whether or not you were exposed to mercury—we all have been to one degree or another. It is more a question of how well your body eliminates the mercury it comes in contact with on a daily basis. Some people have the genetic ability to easily detoxify mercury and eliminate it from the body, while others are genetically susceptible to its accumulation even from low-level, everyday exposure.

Mercury and Lyme Disease: partners in the destruction of your health

Mercury should be given utmost respect and requires entirely different approaches for removal than do other fat-soluble toxins. Mercury detoxification is a subject that deserves great attention in its own right, and it cannot be overlooked as part of a book on Lyme Disease therapies because the two conditions are often linked. Although not everyone with Lyme Disease has mercury toxicity, evidence has repeatedly shown that having Lyme Disease increases the probability of becoming mercury-toxic. This is the case even when a significant mercury exposure has not been identified—as we have said, mercury is in our everyday environment so a singular point of exposure is not necessary to accumulate mercury in the body.

Why does mercury toxicity often accompany Lyme Disease? Below we will examine possible reasons why Lyme Disease and mercury poisoning frequently go hand-in-hand. We'll also see how the two illnesses adversely impact each other.

Mercury catalyzes infections and severely weakens the immune system, so it is not a big leap to accept that people with mercury poisoning would be more susceptible to chronic infections like Lyme Disease. Conversely, Lyme Disease weakens the body's ability to detoxify poisons, so it is not inconceivable to imagine that people with Lyme Disease are more susceptible to accumulating mercury (even from minuscule exposure). But in people with both Lyme Disease and mercury poisoning, which came first? Did the mercury come first, eventually allowing the Lyme infection to thrive, or did the infection come first, weakening the body enough to cause dysfunction in the mercury detoxification process? If mercury toxicity did come first, why did the person become mercury-toxic?

Here are a few possible scenarios that explain how and why mercury toxicity and Lyme Disease are often companions:

1. A person who does not have Lyme Disease may have a genetic sus-ceptibility to becoming mercury-toxic because of a deficiency in liver function. Should this individual be exposed to mercury and become toxic, a suppressed immune system will inevitably follow, and infections will become established with greater ease. Therefore, if exposed to the Lyme bacteria, the individual would be more likely to develop full blown, chronic Lyme Disease than would someone not mercury-toxic.

2. Or, the converse may happen: A completely healthy person, with no genetic predisposition to becoming mercury-toxic, may acquire Lyme Disease. The infection might weaken the body and its mer-cury detoxification abilities. The body would then no longer be ca-pable of removing the mercury to which it is exposed on a daily basis.

3. Another possibility is based on the fact that, as part of its life cycle and survival mechanism, the Lyme Disease organism itself accumu-lates and sequesters mercury. Many researchers have observed that some infective organisms, once established inside the human body, store or use mercury to create a living environment, a niche within the body, inside which the body's defenses are compromised and weakened due to the presence of this heavy metal. Because mer-cury is an immunosuppressant, it is feasible that the Lyme Disease spirochete sequesters mercury in the body as a tool for continued survival in the host environment. The spirochete would do this by grabbing onto minuscule amounts of mercury circulating in the body due to regular (small) daily mercury exposure. After time, the

Lyme Disease organisms would store up more than just a minuscule amount. Significantly increased body burden of mercury would result.

4. Yet another scenario exists when an individual is unknowingly exposed to a large amount of mercury (such as mercury from an old thermometer or use of old, banned mercury products). This might cause mercury toxicity (even without a genetic predisposition) and thus allow a chronic Lyme infection to become more easily established due to the immunosuppressive effects of mercury poisoning.

Individuals who discover that they have both chronic Lyme Disease and mercury toxicity find it nearly impossible to unravel the mystery of which came first. Regardless of how it happens, mercury toxicity often accompanies chronic Lyme Disease, so many Lyme Disease sufferers must undertake mercury detoxification. Most people who have Lyme Disease complicated by mercury toxicity do not experience significant improvement in their Lyme symptoms until the mercury is removed.

Testing for and treating mercury toxicity

How do you know if you have mercury poisoning and how do you get rid of it? Such topics are subject of great controversy. Dozens of books have been written about testing for and treating mercury toxicity. Mercury "experts" vehemently shout all kinds of contradictory information at each other on a regular basis.

Testing for mercury toxicity is one of the most complicated and controversial aspects of dealing with mercury poisoning. Dozens of different testing methods are advocated. Most of the more common methods do not provide truly useful information about just how mercury-toxic someone is. Urine, stool, and blood tests do not give an accurate indication of the total body burden of mercury, because these methods measure only what are called "shallow" body pools of mercury.

One of the most reliable, painless and convenient methods is hair testing, because it measures a much longer mercury excretion period. But even hair testing is not completely accurate. Sometimes normal or low mercury levels in the hair may not indicate that a person is mercury free, but instead the converse: that the individual has been poisoned so severely that the body can no longer eliminate mercury through the hair. Interpreting hair tests properly is a skill most health care practitioners do not have. For these reasons, mercury toxicity should not be ruled out even if one or several tests show safe levels. People who suspect mercury poisoning but do not have positive mercury tests might reasonably try a mercury removal program to see if their symptoms improve. For more information on interpreting hair tests, see Andrew Cutler's newest book, *Hair Test Interpretation: Finding Hidden Toxicities.*

Mercury detoxification treatment is no less complicated or controversial than testing. Most techniques actually do more harm than good and result only in worsening of symptoms and minimal mercury excretion. Mercury is very difficult to eliminate from the body. Most substances and programs claiming to remove mercury, if they do anything at all, actually just stir it up and redistribute it to critical areas like the brain and liver where it can do serious damage. Using a mercury removal protocol that has a high propensity for redistribution is a very bad idea.

Eliminating mercury from the body is accomplished properly by a special type of chelation therapy. Chelation therapy is a method of binding heavy metals for removal from the bloodstream. Chelators are substances used during chelation that circulate throughout the body, bind to mercury, and are then eliminated along with the mercury they are attached to. In Greek, "chelate" means "claw"—the process of mercury removal is so named because chelators metaphorically claw out toxins from where they are bound in the body. There are many different schools of thought and ideologies about how to properly accomplish mercury chelation. Most methods are dangerous and incorrect. Below we will examine three main problems occurring in most common mercury chelation protocols and appropriate solutions for each.

1. The first problem that can render chelators nonproductive and dangerous is that the chelator used does not bond strongly enough with mercury to remove it. Instead, the mercury is merely dislodged from its resting places in the body and sent into circulation, where it quickly bonds to tissues elsewhere. This is called mercury redistribution. It can have seriously damaging effects and can dramatically increase symptoms of toxicity. Body tissues themselves have a high affinity for mercury. If the chelating agent used creates only a weak bond, the mercury will be dropped by the chelator and grab onto other body tissues on the way out of the body. An ideal mercury protocol minimizes redistribution. Substances that are not proven to be appropriate chelators (even though they are quite popular) include cilantro, chlorella, and MSM, to name a few. These substances are not ideal mercury removal agents. Nor are many of the "mercury detoxification" herbal preparations sold in health food stores and by various healthcare practitioners. In some cases, these substances and products can be very dangerous and often do more harm than good. Such substances and products typically create a strong enough bond to move mercury around in the body and cause mercury redistribution, but not a strong enough bond to actually usher mercury *out* of the body.

DMSA (dimercaptosuccinic acid), DMPS (dimercaptopropane-1-sulfonic acid), and ALA (alpha lipoic acid) are three effective, appropriate mercury chelators that create a bond strong enough to successfully usher mercury out of the body and not just redistribute it. These substances have a long, established track record, and also have a great amount of supporting research. DMPS and DMSA are water soluble, while ALA is fat soluble. In a mercury removal program, both a water soluble and a fat soluble chelator should be used.

DMPS is a better choice than DMSA. DMPS or DMSA (DMPS is preferred) can be combined with ALA as part of a comprehensive mercury treatment plan. Oral DMPS capsules are much safer and more effective than the commonly administered IV/injected form of DMPS, reasons for which will be explained over the next several paragraphs. Oral chelators are *always* preferred over IV chelators. Oral DMPS capsules are fairly difficult to locate but can be purchased with a prescription in compounded form from The Falls Pharmacy, Snoqualmie, WA, www.thefallspharmacy.com, (877) 392-7948. The Falls Pharmacy offers mail order prescription fulfillment. DMPS dosing should be approximately 10mg-30mg, every eight hours, as described in the book *Amalgam Illness: Diagnosis and Treatment* written by Andrew Cutler, Ph.D. This book also provides instructions for combining DMPS or DMSA with ALA to build a comprehensive mercury treatment plan. More information about this book will be provided in a few pages.

2. Another problem commonly encountered in an inept mercury removal program is that the chelator is not dosed with sufficient frequency to ensure that a consistent supply of it is available in the blood to "sop up" the mercury knocked loose by the last dose of chelator. Because even proper chelating agents (DMSA, DMPS, and ALA) do not create perfect bonds with mercury, they sometimes drop the mercury on its way out of the body. Thus it is essential to have a constant, fresh supply of chelator in the blood to pick up the dropped mercury and carry it the rest of the way out. Proper mercury chelating substances have a short half-life in the blood which necessitates frequent dosing (sometimes requiring middle-of-the-night doses) to maintain blood levels. A valid chelation schedule requires dosing several times per day. Improper and inappropriate dosing schedules include:

   a. Schedules in which a large dose of chelator is taken infrequently, such as a DMPS injection or IV once every week or month.

   b. Schedules in which a full dose of chelator is taken only daily or every other day.

   c. Schedules in which mercury chelators are taken on an irregular basis, such that there is no consistent dosing pattern.

3. Even if a proper chelating agent is used on an appropriately frequent schedule, a mistake often made is using too large a dose. It is not uncommon for mercury chelation protocols to use doses that are 10 times higher than they should be. The reason for using very low doses of chelator is that the eliminatory system of the body can handle only a small amount of mercury at a time. Mercury is highly toxic, and as you remove it you must ensure that the body has to deal with it in very small portions. If you take large doses of a chelator, lots of mercury gets mobilized, but only a small amount gets excreted. The rest gets redistributed and attaches to other tissue in the body, causing damage and increased symptoms. Larger doses do not get the mercury out faster, they simply make you more miserable during the process. A proper chelation protocol uses a small dose of chelating substance so that the amount of mercury knocked loose is easily handled by the eliminatory system instead of being simply redistributed throughout the body.

To summarize, productive and beneficial chelation protocols use small doses of proper chelators taken frequently. Dangerous protocols use large doses of inappropriate chelators taken infrequently. Productive chelation campaigns result in mercury removal and symptom improvement. Improper, dangerous protocols result in mercury redistribution and damage to the body with very little mercury removal or symptom improvement.

These principles of mercury chelation were discovered by Andrew Cutler, Ph.D. His book, *Amalgam Illness: Diagnosis and Treatment*, is the source from which to learn more about how to safely remove mercury from the body. Cutler's approach to mercury testing and removal relies on sound science and has been used successfully by dozens of Lyme Disease sufferers. The book explains exactly how to remove mercury safely. I personally used Dr. Cutler's methods to successfully cure my own severe mercury poisoning after several other popular mercury programs failed to heal me. My hair test mercury levels were the highest my health care practitioner had ever seen.

The methods described in *Amalgam Illness: Diagnosis and Treatment* are not only effective in removing mercury from the body and reducing side effects during the process, but are also fairly affordable and can be used at home with minimal help from a physician. Anyone considering mercury detoxification should read Dr. Cutler's book before decisions are made. Even your trusted alternative medicine doctor, whom you see for all your needs, is probably wrong about mercury chelation. Mercury chelation is one of the riskiest and most complicated medical therapies you can undertake. Mistakes can cause serious suffering and sometimes permanent damage.

Although the methods described in *Amalgam Illness: Diagnosis and Treatment* will help remove mercury from the body, the process can take months or years. Anyone embarking on a mercury detoxification program needs to know what to do, and what it feels like, in the meantime.

Concurrent mercury toxicity and Lyme Disease

Lyme Disease sufferers need to be aware that having mercury poisoning and Lyme Disease at the same time can be a confusing, frustrating, scary experience. As mentioned before, there is evidence that the Lyme Disease organism intentionally stores and sequesters mercury. This activity results in increased mercury concentrations in and near Lyme Disease colonies in the body—mercury and Lyme Disease are together in close quarters. For anyone afflicted with both mercury toxicity and Lyme Disease, the experience can be a frightening roller coaster ride. The following factors contribute to this experience:

1. Mercury symptoms can be very similar to Lyme Disease symptoms. Because the Lyme Disease bacteria and mercury typically occupy the same places in the body, the symptoms of each are very difficult to distinguish. Someone with Lyme Disease may not be aware that they have mercury poisoning and thus assume that all of their symptoms are Lyme Disease-related, when in reality, some are mercury symptoms. A person who knows they have both mercury tox-

icity and Lyme Disease finds that the next challenge is to separate the symptoms and determine which are caused by which problem.

2. The confusion is compounded by the fact that as mercury chelators mobilize mercury, the Lyme Disease organism reacts. The presence of mercury in the living environment of the bacteria is advantageous to the bacteria. As the mercury-rich environment is altered, the infection responds with self-protective activities. This means that anyone undertaking chelation treatments will not only experience the symptoms and side effects of mercury mobilization and removal, they will also experience the effects of altered Lyme Disease symptoms.

3. To make matters even more complicated, when Lyme Disease organisms are being killed or attacked, mercury symptoms may be altered as well. As you manipulate the Lyme bacteria's living environment and kill Lyme Disease organisms, mercury is mobilized and released. Sometimes mercury is actually stored inside a spirochete or bacterial colony itself. When that colony is disrupted or eradicated (with antibiotics or rife machines or some other anti-Lyme treatment), mercury is released. This results in an outbreak of both herx reaction symptoms and mercury mobilization symptoms. In fact, many herx symptoms commonly experienced by Lyme Disease sufferers are actually symptoms of mercury mobilization. Because dying Lyme Disease organisms can release mercury, it is important to use a mercury detoxification protocol while undertaking anti-Lyme therapy to sop up the mercury that is released during the killing of Lyme Disease bacteria.

4. Mercury is a very strong immunosuppressant, and its presence in the body may mask inflammatory Lyme Disease symptoms. Lyme Disease patients may actually feel that their Lyme Disease symptoms are better when they are mercury-poisoned because the inflammatory response to Lyme Disease is reduced. When mercury is removed from the body, an individual may experience increased Lyme Disease symptoms and herx reactions because the immune system has begun to function properly again.

These are just a few of the confusing elements involved in experiencing mercury toxicity and Lyme Disease (and the treatment of both) simultaneously. Further details are beyond the scope of this book, but by recognizing that the subject can be very complicated and by treating it with respect, you have taken the first step toward figuring out what is taking place in your body and what you can do about it.

As a final point before closing this mercury discussion, it should be noted that mercury chelators are not able to reach mercury stored inside Lyme Disease organisms until the organisms are killed and the mercury is released into circulation. Therefore, as long as there continues to be an active Lyme Disease infection, it is also likely that additional mercury is sequestered throughout the body. For this reason, mercury detoxification should not be considered to be finished until all Lyme Disease bacteria are completely eradicated. A mercury removal program is often needed for quite a long time, sometimes even years.

Lyme sufferers should consider carefully the possibility of mercury poisoning and that any stagnation in their healing progress may be, at least partially, a result of the presence of mercury in the body. It is essential first to find out if mercury is a problem, and then decide how to get rid of it. Most cases of Lyme Disease will not show satisfactory improvement (regardless of which anti-Lyme therapies are used) unless mercury toxicity is addressed. *Lyme Disease and Rife Machines* includes a helpful chart that provides additional mercury detoxification resources, including contact information for a health-care practitioner who is willing to work with Lyme Disease sufferers toward the task of mercury detoxification.

Fish, mercury, and omega fatty acids

Seafood is one of the most nutritious foods on the planet. It has served as a staple food for numerous cultures around the world. It is rich in many important nutrients, the most important of which are omega fatty acids, which play an important role in numerous body functions. Of particular note is the crucial role omega fatty acids play in modulating inflammatory processes, strengthening the immune system, maintaining brain and nerve health, and healing or reversing toxic/chemical imbalances in the brain that can lead to a plethora of psychiatric symptoms.

Because Lyme Disease has deleterious effects on all of the organs and body systems mentioned above, omega fatty acids are critical in the recovery process. Not only do they facilitate deep healing in the body, they also provide relatively fast symptom reduction and increased energy. Omega fatty acids can reduce depression, promote brain healing, and bolster the immune system in fighting Lyme Disease.

Unfortunately, getting your omega fatty acids from fish has become a dangerous game of Russian roulette due to the fact that a large percentage of commercially available fish is contaminated with the toxic heavy metal mercury. Although some types and sources of fish have a lower risk of being contaminated with mercury, it can be difficult or impossible to tell which fish is safe and which is contaminated. Even a small amount of mercury can cause serious, long-term damage and increased symptoms. As we have seen earlier in this chapter, mercury itself causes major damage inside the body and even worse, it helps Lyme Disease bacteria survive and proliferate. The potential damaging effects of mercury poisoning are just too serious to ignore. Regrettably, the best course of action is simply to avoid fish consumption until recovery has been fully achieved. In some cases, maintaining a state of recovery may require forgoing fish consumption for the rest of your life.

An additional reason to avoid fish is that most fish has very high Vitamin D levels. As you can see by reading Chapter 2, Vitamin D can be very damaging to the Lyme Disease healing process.

The problem with avoiding fish in your diet (other than the obvious fact that you will simply miss it!) is that it can be difficult to consume adequate quantities of omega fatty acids without eating fish. There is, however, a workable solution. Flax seed oil, which is derived from the flax plant (also known as linseed) and is a completely vegetarian product, is rich in omega-3, omega-6, and omega-9 fatty acids, and can be used in the diet as a substitute for fish. Flax seed oil can be purchased at most health food stores and some grocery stores. It must be kept refrigerated. It has a strong taste and can be consumed alone but is more palatable when used as part of a recipe (note, though, that flax oil cannot be heated). One tablespoon of flax seed oil per day provides ample supply of omega fatty acids. One way to get your daily dose of flax seed oil is to use one tablespoon of it mixed with lemon juice as a salad dressing. Flax seed oil does not replace all the nutrients in fish, but it does supply the important omega fatty acids.

In addition to fish, it can be important to avoid other sources of marine mercury. Glucosamine chondroitin is one supplement that may be contaminated with mercury because it is made from shellfish shells. If you look around you can find safe, vegetarian glucosamine chondroitin supplements without seafood ingredients. Chitosan and chitosan oligosaccharide supplements, which were discussed in my first book, are also derived from the shells of shrimp and other sea crustaceans, and may carry the risk of mercury contamination. Chlorella, a popular supplement for mercury removal (which in my research is still unproven for this purpose) may also be contaminated.

One Lyme Disease sufferer recently told me that he knows of several brands of Omega fatty acids which claim to be heavy-metal free. If these supplements are indeed clean, they may be appropriate for use. The difficulty, I believe, is in verifying the veracity of such claims.

As a precautionary note, Dr. James Schaller has observed that in some individuals, omega-6 and omega-9 fatty acids can increase inflammation; so, be alert for this possible side effect.

EXERCISE

Many people with Lyme Disease seek advanced, fancy therapies and overlook simple, time-proven methods of maintaining health—like exercise. Lyme Disease sufferers often have a hard time exercising because of joint inflammation, fatigue, and other exhausting problems associated with having Lyme Disease. If exercise is undertaken, the Lyme Disease patient might feel OK during exercise but then experience serious fatigue or other symptoms shortly after or the next day.

Despite these difficulties, research indicates that exercise is a critical component of a complete anti-Lyme program. It accelerates the process of getting well. Needless to say, exercise should not be done to the point of debility. Exercise should be approached with extreme caution by Lyme Disease sufferers with severe weakness or, especially, heart complications. In cases of extreme weakness and debilitation, an exercise program can begin with walking back and forth across the living room several times with the help of a family member. Exercise intensity should be increased slowly.

The important component of an exercise program for a Lyme Disease sufferer is not how much exercise is done, but simply that exercise is done. If nothing more than a 30 second walk is accomplished, it is still beneficial. Many people find that their Lyme-related aches and pains actually improve (instead of worsen) following exercise. Lyme Disease joint problems result from destructive inflammation similar to the damage done by a physical sports injury, such as falling on a soccer field and landing hard on the knee. In cases of sports injury rehabilitation, a physical therapist typically prescribes activity to rehabilitate a joint, not rest. Similarly, a sick, tired body will recover only if it is exercised and challenged (within reasonable limitations). A sedentary lifestyle is unhealthy for all of us, sick or well.

Exercise has been proven to alleviate depression, lift mood, sharpen mental abilities, balance hormones, increase metabolism, and raise body temperature. These are but a few known benefits. Exercise and activity do not mask symptoms, instead they actually repair fundamental imbalances in the body. Until modern times, exercise was an unavoidable part of life. Before cars and desk jobs and inactive forms of entertainment like TV and movies, people were required to use their bodies for daily survival. The human body needs exercise in the same way it needs food, water, nutrition, and sleep.

In addition to general health benefits, exercise specifically benefits Lyme Disease sufferers in several ways:

1. It induces production of Co-enzyme Q-10, a nutrient typically deficient in Lyme Disease. Deficiency of this nutrient is often responsible for many of the heart problems seen in Lyme Disease patients. Tissue samples from the hearts of Lyme Disease sufferers have shown dramatically low levels of Co-enzyme Q-10.

2. It oxygenates tissues and increases circulation to all parts of the body, including the brain. Increased circulation to the brain alleviates Lyme-related depression, memory problems, and mental confusion.

3. It helps digestive processes and reduces the predisposition towards constipation.

In relation to detoxification, exercise is the therapy that supports all other therapies. Increased circulation, metabolism, and energy consumption can literally burn off Lyme Disease neurotoxins in the same way that calories can be burned. The actual physical motion involved in exercising, including contractions of the muscles, causes toxic substances to be shaken loose into circulation in the bloodstream and lymphatic system. These toxins are then more quickly eliminated as all organs in the body are stimulated by exercise.

Think of exercise in terms of this analogy. If you have ever walked by a pond full of standing water, you have noticed that it is stagnant, dirty, murky, often smelly, and full of sediment and algae. In contrast, moving water, such as that found in a rapidly flowing river, is clean, clear, and fresh. In the same way, exercising the body acts to refresh and purify body systems and circulation. Even people without Lyme Disease cannot expect to feel completely healthy without including exercise in their lifestyle. It is a simple fact that the human body needs exercise to stay healthy. Do not overlook this important aspect of the recovery process.

Detoxification reactions

When undergoing any type of detoxification program, the toxins released from stored body tissues cannot exit the body without first passing through the blood. Whether eliminated by the liver, kidneys, or skin, toxins first enter circulation on their way to the appropriate organ. This means that a person who is detoxifying will experience intensified symptoms of toxicity while the toxins are in transit in the bloodstream. The specific symptoms experienced depend on which type of toxin is in circulation at a given time. Symptoms can range from physical ailments like muscle soreness and fatigue to mental dysfunction such as depression, hyperactivity, or even paranoia.

This intensification of symptoms is often known as a "cleansing reaction," "healing reaction," or "detoxification reaction." Such a reaction can be quite uncomfortable and in some cases dangerous or debilitating. For this reason, detoxification must be undertaken slowly and moderately, and its reactions must be controlled. Only one detoxification therapy should be utilized at a time. Simultaneous use of multiple detoxification therapies can lead to greatly intensified detoxification reactions. Detoxification should never be done to the point of causing an unmanageable or out-of-control reaction. As your recovery progresses and your body becomes less toxic, your tolerance for detoxification therapies will increase.

Detoxification reactions are not to be confused with herx reactions (see Chapter 4 in *Lyme Disease and Rife Machines* for an explanation of the herx reaction). They are similar to, and certainly feel similar to, herx reactions because both types of reaction involve increased circulation of toxins. But it is important to remember that herx reactions result from the use of antibacterial therapies and associated bacterial load reduction. Detoxification reactions, on the other hand, do not involve bacterial load reduction.

Although detoxification reactions are different from herx reactions, remedies which alleviate herx reactions can also help detoxification reactions because both reactions result from the effects of increased toxin circulation. The following therapies are helpful in controlling and minimizing both herx reactions and detoxification reactions. These therapies are especially helpful in cases of out-of-control reactions characterized by intolerable symptoms. Because symptoms of a toxic reaction result mainly from the toxins' acidic state, the therapies listed below are primarily intended to alkalize the body. You will notice that some of these therapies are actually the same therapies that can cause detoxification reactions in the first place. So, in certain cases, additional detoxification is the right action to take if a detoxification therapy caused intolerable symptoms.

1. Alka Seltzer Gold—this product contains alkalizing substances without aspirin or other medications and can quickly reduce symptoms. The "Gold" Alka Seltzer is recommended because it is the only one in the product line that does not contain other medicines. Alka Seltzer Gold, because it is conveniently packaged and inexpensive, can be taken on vacation or stored in the medicine cabinet to combat nasty herx or detoxification reactions.

2. Increased water consumption—drinking lots of purified water is one of the simplest and most helpful ways you can minimize symptoms. Water quickly cleans out both the blood and the digestive tract. Be careful to drink only clean, filtered, or purified water.

3. Mineral supplementation—increased mineral consumption, especially molybdenum, as per the information presented earlier in this chapter, can confer substantial relief by neutralizing Lyme Disease neurotoxins.

4. Lithium supplementation—lithium, as presented in Chapter 8, has a powerful ability to protect the brain and other cells throughout the body from the effects of toxins circulating in the bloodstream. Rapid relief of symptoms can be attained with lithium supplementation.

5. Sauna/bath therapy—a sauna treatment or hot bath can be taken for immediate symptom relief.

6. Exercise—exercise quickly increases circulation, oxygenates tissue, stimulates detoxification processes, elevates mood, and triggers sweating which further expedites toxin removal. Exercise is one of

the most valuable detoxification therapies and should be considered a foundational activity.

7. Oral charcoal supplements—charcoal has incredible absorptive properties and can reduce symptoms by sopping up toxins in the digestive tract.

8. High-fiber foods—because the bottleneck of toxin removal is often the digestive tract, high-fiber foods can both accelerate digestive transit time and at the same time, absorb toxins in the digestive tract.

9. Anti-inflammatory and anti-allergy medicines—if a reaction involves inflammation or an allergic response, these medicines can provide relief. Benadryl can control an allergic response to toxins. Quercetin is a flavonoid that is responsible for many of the healing actions of various herbal remedies. Quercetin can be purchased at most health food stores and can be used as a substitute for Benadryl to achieve relief from an allergic-type response. It should be noted that one doctor in Virginia has observed that Lyme sufferers are more likely to develop a dependency on antihistamine drugs than are people not suffering from Lyme Disease. This doctor does not recommend continued use of antihistamines for Lyme Disease or other chronic illness due to the potential for this dependency and also the fact that antihistamine drugs can be immunosuppressive.

Non-steroidal anti-inflammatory (NSAID) medicines, such as Ibuprofen, may help reduce symptoms of inflammation. NSAIDs should obviously be used sparingly. Their use can be warranted when a reaction involves intolerable symptoms and immediate relief is sought, i.e., in the case of a herx-related headache that will not go away. Steroidal anti-inflammatory drugs such as cortisone and prednisone **MUST BE COMPLETELY AVOIDED** unless the reaction is life-threatening. Steroidal anti-inflammatory drugs debilitate the immune system and can cause permanent worsening of Lyme Disease symptoms.

Detoxification reactions (and herx reactions) are your ally and will lead to improvement if they are induced in controlled moderation. These reactions are necessary in the recovery process. However, in excess, both types of reaction can be not only very uncomfortable, but can actually be destructive to the healing process. Ensuring that detoxification therapies are used moderately and carefully will prevent out-of-control detoxification reactions. Similarly, applying antibacterial therapies in moderation will prevent out-of-control herx reactions. Moderation is one of the most important aspects of a Lyme Disease treatment program. Remember, recovering from Lyme Disease is a marathon, not a sprint. Taking a sprinting approach will lead to frustration and stagnated progress. Taking a slow, steady, sustainable marathon approach will lead to smooth, consistent, predictable progress.

Chapter 5:
Electromedicine
(Rife Machine Therapy)

Preface

My first book, *When Antibiotics Fail: Lyme Disease and Rife Machines,* was published in January of 2005. This book described how rife machine therapy is one of the most promising treatments available for Lyme Disease. Since *Lyme Disease and Rife Machines* was published, additional evidence, including new user reports, has confirmed that rife machine therapy is indeed an extremely valuable core therapy, essential to ensuring that continuous healing occurs. It has been repeatedly demonstrated that rife machine therapy takes people from being bedridden and dysfunctional to living productive, happy lives. This progress is possible even after standard antibiotic therapy fails.

However, many people have noticed that while they are able to quickly get to about 90% well using a rife machine, the last 10% of the healing process is slow and difficult. Achieving a full, 100% recovery with a rife machine alone is possible—but it is slow. The most logical explanation for this slowed progress is simply that, while rife machine therapy addresses a very important aspect of the Lyme Disease complex, it is not a silver bullet and there are yet other aspects of the complex which it does not target. For this reason, my second book, the one you now hold in your hands, was written and published—to share information about other valuable therapeutic approaches to healing Lyme Disease. The breakthrough therapies in this book are in no way intended to replace rife machine therapy. I do not believe that any adequate replacement therapy exists. Instead, the therapies in this book are intended to support rife machine therapy. This is a key statement and bears repeating: the information in *Lyme Disease and Rife Machines* is still accurate and applicable. New information presented in this book should support and enhance rife machine therapy, *not replace it.*

If you are currently using a rife machine and experiencing good results, there is no need change what you are doing. Some people do get to 100% with rife machine therapy alone. Doug MacLean, the father of modern rife machine therapy as used for Lyme Disease, is one example, as are many people who regularly participate on the Lyme-and-rife online discussion group.

So how does rife machine therapy fit into the new information provided in this book? Rife machine therapy should be the core of a Lyme Disease treatment protocol. Without rife machine therapy, the treatments and protocols discussed in this book are rendered much less effective. However, when combined with rife machine therapy, the treatments and protocols in this book are highly beneficial and synergistic. The two books are not in competition with each other, but instead fit together like puzzle pieces. Rife machine therapy complements the treatments in this book, and the new treatments in this book complement rife machine therapy.

For a complete explanation of rife machine therapy as used to fight Lyme Disease, read *Lyme Disease and Rife Machines*. This chapter does not provide a thorough treatment of this subject but instead only an introduction.

Readers who have already read *Lyme Disease and Rife Machines* will find the first section of this chapter redundant. Updated rife user tips and other hot-off-the-press information will be of more interest to you and can be found in the latter portion of this chapter.

What is a rife machine?

The human immune system uses electricity to ward off invading microorganisms. Science & Vie Magazine reports that human leucocytes kill bacteria and pathogenic fungi by electrocution. So, it is surprising that most people have not heard of rife machines—an electrical treatment for infections. Lyme Disease is one infection that responds exceptionally well to electrical therapies, so it is even more surprising that many Lyme Disease sufferers have not heard of rife machines. Yet, surprising or not, if you don't know what a rife machine is you represent the majority of the population.

Rife machines get their name from Dr. Royal Raymond Rife, an American scientist whose early 20th century experiments and discoveries were groundbreaking. Rife had his own microbiology laboratory that was among the most well equipped in the world. He designed and built a microscope that was 50 years ahead of its time, identified many microorganisms that had never been seen before, and discovered that exposing microorganisms to certain electromagnetic frequencies resulted in their death. The significance of Rife's discoveries is comparable to that of any major invention, such as the telephone or automobile. His brilliant research resulted in the ability to eradicate life-threatening infections.

Although Rife's pioneering biomedical discoveries were numerous, spanning the gamut from microscopy to biochemistry, the most significant of them was unquestionably the rife machine. How did Rife's machine work? Microorganisms (including bacteria, viruses and fungi) each have a specific vibratory frequency, or "mortal oscillatory rate" (MOR) to which they can be exposed, resulting in their deactivation or death. A rife machine is the electronic apparatus used to deliver the frequency (MOR) to the body. A rife machine delivers this frequency by applying an invisible electromagnetic field to the body. The field passes through the entire body and disables targeted microorganisms.

At one time Rife was considered a medical genius. In the 1930's, many doctors had rife machines in their offices and were successfully treating patients with them.

But it isn't so today.

Despite the scientific validity substantiating Rife's approach to ridding the body of infectious microorganisms, his 1930's research is wrought with controversy and mystery. Modern researchers, authors and historians have suggested that his work was suppressed or ignored by those who stood to lose money or other gain if his ideas got traction. For example, penicillin (the first antibiotic) was released near the time Rife's work went underground. The rife machine would have been direct competition for penicillin.

Whether his work was suppressed or just ignored, today doctors do not use rife machines, and sadly, we do not even have a complete record of Royal Raymond Rife's story. Historical documents prove that Rife was able to kill microorganisms and alleviate disease with electromagnetic frequencies. But there is a void in the record of exactly which electronic setup, or machine, he used. It has been over 70 years since Rife conducted his research. That is a long time for records to be kept accurately, especially if people feel threatened that the records might cause a forced paradigm shift in how medicine is practiced. Numerous historical examples illustrate that medical paradigm shifts are resisted for as long as possible.

But fortunately the missing links have been cause for more than just confusion. They have motivated modern researchers to develop new machines in an attempt to duplicate Rife's results and recreate the Rife machine. Newly invented and currently available machines should be thought of as modern rife machines to distinguish them from Rife's original. Today many modern rife machines are available, each of which significantly varies from the others due to lack of a clear model upon which their designs are based.

As would be expected given the uncertainty surrounding rife machine technology, modern rife machines are inconsistent in their ability to kill infectious microorganisms, both in the laboratory and according to reports from people using them to treat various infections. Some people fully recover, others get a lesser degree of help, while still others don't benefit at all. Modern rife machine technology can be hit-or-miss. Fortunately, Lyme Disease is one infection that responds exceptionally well to certain types of modern rife machines.

For an excellent account of the Royal Raymond Rife story, read *The Cancer Cure That Worked* by Barry Lynes. Barry's was the first book written about rife machines and not only tells the full story but also provides a detailed history of rife machine technology from Royal Raymond Rife's day to the present. Nenah Sylver's book, *The Handbook of Rife Frequency Healing* (also written under the name Nina Silver), is also an excellent resource and is helpful for further clarification of rife machine principles.

Rife machines vs. Lyme Disease: A new application of an old discovery

Lyme Disease was not a recognized illness when Rife conducted his experiments, so he never studied the bacteria. The effectiveness of electromagnetic frequencies against Lyme Disease was discovered more than fifty years after Rife's studies, ironically by a researcher who was not even aware of Royal Raymond Rife. Doug MacLean (from now on, simply "Doug") was an engineer who himself suffered from Lyme Disease and was not getting well with conventional therapy. When antibiotics failed him in the late 1980's, he began the search for a better treatment.

His search turned to electromagnetic machines when he happened to speak with a relative who told him something vague about electromagnetic frequencies having the ability to disable microorganisms. Doug was never told about Royal Raymond Rife, or actually how to do this, but he was eager to investigate. His background as a manufacturing engineer gave him the tools and knowledge to proceed. He converted his basement to a makeshift microbiology laboratory (not so different from Rife's) and acquired live Lyme Disease spirochetes through a colleague who worked at a biomedical research facility.

After carefully setting up his laboratory (including a dark field microscope) Doug was able to observe spirochetes being killed as he applied certain electromagnetic frequencies to them. He even captured the bactericidal effects of electromagnetic fields on videotape.

Doug's research was phenomenal because it objectively proved that Lyme Disease spirochetes could be destroyed with electromagnetic frequencies. But watching spirochetes die under the microscope was not Doug's only indication that his research might hold promise.

As he peered into the microscope to watch spirochetes get ripped apart by the electromagnetic field, he was himself inadvertently exposed to the treatment frequencies. From this indirect and unintentional exposure, he gave himself an accidental treatment. This caused the biggest herx reaction he had ever had. Now he knew these frequencies worked in vitro and in vivo (in a test tube as well as in a human being).

He knew he was on the right track.

These victories gave him the strength and perseverance to keep at it. He built a bigger machine that could treat the whole body instead of just a small test tube. Over the course of a few years, with various machine design changes, Doug invented a modern rife machine that he used to attain remission from his Lyme Disease.

Today Doug has been symptom-free and antibiotic-free for more than 15 years. Doug's case of Lyme Disease was the first in known history to be successfully cured with specific electromagnetic frequencies.

After Doug got well, many Lyme Disease sufferers followed in his footsteps and built their own machines according to his design (which he graciously made available, free of charge, to anyone interested). The news about rife machine success against Lyme Disease spread like wildfire through Lyme Disease support groups. Most of the modern information about and interest in rife machine technology for Lyme Disease can be traced back to the humble, life-saving experiments Doug conducted in his basement. The latest and most effective version of Doug's machine is known as the Coil Machine, also sometimes referred to as the Doug Device. It is thoroughly discussed in *Lyme Disease and Rife Machines*.

Doug's discoveries were not just a contribution to the Lyme Disease community. They serendipitously validated the work of Royal Raymond Rife himself. Over 70 years ago, Royal Raymond Rife discovered the incredible usefulness of electromagnetic frequencies against infections, and just 15 years ago, Doug (unknowingly) independently verified this truth with his own laboratory experiments.

At the 2006 Rife International Health Conference, held in Seattle, Washington on October 20-22, I interviewed Doug MacLean. Amazingly, this was Doug's first-ever public appearance. You can order a DVD that includes both this interview and my presentation at the conference by visiting www.lymebook.com/conference.

Why don't doctors use rife machines?

The following letter from a Lyme Disease sufferer illustrates why physicians do not use rife machines and why they are not considered a part of mainstream medicine.

I have been amazed by the success stories I've heard about rife machines. I met with a group near my home which has been using a plasma rife machine, and they say it is the only thing that helped them. Needless to say it got me quite excited. The thought of having a clear mind and strength to go out and do what I used to seemed pretty good.

I met with my LLMD [Lyme Literate Medical Doctor] and he asked how my antibiotic treatment was going. I told him the same thing I've said before....some bad days and some really bad days...you know the routine. Then I brought up rife machine therapy and told him my brief story about meeting with people who had great luck with it, as well as my own limited experiences with it.

As soon as I mentioned it he pulled out a pad of paper and jotted down the website address of the Lyme-and-Rife Yahoo! online support group (access the group at www.lymebook.com/resources), and told me the name of the machine to get. He also talked about some remedies I would need for the severe herx reactions I was going to have. He then told me about a patient of his who is an electrical engineer and has had Lyme for about a year. She researched rife machine therapy and found the best way to go with it. She has had great success in the few months she has used it.

My doctor seemed pretty excited that I brought it up and had info ready for me when I did. From what I gathered he cannot bring up the subject because it is not FDA approved. This seems somewhat perverse to me, that there is an effective treatment out there and doctors cannot mention it to their patients because of legal reasons. He seemed pretty frustrated with the system. In the meantime, people suffering from Lyme Disease are left to research their own means of a cure.

Peace,
Eric

According to a survey conducted by the Lyme-and-Rife online discussion group asking patients if their doctors know about rife machines, 39% of LLMDs know about them and of those 39%, 77% suggest they are helpful for treating Lyme Disease. Both LLMDs and Lyme patients are aware that rife machines work. Yet, doctors cannot recommend or use them. Why?

When the medical profession was established a doctor's goal was to help a patient by using the best therapies available. Although most doctors still have this goal, a doctor's toolbox of therapies has become limited. Doctors are only licensed to practice medicine by using treatments that have been deemed by the U.S. government to be safe and effective. This would not be a problem if the governing authorities really approved the most effective medical therapies. But we must examine how new medical therapies get approved. Are they really the best therapies?

The governing authorities decided that approval for new medical treatments requires long, expensive clinical trials that are intended to protect the public from potentially dangerous, unproven medical treatments. The trials require millions of dollars and thousands of technical man hours. Are clinical trials a good idea? Of course! They ensure that new therapies are thoroughly studied before being released.

The problem is that clinical trials are entrusted to private, for-profit companies. Although the government conducts a significant amount of not-for-profit medical research through organizations such as National Institutes of Health (NIH), the research data that gets converted into medical products and services is assigned to profit-driven companies. These companies are motivated by the same force that drives other businesses in America—profit.

But all too often, the medical products that bring in the best cash flow are not actually the safest or most effective products. This is a big problem and creates a major conflict of interest. The companies we trust to research and produce life-saving medicines are daily faced with the question of, do we research the most effective medical therapies or the most profitable medical therapies?

When faced with this question, many companies choose high-profit research opportunities regardless of whether they offer the greatest potential benefit. Companies actually do not have a choice in this decision. The American economy is just too efficient and brutal to allow the survival of companies that do not put profit first. Most medical research companies are publicly traded and have thousands of stock holders, each of whom has a financial interest in the company. These stock holders own the company. They buy stock hoping to make money. Companies making less money or too little money get overtaken by companies willing to do what it takes to stay on top. It's a business thing. It's the law of capitalism. The companies that don't like this way of doing business don't last very long. So, the medical research companies that survive in our economy are the ones that put profit first.

If companies produce the most profitable products, we must ask: What is the most profitable means of medical care and how profitable is rife machine technology in comparison?

Drugs are significantly more profitable than rife machines. Look at what Fortune Magazine, April 15, 2002, said about the pharmaceutical drug industry: In 2001, the ten American drug companies in the Fortune 500 ranked far above all other American industries in average net return. Average net return as a percentage of sales for the pharmaceutical companies was 560% higher than that of all other industries across the gamut of American commerce! The Bolen Report made a similar observation:

> *"The most startling fact is that the combined profits for the ten drug companies in the Fortune 500 ($35.9 billion) were more than the profits for all the other 490 businesses put together ($33.7 billion). When I say this is a profitable industry, I mean really profitable. It is difficult to conceive of how awash in money big pharma is."*
>
> *-The Bolen Report*

Looking at the profitability of drugs in comparison with rife machines, consider that rife machines use electricity to function, and just as water, air and fire cannot be patented, neither can electricity. Electricity is a natural force and is available to those who need it. Of course, electrical companies do make money by providing electricity, so electricity can be profitable. But the cost of electricity to the consumer is very low in comparison to the price of drugs. To run a rife machine enough to allow for a reasonable treatment schedule costs less than $5/month in electricity. It simply does not make sense for profit-driven companies to spend millions of dollars researching medical treatments that would be difficult to patent.

In a country where medical therapies are determined by free market forces, drugs get researched, produced and sold more than any other therapy.

Less profitable products and services get demoted to "alternative medicine" status because companies do not spend money to get them officially FDA approved. These low-profit therapies get relegated from the pharmacy to your alternative health food "shop." It does not matter how effective they are, it only matters how profitable they are. This answers our original question. Because doctors cannot recommend or use medical devices that are not FDA approved, doctors do not treat their patients with rife machines, regardless of whether rife machine technology is the best option for the patient.

Are rife machines the cure for Lyme Disease?

There is clinical evidence that rife machines work: People get better when they use rife machines. There is laboratory evidence that rife machines work: Doug's experiment provided objective confirmation that rife machines kill spirochetes. Thus, rife machines can be scientifically viewed as a useful treatment for Lyme Disease. But the question still remains: are rife machines a helpful treatment, or are they the cure?

New information available since I published my first book indicates that about 30% of rife machine users get completely well with rife machine therapy alone. However, 70% of users find that while rife machine therapy is beneficial, it does not take them all the way out of the woods. These Lyme Disease sufferers typically report that rife machine therapy is anywhere from the most helpful treatment they have ever used to just a beneficial treatment that ensures continuous progress is made. In some cases, rife machine therapy may be a cure, but in the majority of cases, it does not lead to 100% remission of symptoms.

Hence the reason for writing this book. With the added benefit of the other healing therapies discussed throughout this book, many people have reported that, while continuing to use rife machine therapy as a core treatment, they are able to make further progress toward a complete recovery.

Variables affecting rife machine treatment outcome

There are many variables that influence how successful a Lyme Disease sufferer will be with rife machines. The complicating variables in rife machine therapy include the following factors:

1. There are hundreds of strains of the Lyme Disease bacteria.

2. Some people may have co-infections while other people may not. Some co-infections are more serious than others. Some respond better to rife machine therapy than others.

3. The genetic constitution of a person; for example, their ability to remove Lyme biotoxins from the body.

4. A person's commitment to be disciplined with lifestyle factors that support recovery.

5. Whether a person has concomitant health problems in addition to Lyme Disease that are preventing a full recovery.

6. Whether a person used rife machines long enough to ascertain if they work.

7. The technical and experimental nature of rife machine therapy: Because these machines are not regulated or quality-controlled and there is no standard for treatment details and schedule, there are literally hundreds of variables involved in achieving a successful result, including:

    a. Do you have the right machine?
    b. Is it working properly?
    c. Are you operating it properly?
    d. Are you running the correct frequencies for an acceptable period of time?
    e. Are you doing treatments often enough or too often?

8. Lack of communication between rife machine users. The people who began treatment years ago are hard to track down. Many of them have gone back to the business of life and are not connected to Lyme Disease communities.

9. Whether being symptom free from Lyme Disease means you are cured.

10. Whether or not an individual has indoor mold exposure from homes, schools or offices. According to Dr. James Schaller, 30% of United States structures have indoor mold which produces mold biotoxins. Simply stated, he says, if you can see or smell mold, then you are being exposed to mold biotoxins which are found on the surface of the mold spores. The presence of these toxins greatly reduces the body's ability to fight Lyme Disease.

These variables also apply to many other types of Lyme Disease treatment. An additional variable that affects success with rife machines is misdiagnosis. If someone does not respond to rife machines, it is possible they may not really be suffering from Lyme Disease. Or, Lyme Disease may not be the cause of their primary symptoms. This may seem surprising in light of the fact that Lyme Disease is often under-diagnosed, not over-diagnosed.

But the pendulum is beginning to swing the other way. Many doctors and alternative health care practitioners are using Lyme Disease as a garbage bag diagnosis, slapping the Lyme Disease label on anyone who walks in their office with mysterious and undiagnosed health problems. In this way, someone who does not have Lyme Disease may pick up the diagnosis and go around trying Lyme Disease therapies without much success. The three most accurate predictive indicators that a person will not respond to rife machines are:

1. No herx reaction has ever been experienced in response to any Lyme Disease treatment, including antibiotics.

2. No significant and defined improvement or change in condition has ever been experienced in response to any Lyme Disease treatment.

3. Primary disease symptoms are not consistent with Lyme Disease, and/or symptoms are suggestive of some other health problem.

In the event that one or more of these predictive signs is present, the likelihood of responding to rife machine therapy decreases significantly. In these cases, it would be prudent to reconsider diagnosis or at least allow for the possibility that primary symptoms may be due to something other than Lyme Disease, for example, mercury poisoning or exposure to indoor mold toxins.

This chapter is intended only to be an introduction to rife machine therapy. For more information, including guidelines for selecting a machine, details of planning a rife treatment campaign, and other related discussion, see *Lyme Disease and Rife Machines*.

Updated rife user tips

The vast majority of the information presented in my first book, *Lyme Disease and Rife Machines*, has not changed (to the best of my knowledge) since I published that book. Accordingly, there are no plans for an updated or revised edition. However, there are a few tidbits of new information regarding rife treatment which are presented below.

To fully understand the following information, it is necessary to have a grasp of basic rife machine principles as described in *Lyme Disease and Rife Machines*.

TRAVEL AND RIFE TREATMENTS

When very sick with Lyme Disease, most people do not and cannot travel very much. Road trips, vacations, air travel, and other excursions are often not possible. There are several reasons for this. First, and most obviously, someone will probably just feel too sick. Second, and less well-known, is the propensity for flareups to occur during and after travel. It is quite common for normal Lyme Disease symptoms to become out of control during travel. Lyme Disease organisms are more active during travel because they sense changes in the environment and respond to those changes with bolstered survival activities.

However, as someone begins to feel better, travel is more appealing and becomes possible. But even when feeling better, travel presents some special problems for which several potential solutions are available.

The first problem is that, as mentioned, flareups are more common during travel—even after a person has made significant healing progress. The best way to prevent a flareup during travel is to perform a rife machine treatment the day or night before leaving for a trip. Although this requires dealing with the unpleasantness of a herx reaction on the first day of travel, it is the best solution because it allows for maximum bacterial suppression during the trip, and it pushes the timing of your next treatment as far back as possible. Essentially, doing a rife treatment the night before you leave gives you the best chances of not feeling the need for another treatment during your trip.

The problem is that your travel plans will rarely cooperate with your rife machine treatment schedule, and more likely than not, you will not be due for a rife treatment the night before you leave for your trip.

To solve this problem, plan your trip as far in advance as possible. Then, after you know the dates of your trip, look ahead over your rife machine treatment schedule. If you typically apply a rife machine treatment every seven days, and you notice that you will be due for a treatment right in the middle of your trip, try to adjust your treatment schedule so that you will be due for a treatment the day before the trip instead of in the middle of the trip. This can be done by slightly shortening or lengthening the time which elapses between treatments. For example, by treating every six days instead of every seven days until your trip, you may be able to adjust your schedule such that you are due for a treatment the day before you leave. If you are unable to accomplish this for any reason, you should still do a rife machine treatment the night before your trip even if you are not due for one.

Unfortunately, even when following the above instructions, many people still notice a symptom flareup while traveling. This is because, inevitably, Lyme Disease is more active during travel.

Therefore, having a rife machine available wherever you are going is a helpful measure. This might mean bringing one with you (the GB 4000 + amplifier fits nicely inside a small, carry-on suitcase with room to spare for a couple days worth of clothing and necessities) or having one available to use at your destination. If you travel to the same destination often, you might decide to purchase a machine and keep it there, or locate another Lyme Disease sufferer in that city who will let you use their machine. Having a rife machine available at your destination will be very beneficial and contribute greatly to your peace of mind.

Another way to deal with travel flareups is to bring antibiotics with you to calm a flareup should it happen. You may have to deal with a herx reaction as the result of using antibiotics, but this is often less uncomfortable than the feeling of an uncontrolled flareup. To ensure that herx reactions are as mild as possible, you should only bring an antibiotic that you have previously used—herx reactions to new antibiotics are often much more severe. Additionally, you may wish to bring a non-pharmaceutical antibiotic because these typically have fewer side effects than pharmaceutical antibiotics. You do not want to be caught with diarrhea when traveling.

You may want to take several antibiotic choices in case you have a tough flareup that does not easily respond to antibiotics. For example, you may choose to bring Samento and olive leaf extract. In any case, you should not use the antibiotics unless you actually feel a need for them on the trip. If you do need them, it is possible that a couple doses will take care of the problem—do not feel the need to continue antibiotic use for the remainder of the trip. In comparison with antibiotics, rife treatments are generally preferred when traveling.

Be absolutely sure that the antibiotics you bring on the trip have a relatively short half-life. Zithromax has a half-life of over 68 hours! Using antibiotics with a short half-life (three to 12 hours) has no therapeutic disadvantages but ensures that you have control, and that you will not be stuck with an endless herx reaction on your treasured family vacation. Non-pharmaceutical antibiotics typically have appropriate, short half-lives.

Regardless of which steps you take to prepare for your trip, one strategy that can make your life easier is to plan short trips. Unfortunately for travel-happy people, planning short trips is a reliable way to ensure that the travel experience is pleasant. As a general rule, an acceptable length trip is half the time that normally elapses between your rife machine treatments. So if you normally treat every six days when you are at home, a three-day (three night) trip will probably not be excessively stressful.

Avoid trying new therapies or using treatments you know will cause significant herx/healing reactions prior to a trip. If you want to try a mercury chelation program and you are planning a trip in four weeks, wait until you get back from the trip.

By following these simple guidelines, traveling while recovering from Lyme Disease can be pleasant and feasible. Obviously, everyone is different, and your personal wisdom and circumstances should be considered more accurate than these guidelines.

WHEN TO DO RIFE MACHINE TREATMENTS: MORNING, AFTERNOON, OR EVENING?

One question which is often asked on the Lyme-and-Rife internet discussion group is what time of day rife treatments should be done.

The most important consideration is convenience. Do a rife treatment whenever it best fits into your schedule. One of the advantages of rife machine therapy which makes it an ideal treatment for Lyme Disease is the flexibility inherent in the ability to plan your own treatment schedule.

All things equal, applying a rife machine treatment before bed seems to be the most convenient and practical solution. Many people find that this allows them to sleep through the worst of the herx reaction, and, in addition, rife machine therapy tends to have a relaxing, sleep-inducing effect. Additionally, the treatment can be done while falling asleep with a good book or catching the nighttime news. Some people even leave the machine by their bed and sleep through the treatment. However, if you plan to do this, ensure that you set your alarm and wake up to turn the machine off before sleeping through the night. Rife machine treatments should be less than an hour long. Also, this requires a machine that can be preprogrammed to automatically run through an entire treatment sequence.

Some people may find it more convenient to treat in the morning while reading the paper or a favorite magazine.

The time and place for a rife treatment also depends on the type of machine you have. Some machines are completely hands-free and can be used while checking e-mail, reading a book, or watching TV. If your machine is hands-free, make sure that you do not operate other machinery which could potentially interfere with the treatment, such as a cell phone or microwave, during the rife treatment. Additionally, do not move around while taking a treatment—stay still and sit or stand about a foot away from the machine (certain more powerful machines may require sitting or standing further away from the machine, such as six feet).

Certain machines require hands-on operation which renders it difficult to check e-mail or read a book during the treatment. In these cases, it may be possible to read short excerpts from a magazine article between switching frequencies and changing the machine set up. Doing this will make the treatment a little more friendly and fun.

OVER-TREATMENT: TOO MUCH OF A GOOD THING

Lyme Disease and Rife Machines describes numerous reasons why a person should not over-treat. However, I would like to reinforce the necessity of using a moderate rife treatment schedule and the importance of avoiding over-treatment. I still read stories of people using their rife machine far too often.

First, rife machine therapy is experimental. All potential positive and negative effects are not known. Before you panic because you think I'm telling you that rife machine therapy is dangerous and has side effects, let me say that my opinion on the safety of rife machine therapy has not changed since I wrote *Lyme Disease and Rife Machines*. I have no new information to indicate any negative side effects. However, every medical therapy in existence, including herbs, nutritional supplements, drugs, and surgery, can be overused to the point of harm. Too much of a good thing is always a bad thing. At the time this book was written, it is not known precisely when that point is reached with rife machine therapy. However, it is logical to stay as far away as possible from the point at which rife treatments become excessive and harmful.

The cost/benefit ratio of rife machine technology as a treatment for Lyme Disease is acceptable only when the machines are used moderately and rationally. To use rife machine therapy "rationally" means to use it as little as possible yet still gain the positive results it offers. By reading *Lyme Disease and Rife Machines* you will see that rife machine therapy does not work better the more it is used. Someone who treats every week will not recover faster than someone who treats twice a month. This is a critical point. It is not rational to use rife machine therapy more than it is needed—treating every day is, in all cases, *excessive*. Treating once a week but performing an unnecessarily long treatment session (such as two to four hours) is also *excessive*. Rife treatment should be taken as infrequently as possible without going so long between treatments that symptoms worsen. This rule is only common sense—the same common sense that tells you not to take 8 Advil if 2 will do the job.

Using rife machine therapy rationally can also mean employing other therapies throughout the healing process, thus allowing rife machine treatments to be done less frequently. For example, when pharmaceutical or non-pharmaceutical antibiotics are in use, rife machine treatments are needed less. In the same way, because of rife machine therapy, pharmaceutical and non-pharmaceutical antibiotics are needed less. By this way of thinking, rife machine therapy and antibiotic therapy can be used in conjunction with each other, on a rotation schedule, with breaks in between, such that total use of each therapy is minimized. Optimizing use of any medical therapy to avoid side effects is simply the only course of action that makes sense. In addition, rotating therapies like this also increases antibacterial effect as you hit the elusive and resilient bacteria from different angles. Obviously, you may need to alter or fine-tune these recommendations according to your situation and intuition. Your own observations and experiences far outweigh the value of information found in a book.

It is absolutely critical to avoid over-treatment. This is one of the most important guidelines in a successful rife machine treatment campaign.

EFFECTIVENESS OF VARIOUS MACHINES

Since *Lyme Disease and Rife Machines* was published, the only new information with regard to comparative effectiveness of various machines is that individual responsiveness must be considered. For some people, the EMEM machine may be sufficient to provide complete healing. For others, it may not be enough. The most powerful and helpful machine to date, based on user reports and historical reliability, is still the Coil Machine (AKA the Doug Device or QSC1850HD Machine ["QSC1850HD" is simply the name of the amplifier used in this machine]). Therefore, if someone is using a different machine and results are diminishing, a Coil Machine should be considered. This is an important point to recognize because the full value of rife machine therapy may not be evident until you have used the most helpful machine. If someone concludes that rife machine therapy is not helpful but they have not used the Coil Machine, their conclusion is unfounded.

In all cases, it is beneficial to try as many machines as possible, especially all of the primary four machines described in *Lyme Disease and Rife Machines*. By trying new machines, you will gain a better understanding of how well each machine works, whether you should upgrade your current machine (assuming you have one), and if you should consider using multiple machines in your treatment campaign. Obviously, your financial situation will strongly influence your decisions in this area.

I have made a fairly strong effort to research further the comparative effectiveness of various machines. However, despite quite a bit of energy spent, I have been unable to reach conclusions that are different from those in *Lyme Disease and Rife Machines*. So the bad news is that there is not much new information (at least that I can provide). The good news is that, in my opinion, everything I wrote on this subject in *Lyme Disease and Rife Machines* still applies.

NEW RIFE MACHINE MANUFACTURERS

Some of the machines which *Lyme Disease and Rife Machines* indicated require assembly are now available for sale already built. This is because various companies have noticed increased demand for certain types of rife machines and subsequently have begun producing them. While this is obviously beneficial for people who do not wish to construct their own machines, there are some considerations which must be acknowledged.

First, some companies have begun making machines discussed in *Lyme Disease and Rife Machines*, yet made changes to the machine design. In some cases, these changes may not affect machine function. In other cases, changes may be the brainchild of engineers who think they can improve the design and function of the device. Some of these devices may in fact be better built and may even provide better results. However, in changing the design of a tried-and-true rife machine that has been successfully used by the Lyme Disease community for decades, there is an inherent risk of creating a less helpful, and potentially more dangerous, machine. For this reason, it is recommended that anyone considering purchasing a machine conduct adequate research to insure that the machine they purchase is actually the machine they want. Just because the manufacturer labels it as it is labeled in *Lyme Disease and Rife Machines* does not mean it is actually the same machine. Because there are no wide-scale clinical trials of different machines, it may take decades for new designs to prove themselves through the test of time.

Second, machines produced by companies will be more expensive than the cost of building a machine yourself. This is not necessarily a disadvantage if you have adequate financial resources, but if you do not, you may wish to consider building a machine yourself.

Third, if you purchase a machine from a manufacturer, you will be less independent. If the machine breaks, you will need to rely on the manufacturer to fix it. In some cases, the manufacturer may charge to repair the machine. The manufacturer may, at some point, go out of business. In contrast, if you construct a machine yourself, you will be educated about how it works and prepared to make any repairs necessary. For those who want to be independent in this way, building a machine yourself is a good option.

All things considered, the availability of new, ready-built machines is an advantage to the Lyme Disease community. There will always be the option of building a machine, but many people are simply too sick to build their own machine, so the option to purchase one opens the door for rife machine ownership to many people who would otherwise be excluded. By educating yourself and doing your homework, you can ensure that your dollar is not wasted on unproven equipment.

This book will not provide manufacturer contact information, but you can find this information at www.lymebook.com/resources.

Note: In *Lyme Disease and Rife Machines*, the Coil Machine was said to have some very significant disadvantages due to the fact that it requires assembly and is fairly difficult to operate. Now that the machine is available to purchase pre-built, this has changed: tedious construction is no longer required and some of the newer Coil Machine models are easier to use. For this reason, when you take into account the fact that the Coil Machine is arguably the most helpful rife machine for fighting Lyme Disease, owning and using a coil machine becomes very appealing. If you have been considering upgrading to a Coil Machine, this may be a good time. The primary drawback to purchasing a Coil Machine is the financial cost. At the time this book was written, purchasing a ready-built Coil Machine will cost you about $2500, in contrast to the $1100 or so you would spend building it yourself.

Please note that Bryan Rosner does not endorse any machine manufacturer. This book and Bryan Rosner make no medical claims about health benefits of rife machines. Consult a physician before using any new treatment.

Part II:

The 5 Supportive Supplements

Introduction to the five supportive supplements

S upplements play an important role in treating chronic Lyme Disease. However, although extremely beneficial, the breakthrough supplements discussed on the following pages are not sufficient to be core therapies in the treatment of Lyme Disease. Instead, the protocols discussed in Part I should be used as the core of a Lyme Disease treatment protocol, and the supplements presented hereafter should be employed in support of those core protocols.

With that caveat, let's move on to examine how the 5 supportive supplements were chosen. Thousands of supplement products line the walls of health food stores and the selection is growing with each passing year. Supplements are a business just like any other business. Hyperbolic marketing tactics and flashy labels compete for your attention and ultimately, your dollar. The upside to the recent explosion in the alternative health field is that every supplement you need is available. The downside is that every supplement you don't need is also available. The challenge is to tell the difference.

There are some pretty good reasons to be very selective about which supplements you take and which you avoid. The first reason, and one that applies to most people, is financial cost. The second reason is inconvenience—taking lots of different supplements results in a difficult routine to comply with and often leads to frustration and abandonment of the program. Dr. James Schaller refers to this phenomenon as "pill fatigue."

But even if you have all the money and time in the world, supplements should still be chosen carefully. All supplements take a toll on the body. Even the mildest of supplements contain potent substances which require energy to process and which also place stress on the eliminatory organs such as the liver and kidneys. Because these organs are already burdened due to chronic inflammation and toxin removal responsibilities created by Lyme Disease, it is necessary to avoid superfluous supplementation. In addition, most supplements have preservative ingredients, gelatin (or other types of) coating, or bonding material to hold the pill together. All three of these are undesirable ingredients and potentially harmful.

Another reason to avoid excessive supplementation is that the human body is simply not designed to process concentrated, supplemental forms of nutrients. Eating a balanced diet is the best way to get nutrients. Supplements should not be used as a substitution for a healthy diet by people too undisciplined to eat right.

So, when is supplementation appropriate? The decision to consume nutrients in supplement form should be made based on the following criteria.

The first criterion upon which to base supplement selection is necessity. There should be a clear need for whatever it is you are considering taking. You should know exactly what the supplement does and why your body isn't already accomplishing that function on its own. It should be clear that the nutrient in question is not attainable in the necessary quantities in a healthy diet. You should not take new, faddish supplements just because someone said they help Lyme Disease. For example, coenzyme Q10 (recommended in Chapter 9) is necessary because it has been proven that this nutrient not only plays an extremely important role in normal body functions but is also found to be deficient in most Lyme Disease sufferers. Additionally, the amount of coenzyme Q10 necessary to restore this deficiency is not readily available in a healthy diet. Therefore, supplementing with coenzyme Q10 is a justified decision.

Second, supplements should address the root cause of issues in the body, not cover symptoms. Systemic enzyme supplements, which are recommended in this book, are natural, nutritious, and provide the immune system with important support that helps strengthen and direct immune activities. Additionally, systemic enzyme supplements naturally reduce inflammation by actually eliminating the cause of inflammation (as you will read). In contrast, steroidal anti-inflammatory drugs, which also eliminate inflammation, do not strengthen the immune system but instead weaken it and mask symptoms. Both systemic enzyme supplements and steroidal anti-inflammatory drugs can have a similar effect on *how you feel*—they make you feel better. However, steroids cause serious damage to the healing process and should not be used, while systemic enzyme supplementation actually supports the healing process.

As an aside, it should be noted that non-steroidal anti-inflammatory drugs (NSAIDS) such as Ibuprofen are permissible for use on a limited basis to alleviate inflammation—particularly the severe instances of inflammation such as a bad headache resulting from a herx reaction.

Third and not least of the criteria for selecting supplements is individual tolerance. The fact is that we are all different and so are our bodies. One Lyme Disease sufferer's medicine is another's poison. Everyone with Lyme Disease has in common an out-of-control bacterial infection, and not much else. Your individual response to a given supplement should be the final factor that determines whether or not you use it. Do not let a "one-size-fits-all" recipe determine your treatment program. Doctors or practitioners who ignore your knowledge of your body and intuition should not be trusted. Your knowledge of your body and your intuition are not just important during the healing process, they are actually your most valuable assets. You should guard and grow these assets as much as possible.

Healing and cleansing reactions are normal when taking a new supplement, however, not all reactions fall in this category. Some reactions can simply be the body rejecting a given supplement. Only you live in your body so only you can tell the difference. Learning to tell the difference can take a long time, but eventually, you will learn. Supplements that cause non-beneficial adverse reactions should not be used, regardless of who recommended the supplement and how great they said it is.

Because Lyme Disease is a bacterial infection, supplements which have antibacterial activity are permissible for use. For example, mangosteen supplementation (recommended in Chapter 7) was chosen for its antibacterial activity. However, antibacterial supplements should be used in moderation, according to the same guidelines set forth for pharmaceutical antibiotic use presented in Chapter 1.

Somewhat controversial is the subject of how long a given supplement should be used. Some researchers believe that nutrient-based supplements such as coenzyme Q10 should be taken indefinitely. Other researchers believe that there comes a point of diminishing returns when benefit does not outweigh financial and other costs. Generally, I subscribe to the latter position and believe that most supplements should be used for a while to bring nutrient levels up out of deficiency, and then the supplement can be discontinued. It should probably be used again periodically as long as the infection remains to cause the deficiency. As mentioned, antibacterial supplements should also be taken only intermittently, as explained in Chapter 1.

Obviously, this book does not contain a complete list of beneficial supplements. You should consult your physician and also stay up to date with current Lyme Disease research to ensure that your supplement regimen is optimized. The above criteria should help you evaluate other supplements not included in this book to determine whether or not they should be added to your protocol. Additionally, *Lyme Disease and Rife Machines* describes several supplements not included in this book that are critical to successfully treating Lyme Disease. If in doubt when considering a new supplement, as long as the supplement is relatively affordable and non-toxic, just try it. If it helps you, use it for a while until it stops helping, discontinue it, and then consider using it again periodically.

You should only add one new supplement at a time to your treatment program. It is essential that you are able to recognize and analyze your response to a new supplement so that you can determine whether it is harmful or beneficial. This is only possible when you add supplements one at a time.

When purchasing supplements, consider price-checking online at www.iherb.com and www.vitacost.com, where you'll often find that prices are half those found in health food stores. With the interconnectedness that the internet provides, it is becoming more and more difficult for retailers to charge full retail price for supplements. You should be able to find good deals on most supplements from various internet sources.

Chapter 6:
Systemic Enzymes

Introduction

Systemic enzyme supplementation is one of those little-known yet highly effective natural remedies for a very common health problem involved in a myriad of disease or trauma conditions: inflammation. Dozens of ailments involve inflammation, and, consequently, systemic enzymes have application in a wide variety of illnesses. Lyme Disease is one such illness. Usually managed by pharmaceutical interventions, inflammation is a defining feature of the Lyme Disease complex and is responsible for many of the symptoms and disease processes which occur during the course of the infection.

But the benefit of systemic enzymes does not stop with inflammation. These enzymes have application to a wide variety of pathological conditions because they are capable of producing multiple physiological effects in the body. According to studies indexed by the U.S. National Library of Medicine, systemic enzyme supplementation has been proven beneficial in immune system disorders, digestion, energy production, prostate problems, bronchitis, physical trauma, wound healing, excessively thick blood, heart disease, liver disorders, and detoxification. Of particular note is the benefit systemic enzyme supplementation offers in the treatment of cancer. According to a study conducted in the Ukraine, systemic enzymes are capable of not only attacking cancer tumors but also protecting the patient from the adverse effects of radiation therapy by preventing fibrous changes in the lungs, skin, fatty tissue, soft tissue, liver, and kidneys during therapy.

You can read the studies for yourself by visiting the U.S. National Library of Medicine at www.ncbi.nlm.nih.gov/entrez. As of October, 2006, a search for "Wobenzym" (the brand of systemic enzymes recommended in this book) brings up 49 relevant published scientific studies.

Although some of these studies were done in the United States, most of them were conducted by researchers in countries outside of the U.S. such as Germany, Russia, Spain, Ukraine, and the Czech Republic. Unfortunately, as is often the case with low-cost, natural remedies, the countries most interested in studying them typically have pressing needs for affordable, practical healthcare solutions and do not have the time or resources to chase after complicated patents and synthetic pharmaceutical concoctions. For this reason, countries other than the United States are often the best sources for reliable data gathered by professionally trained scientists on natural remedies.

What is an enzyme?

Enzymes are proteins that catalyze (speed up) chemical reactions. Produced in the body and present in all foods, enzymes are an essential part of human physiology and health. There are hundreds of different kinds of enzymes, each with a different purpose. Some enzymes rearrange molecules, others synthesize chemicals, and yet others break down compounds. Life would not be possible without enzymes to facilitate the thousands of chemical reactions that sustain life. Our discussion will focus on proteases, a specific category of enzyme that breaks down proteins. Protease enzymes are also known as proteolytic enzymes. "Protease" and "proteolytic" mean "protein-digesting."

United States Versus Foreign Research: A Global Perspective

One of the biggest problems with systemic enzyme therapy (as well as with most alternative healthcare) is that most people in the United States will never hear about it. Regardless of its effectiveness, this therapy is not considered a valid treatment option in the United States. The properties which make systemic enzyme supplementation valuable and effective are the same properties that make it an unappealing research option in the United States: affordability, non-patentable ingredients, and poor profit potential.

The United States' focus on profit-producing health care products stands in stark contrast to the preference by many other countries for natural, affordable remedies. This is evident when one compares accepted Lyme Disease treatments in the U.S. to those commonly utilized abroad. In the United States, doctors almost exclusively recommend synthetic, patented pharmaceutical antibiotics to Lyme Disease patients. In much of Europe, Africa, and other parts of the world, where resources are scarce, doctors simply choose the treatments that work, without giving consideration to profit potential. In some cases, pharmaceutical drugs are still chosen. However, in many cases, especially when antibiotics fail, natural, non-toxic, affordable alternatives are applied. Examples of such Lyme Disease treatments include rife machine therapy (which has been officially approved for medical use in Europe and Canada for certain disorders), sauna therapy (which is readily recommended by mainstream hospital physicians in Italy), ozone therapy, homeopathy, herbs, acupuncture, and other similar therapies.

A comparable pattern can be seen when looking at treatments for many types of diseases other than Lyme. Cancer, for example, is treated in the United States by use of expensive, patented, and very toxic pharmaceuticals. In other countries, alternatives are often used—much of the time with a higher success rate and far fewer adverse side effects.

Not only is there a lack of information and excitement about affordable, natural remedies in the United States, there is also unabashed persecution of them. In fact, while those who control the regulatory infrastructure in the United States will not directly admit it, guidelines for studying and approving new medications and therapies are highly biased and hostile with regard to new treatments that would not fare well in a commercial environment. *(continued)*

Why are enzyme supplements needed?

Why can't we get enough enzymes from our food and/or from our body's native manufacturing processes? There are several answers to these questions:

(continued) How does this information impact Lyme sufferers? The fact that quality Lyme Disease research and treatments are often heavily weighted to foreign countries means that Lyme Disease sufferers relying solely on U.S. research will not have full access to the broad range of resources that are actually available. Residents of the United States are continuously bombarded by and directed toward overused and understudied pharmaceuticals. Natural, affordable, non-toxic alternatives are overshadowed by the monstrous commercial business of, and hyperbolic marketing campaigns for, synthetic drugs.

If you want access to the best information and treatment options, you must expand your research horizons to include other countries. Doing just that is one of the focuses of this book—some of the most effective treatments that this book brings to light are popular and commonplace in foreign countries but obscure or unknown in the United States. To this end, treatments discussed in this book represent a cross-section of therapies from numerous parts of the world, not just the United States. Systemic enzyme supplementation is one example. In the U.S. systemic enzyme supplementation is often described as mere "unsubstantiated, unstudied alternative therapy." In Germany it is mainstream—systemic enzyme formulations sell almost as well as aspirin.

Pharmaceutical antibiotics are a valuable tool in treating Lyme Disease (see Chapter 1). They should not be tossed out. Instead, they should be used moderately and systematically alongside other valid approaches found around the globe. A global perspective will allow you to make educated Lyme Disease treatment decisions based on full knowledge of your options.

1. Although some enzymes are manufactured by the body, we also need enzymes which are acquired exclusively as a part of our diet. This source can be lacking because cooking and processing of foods destroy enzyme content. Because processed foods are the primary component of our diets, we do not consume an adequate quantity of enzymes in order to stay healthy. Further, even if we did attempt to consume a completely raw, unprocessed diet, it would still be difficult to get adequate enzyme intake because many beneficial enzymes are found in high quantities only in raw meat, which can be dangerous and undesirable to consume. Enzyme supplementation can compensate for inadequacies in our diet.

2. Individuals suffering from an illness or disease require even more enzymes than do healthy people. To facilitate healing, the body requires considerably more available enzymes than are necessary

when it is not battling disease. Taking enzyme supplements can have a great impact on the speed and success of the healing process.

3. Due to the very nature of the infection, those who are afflicted with Lyme Disease have a greater need for enzyme supplementation, making it all the more difficult to consume or synthesize sufficient quantities. As you will read, enzyme supplementation has many disease-specific benefits for Lyme Disease sufferers.

Systemic enzyme supplementation vs. digestive enzyme supplementation

There are two ways to supplement enzymes. The first use for enzyme supplementation, and the one which is most popular and well-known, is to aid digestion. The pancreas itself secretes digestive enzymes which break down the three categories of food (proteins, carbohydrates, fats), but people with digestive difficulties often notice great improvement when they take enzyme supplements along with a meal. When taken with food, supplemental enzymes join forces with pancreatic enzymes to ensure that food is digested completely. Undigested food (which can occur due to a weak pancreas) causes bloating, constipation, diarrhea, gas, malabsorption of nutrients, food allergies, and other digestive ailments. Supplemental enzymes can completely eliminate these problems. Digestive enzyme supplement formulations often include more than just proteases (enzymes that break down proteins)—enzymes that break down carbohydrates and fats are also typically included. One of the best supplemental enzyme products designed to aid digestion is ParaZyme which is manufactured by RenewLife (www.renewlife.com).

Although taking supplemental enzymes to aid digestive processes can be beneficial in Lyme Disease and other conditions, it is not the focus of this chapter. In this chapter, we turn our attention to another kind of enzyme supplementation.

The second and less well-known use for supplemental enzymes is not to consume them at mealtimes, for the purpose of aiding digestion, but instead to allow them to be systemically absorbed and circulate throughout the body via the bloodstream. To accomplish this, enzyme supplements must be taken not with food but instead between meals on an empty stomach. Enzyme supplement tablets or capsules used for this purpose must have an enteric coating, which is a protective layer placed on the product during manufacturing that prevents the supplement from being broken down by stomach acid. Enteric coated supplements, when taken on an empty stomach, pass through the damaging acids found in the stomach and move safely into the small intestine where they are absorbed into general circulation. Protease (protein digesting) enzymes are the preferred type of enzyme for use in systemic enzyme supplementation.

The procedure of taking enteric coated protease enzymes on an empty stomach is known as "systemic enzyme supplementation," this chapter's topic. As we have said, although not widely known in the United States, systemic enzyme supplementation is a mainstream treatment modality in many other countries, including, for example, Germany. In fact, enteric-coated Wobenzym, the most reliable and well-known systemic enzyme product (and the one recommended in this book), is made in Germany.

Before looking at the specific benefits of systemic enzyme supplementation in Lyme Disease, it is necessary to note that there is controversy surrounding the ability of enzymes to be absorbed intact, enter circulation, and have systemic effect. Conventional belief is that enzyme supplements are broken down in the digestive tract and cannot enter circulation (even if they make it past the stomach via protection by an enteric coating). However, again, we must turn to research conducted outside of the United States to clarify the issue. A study conducted in the Czech Republic indicates that enzyme supplements are in fact absorbed and do have systemic effect. Here is an excerpt from the study:

> "Systemic enzyme therapy represents a special therapeutic approach consisting in the oral application of high doses of hydrolytic animal and plant enzyme combinations. This originally empirical method was, by detailed experimental analyses and successful clinical studies, transformed into a widely appreciated therapeutic method for

various pathologic processes. In spite of this fact, systemic enzyme therapy has been repeatedly questioned by referring to an almost hundred year old dogma claiming the unabsorbality of enzymes in the macromolecular form. The authors present arguments denying the unexceptional validity of this dogma. The histological, radiological, biochemical (chromatographical, enzymological), immunological and biological methods have convincingly proven that a part of swallowed enzymes may pass the intestinal barrier in an undamaged macromolecular form and realize their activities in the body. The most important elements able to absorb macromolecules seem to be so called "M-cells" (FAE) which cover lymphoid foci of the organized gut lymphoid tissue. Other mechanisms of enzyme resorption are under discussion. The absorbed enzymes are rapidly complexed with naturally occurring blood antiproteases. In these complexes the potential immunogenicity of enzymes is restricted and they are concentrated into pathologically affected areas of the body. Complexes in addition display important immunoregulatory activities."

Another study, conducted by the Institute for the Care of Mother and Child in Praha, Czech Republic, concludes that:

"Systemic enzyme therapy (SET) represents a specific therapeutic approach consisting in peroral application of blends of animal and plant hydrolytic enzymes. A significant part of the swallowed enzymes (about 25%) is resorbed in the intestine in functionally active form. After being complexed with natural antiproteases, enzymes are concentrated in wounds, inflammation sites and immunopathological foci. SET has many important indications in traumatologic, thrombotic, infectious, inflammatory, immunopathologic and even tumorous processes. Rheumatoid arthritis, Bechterew's disease, activated arthrosis and extraarticular rheumatism represent important and sensitive targets of SET. In situ and in vivo studies continue to elucidate selective interferences of absorbed proteolytic enzymes with the crucial pathogenic mechanisms of rheumatoid processes."

It is important to pause for a minute and consider just how ground-breaking these studies are. If the United States integrated the truths discovered in the above studies into conventional medical practices, people with a wide spectrum of diseases would be given a new, very powerful weapon to add to their medicinal toolboxes. Basically, what these studies report is that protease enzymes, after being absorbed from the small intestine, complex (attach to; combine) with blood and are transported to disease-ridden sites throughout the body where they exert their effects. This is groundbreaking research yet it is largely ignored in Western medicine. Let's now examine exactly what the effects of this therapy are with specific focus on pathology found in Lyme Disease.

Systemic enzymes in the treatment of chronic Lyme Disease

INFLAMMATION

One of the primary benefits of systemic enzymes, as alluded to earlier, is their anti-inflammatory properties. Unlike both steroidal and non-steroidal anti-inflammatory drugs (NSAIDs), systemic enzymes fight inflammation by actually eliminating its cause instead of suppressing or masking symptoms.

To understand how this occurs, it is necessary to define what inflammation is. Inflammation is a response of the immune system to the presence in the body of a foreign substance (e.g., a bacterium, virus, allergen, or another type of extraneous particle). In cases of infectious disease (such as Lyme Disease), inflammation is caused by circulating immune complexes (CICs), which are residual protein clumps left over after a battle between the immune system and Lyme Disease bacteria.

CICs are primarily composed of a coupling of one antibody and one antigen. Antibodies are immune system cells produced by the human body and sent into the bloodstream to attack and destroy invaders. Antigens are proteins located on allergens and microorganisms that alert the immune system to the presence of the foreign substance. Long after the battle has taken place between the immune system and the invader, antibody-antigen pairs can remain in circulation throughout the body, as a byproduct of immune system activity. Essentially, a CIC is a piece of debris, or toxin, that should be removed by the body's detoxification system but sometimes ends up floating around and getting caught up in various tissues.

This CIC, if it remains in the body, will continue to elicit superfluous immune system response (inflammation) even if the offending invader has long since been eradicated. In the case of Lyme Disease, the constant battle between bacteria and the immune system means that a multitude of CICs are being produced at all times. Some of these CICs are successfully removed via the body's detoxification processes. However, a significant quantity of circulating immune complexes end up bouncing around the body and getting caught up in joints and other places. This results in ongoing inflammation and immune system activation, to the point of hyper-immune activity, beyond that which is productive for fighting infection. Lyme-related arthritis is an example of a condition caused by the presence of CICs. It is hypothesized by researchers that other, non-Lyme cases of arthritis (and other types of inflammation, for that matter) are also caused by circulating immune complexes. Hyper-inflammation caused by the presence of CICs is a major contributing factor to many types of chronic, debilitating diseases.

Anti-inflammatory drugs, both steroidal and NSAIDs, do absolutely nothing to remove or pacify CICs. Instead, they simply inhibit the body's inflammatory response to them. There are several problems with this approach. First, many common anti-inflammatory drugs indiscriminately turn off all types of immune system functionality, not just hyper-immune activity. This can have a crippling effect on the entire immune system. Second, because the root cause of the problem is not being addressed, anti-inflammatory drugs have only temporary effect. As soon as the anti-inflammatory chemical leaves the bloodstream, inflammation returns. This leads to a dependence on the drugs. Third, anti-inflammatory drugs typically have dangerous side effects. Steroids are the worst offenders, with a multitude of serious and life-threatening side effects. In Lyme Disease, steroids can cripple the immune system to the extent that the infection may get out of control and cause permanent damage. The problems caused by non-steroidal drugs are less severe but are still somewhat dangerous. Ibuprofen, the active ingredient in Advil, is known to cause stomach and esophagus damage if used long enough. In any case, both steroidal and non-steroidal anti-inflammatory drugs are a less-than-perfect solution to the problem of CIC-caused inflammation.

Although less toxic, herbs with anti-inflammatory properties share some of the same disadvantages as anti-inflammatory drugs. Typically, anti-inflammatory herbs do nothing to actually remove the cause of inflammation; instead, they simply block the inflammatory process. For this reason, while herbs are often better than drugs, they are not an ideal solution.

Enter systemic enzyme supplementation, which is a better remedy than both herbs and drugs. This therapy offers solutions to each of the problems encountered when using anti-inflammatory herbs and drugs. First, systemic enzyme supplementation does not indiscriminately turn off the inflammatory immune response, but instead it goes right to the root of the problem and actually digests and destroys circulating CICs. Remember, this chapter focuses on proteases, enzymes which break down proteins. Circulating immune complexes are comprised of proteins. Relief from inflammatory symptoms gained by systemic enzyme supplementation is a result of eliminating the actual problem instead of covering symptoms—the CIC itself is broken down and obliterated. Second, systemic enzyme supplementation leads to lasting symptom relief, not mere temporary improvement, because the cause of inflammation is being removed—not superficially masked. After systemic enzyme supplementation is discontinued, symptom improvement persists. And third, systemic enzyme supplementation is not associated with any adverse side effects. In fact, the ancillary effects of systemic enzyme supplementation are highly beneficial to Lyme Disease sufferers, as we will see.

Scientific evidence supporting the benefits of systemic enzyme supplementation in inflammation is well established. A 6-month study conducted by Sanford Roth, M.D., medical director of The Arizona Research and Education Center and past president of the American Society of Clinical Rheumatology and the International Society for Rheumatic Therapy, concluded that systemic oral enzymes effectively normalize the inflammatory response to ease joint discomfort. Roth stated that "systemic oral enzyme supplementation was found to be as effective as Voltaren, a commonly prescribed medication, yet without any significant side effects." Additionally, according to the book *Maximizing the Arthritis Cure* by Jason Theodosakis, M.D. (St. Martin's Press, 1998), "the best news about oral enzymes is their long history of use and the quality of clinical data gathered... enzyme preparations have been shown to be as effective as anti-inflammatory drugs, such as NSAIDs, in treating many different conditions, including arthritis."

Circulating immune complexes (CICs) are responsible for many health problems in addition to inflammation. These include, among others, food allergies, autoimmunity, respiratory problems, cancer, and kidney damage. Systemic enzymes are beneficial to at least some degree in all of these conditions. Anti-inflammatory drugs have limited or nonexistent benefit.

DETOXIFICATION

The next benefit of systemic enzyme supplementation is its ability to detoxify the blood, from not only CICs but also many other types of debris that can accumulate as a result of chronic disease and poor diet. In Lyme Disease, hyper-coagulation of the blood (thick blood) is a very common problem caused by circulating debris and other blood-related effects of the infection. Hyper-coagulation results in numerous deleterious effects and symptoms including poor circulation and oxygenation, reduced blood flow to the brain and associated psychiatric symptoms, fatigue, muscle soreness, and joint pain and stiffness. These problems are exacerbated by the presence of circulating Lyme Disease neurotoxins which further impede the blood's ability to deliver oxygen and nutrients to cells. Symptoms can be so severe that debilitation results. In fact, a significant portion of Lyme Disease symptoms are not caused by the actual presence of the bacteria itself, but instead by blood-related conditions that prevent nutrients and oxygen from getting into cells and waste from getting out. The brain often experiences the most extreme manifestations of blood toxicity. The brain is a very sensitive, delicate organ, and small disruptions in blood flow and quality can lead to dramatic symptoms.

Systemic enzymes clean the blood and cells of the body. Aftab Ahmed, Ph.D., vice president of research and development and business development for Marilyn Nutraceuticals, and a former associate professor of neurology at Northwestern University Medical School, refers to systemic enzymes as "pairs of molecular scissors that cut and prune." Because a significant portion of debris circulating in the bloodstream consists of protein (with the exception of, for example, toxins like mercury, which is a heavy metal, not a protein), protease enzymes can be very effective in cleaning up the blood. One example of a toxin which systemic enzymes can break down and eliminate is the Lyme Disease neurotoxin. Reducing the quantity of circulating neurotoxins has significant healing and symptom-reducing value.

Systemic enzyme supplementation is so effective in cleansing the blood that persons taking blood-thinning pharmaceutical drugs are often able to discontinue them when they begin supplementing enzymes. If blood-thinning drugs are used concurrently with systemic enzyme supplementation, the blood can become dangerously thin—thus necessitating warnings on labels of systemic enzyme products to that effect.

One particular disease believed to be caused in part by excessively thick, toxic blood is fibromyalgia. Closely resembling Lyme Disease (and in some cases, a manifestation of Lyme Disease), fibromyalgia is characterized by fatigue, extreme muscle soreness, depression, sleep disorders, chemical sensitivities, and flu-like symptoms. Many of the symptoms manifested in fibromyalgia are thought to be caused by a decreased ability for the blood to deliver oxygen and nutrients to muscles and other tissues, as well as a decreased ability for waste products to be removed. Conventional treatment for fibromyalgia (if treatment is given at all—many physicians erroneously believe the condition to be a psychosomatic disease) includes pharmaceutical anti-inflammatory drugs, blood thinners, and even antidepressants. Many fibromyalgia sufferers who are fed up with relying on toxic drug cocktails to gain superficial symptom relief have turned to systemic enzyme supplementation.

One such person is Gloria Gilbere, N.D., D.A.Hom., Ph.D., author of *Invisible Illnesses.* A fibromyalgia sufferer herself, Gloria healed her own invisible illnesses with the help of systemic enzymes. Gloria turned to alternative therapies after being on an anti-inflammatory drug that caused a lesion to form in the lining of her stomach and led to a downward spiral of other health problems. She comments that "we do not need to continue to poison our bodies with high potency painkillers, anti-inflammatory drugs and other unnatural substances when we have something as effective as systemic enzyme supplementation." Hers is not the only story of a fibromyalgia sufferer gaining victory through the use of systemic enzyme supplementation.

HERXHEIMER REACTION REDUCTION

Another benefit of systemic enzyme supplementation related to cleaning the blood is herx reaction amelioration. Systemic enzymes have a twofold effect. Not only do they digest and eliminate neurotoxins, they also digest and eliminate the immune-activating debris (both CICs and dead bacterial fragments) present after bacteria are killed. This twofold benefit has profound symptom-reducing effect during herx reactions. Many people notice an immediate burst of energy and decrease in symptoms when they take systemic enzymes in the midst of a herx reaction. Systemic enzyme supplementation is one of the most effective ways to reduce symptoms of the herx reaction without short-circuiting the immune system.

ANTIBACTERIAL ACTION

The next attribute of systemic enzymes which we will examine is an amazing, albeit controversial, benefit. There is significant evidence that systemic enzymes actually have the ability to directly attack and kill Lyme Disease bacteria itself. Furthermore, some researchers hypothesize that enzymes have not only a damaging effect on spirochetes but also on cell-wall-deficient bacteria and cysts. These hypotheses are based on the fact that microorganism cell walls, cyst encasements, and cell-wall-deficient bacteria themselves are comprised largely of proteins and peptides. Because systemic enzyme formulations consist of proteases which break down protein, it is likely that these enzymes help destroy the bacteria—or at least weaken it such that other antibacterial treatments will have a stronger effect. Protease enzymes would probably work quite well in conjunction with other Lyme Disease treatments that attack the bacteria. For example, once rife machine therapy (or exercise, antibiotics, mangosteen, the immune system, or any other anti-Lyme treatment) weakens and compromises the bacteria, protease enzymes may serve to finish them off.

Admittedly, further research is needed in order to confirm this hypothesis. However, the ability for enzymes to kill bacteria is not just theory. It has been observed in vitro that protease enzymes can lyse (destroy by means of enzymatic reaction) microbial cells. One study in particular, conducted by Dr. von Haunersches Kinderspital, a German scientist, found that enzyme supplementation doubles the rate of phagocytosis (killing of microorganisms) in blood samples infected with candida albicans. In other words, not only does systemic enzyme supplementation have the many benefits we've already examined, it is also potentially a tool for weakening the Lyme Disease complex itself.

The most convincing evidence that systemic enzymes have direct antibacterial activity comes in the form of patient experiences. Many Lyme Disease sufferers have noticed herx reactions which are followed by improvement (similar to that experienced as a result of other, established forms of antibacterial treatment) during systemic enzyme supplementation. Reportedly, this experience can be quite startling in comparison with the experience of using other antibacterial therapies such as antibiotics or rife machines. Because systemic enzymes not only kill bacteria but also digest the resultant toxins and CICs, the effect can be powerful and very beneficial—systemic enzyme supplementation is one of the only known therapies to both kill bacteria and clean up the resulting mess at the same time. This dual effect can actually prevent (or at least minimize) herx reactions. Further confirming the likelihood that systemic enzyme supplementation has antibacterial effects is the observation that rife treatments are needed less frequently when systemic enzyme supplementation is in use.

A note of caution: If systemic enzymes are in fact antibacterial, they should be used sparingly and intermittently, with scheduled breaks between dosing, similar to the manner in which any other pharmaceutical or non-pharmaceutical antibiotic is administered (as described in Chapter 1).

A final word

Before concluding this chapter, let's answer one of the oft-asked questions relating to systemic enzyme supplementation: if systemic enzymes can digest CICs, toxic debris, Lyme Disease neurotoxins, and even possibly bacteria, how do we know they do not also digest healthy human tissue? Human tissue is, after all, made up of protein.

Fortunately, healthy human cells are protected by protease inhibitors, which deactivate proteolytic (protein-digesting) enzymes on contact. In the same way that the digestive enzymes produced in your pancreas will break down your food without breaking down your stomach and intestinal lining, systemic enzymes circulating in the blood will only break down foreign proteins. Lyme Disease bacteria, CICs, and other debris and unwanted substances found in the blood are not protected by protease inhibitors. Systemic enzyme supplementation is only able to break down certain organic substances—namely, those that we do not want in our bodies.

In some cases, systemic enzyme supplementation *will* break down human tissue—although this can actually be beneficial. While healthy human tissue is protected by protease inhibitors, weak or diseased human tissue may become susceptible to the actions of protease enzymes. Denatured or damaged tissue can be broken down and eliminated, while healthy tissue is left unaltered. As weak and damaged tissue is digested by supplemental enzymes, the body will be prompted to produce new, healthy tissue, leading to accelerated healing and regeneration of previously damaged cells. This process is similar to the process by which oxidative therapies (such as ozone) break down weaker tissues and cause new tissues to be synthesized.

A similar analogy can be made with the task of pruning a plant. While appearing harmful, pruning can actually result in the production of new, more vigorous growth. In the same way, systemic enzyme supplementation not only selectively targets foreign substances, bacteria, and unhealthy human tissue for destruction, it also facilitates the process of healing and regeneration which can help the body recover from chronic disease.

Conclusion and product information

Systemic enzyme supplementation is highly beneficial in the treatment of Lyme Disease. The effects of the therapy—reducing inflammation, eliminating circulating immune complexes, prompting tissue repair, killing bacteria, ridding the blood of debris, modulating and regulating the immune system, increasing circulation, and decreasing pain—combine to bring about considerable benefit to the Lyme Disease sufferer. The cumulative, subjective experience of supplementing enzymes is immediate and profound symptom relief on an ongoing daily basis as well as during herx reactions. The cumulative therapeutic effect is reduced bacterial load, detoxification, and accelerated healing. For these reasons, systemic enzyme supplementation earns its place as one of the top 10 treatments for Lyme Disease. Furthermore, benefits extend beyond Lyme Disease—nearly all health conditions, chronic or acute, can be helped by systemic enzyme supplementation.

There are several different retail products designed to be used for systemic enzyme supplementation. Some of these products are of high quality, some are not. The product selected for recommendation in this book is Wobenzym, manufactured in Germany by Mucos Pharma and distributed in the United States by Naturally Vitamins. This particular brand was selected for three reasons:

1. In most instances, Wobenzym is the product examined in the research studies which investigate the effects of systemic enzyme supplementation. A significant amount of research has identified Wobenzym as a high quality, consistently manufactured, reliable systemic enzyme formulation.

2. Wobenzym is also the product of choice of most of the Lyme Disease patients who have used the supplement as part of their treatment plans and have reported subsequent positive results at the time this book was being written.

3. Wobenzym is manufactured in Germany, a country which not only believes in the benefits of systemic enzyme supplementation but also conducts a significant amount of research into its use.

The Wobenzym enzyme formulation is available in either clear-coated or red-coated tablets. The clear-coated tablets are recommended because they do not contain added sugar and dyes. Suitable dosing can vary. Guidelines on the product label are typically appropriate. Some people find that they do best when systemic enzyme supplementation is utilized continuously, while other people prefer to take breaks. Since systemic enzymes most likely behave to some degree as an antibiotic and are thus governed by the same principles that govern antibiotic use (as set forth in Chapter 1), taking breaks during supplementation is probably the most prudent choice.

Wobenzym is widely available at health food stores and internet supplement sites. Lowest prices may be available at www.iherb.com.

Chapter 7: Mangosteen

Multitalented mangosteen: queen of the fruits

The mangosteen (*Garcinia mangostana L.*) is a type of fruit unfamiliar in the United States but highly prized in many other parts of the world. A tropical fruit, it grows in the warm, wet climates of countries like Thailand, Malaysia, Vietnam, the Philippines, Indonesia, Jamaica, and Brazil. The mangosteen tree is believed to have originated in two groups of Southeast Asian islands, the Sunda Islands and the Moluccas. The tree is evergreen, slow-growing, and can attain a height of between 20 and 82 feet. Its flaking outer bark is dark brown to black; the tree's inner bark contains yellow, gummy, bitter latex. The leaves of the mangosteen tree are short-stocked, leathery and thick, glossy on top and yellowish green and dull beneath.

The mangosteen fruit itself (not to be confused with the mango, an entirely different fruit) is round and dark purple, with a very smooth exterior and a diameter of 4 to 7 cm making it about the size of a tangerine. The hard outer shell is 1 to 2 cm thick. Open the shell and you will find a dark purple, staining juice (often used as a dye) as well as four to eight triangular segments of white, juicy, soft flesh. The flesh is slightly acid but sweet and mild in flavor and is widely acclaimed to be not only exquisitely delicious but also possessive of healing attributes. In Asia the fruit is known as "Queen of the Fruits." Part of the mangosteen's rich folk history is the story that Queen Victoria offered a sizable prize to anyone who could bring the renowned fruit to her.

There are a couple reasons why you may never have heard of the mangosteen. First, mangosteen trees are not found in the United States, with the exception of a very small number in Hawaii and Florida. The tree requires ultra-tropical conditions to grow—a single temperature drop below 45°F will instantly kill it. Second, despite the fruit's legendary flavor and medicinal value, unfumigated whole mangosteens are illegal to import into the United States for fear of contamination with the Asian fruit fly, an insect having the potential to severely damage U.S. crops. Although sometimes sold as a canned or frozen product, the fruit is very seldom found fresh in Western countries. Rarely, fresh mangosteen can be found at Asian markets in the United States. Certain forms of the fruit can, however, be imported legally, and these are used to make various nutritional supplements and juices.

Historically, the mangosteen has been used for centuries in Asian countries as a traditional remedy for many health problems. Today, its use continues in developed and undeveloped nations as both a delicacy and a medicine. Only recently has knowledge of the benefits and delicious taste of mangosteen begun to sweep North America. As more Americans learn of this healing food, interest continues to grow, and so do the companies selling mangosteen products.

Consumption of mangosteen fruit as part of a nutritious diet has been found to offer unrivaled benefit in a wide variety of health conditions, from infection and autoimmunity to cancer and excessive inflammation. Of special note is the mangosteen's ability to provide dramatic relief to sufferers of multiple sclerosis. The healing power of the mangosteen comes from its active ingredients, compounds known as xanthones, which are a type of phytochemical. Phytochemicals are non-nutritive substances found in plants (both vegetable and fruit) which by definition are not required for normal functioning of the body but that nonetheless have a beneficial effect on health or play an active role in the prevention or amelioration of disease. There are over a thousand known phytochemicals, and certain of these have been shown to produce beneficial health effects such as enhancement of the immune system, reduction of inflammation, and antibacterial, anti-carcinogenic, and antiviral activity. The xanthones found in the mangosteen are not readily found in other plant sources, which is why the fruit is considered such a valuable medicine.

Published research

The first scientific article on the mangosteen was written in 1697 by Jaques Garcin, from whom the fruit received its botanical name. Since then, researchers in 11 countries have published numerous scientific studies on the medicinal qualities of the mangosteen. These studies primarily focus on the many xanthones found in the fruit, and, in most cases, were conducted not only to determine their effects on the body but also to discover the mechanism of action behind the reputed medical benefits of mangosteen. Below is a sampling of some of the most recent scientific studies on mangosteen fruit.

ANTIBACTERIAL EFFECTS OF MANGOSTEEN

The Osaka Prefectural Institute of Public Health in Osaka, Japan, published results of a study in which alpha-mangostin (a mangosteen xanthone) was tested for antibacterial activity against vancomycin resistant Enterococci (VRE) and methicillin resistant Staphylococcus aureus (MRSA). Both VRE and MRSA are serious infections extremely difficult to treat even with the most advanced antibiotics. Findings indicated that the mangosteen isolate actively inhibited bacterial growth of both pathogens. Additionally, it was shown that synergistic antibacterial effects could be achieved by combining mangosteen with other antibiotics employed against the two infections.

The Department of Microbiology at Prince of Songkla University, Thailand, conducted a similar study on the bacterial inhibitory effects of 10 traditional Thai medicinal plants on hospital isolates of methicillin-resistant Staphylococcus aureus (MRSA). Of the three plants with the strongest antibacterial properties, mangosteen was found to have the lowest minimum inhibitory concentration (MIC) requirement, meaning that it had the most potent inhibitory effect.

Research on xanthone extracts from the pericarp (hull) of Garcinia mangostana and their effects on intracellular bacteria was undertaken by The Department of Clinical Microscopy, Faculty of Associated Medical Sciences, Chiang Mai University in Thailand. The mangosteen extracts were seen to cause bacterial death by stimulating phagocytes. These are cells that ingest (and destroy) microorganisms or other cellular debris, an important initial response of the immune system to infection.

The Department of Microbiology at Mahidol University, Thailand, tested 13 native Thai plants for their ability to inhibit growth of Propionibacterium acnes and Staphylococcus epidermidis, bacteria known to cause acne. Based on the method used (broth dilution), the research found mangosteen to be the most effective of the 13, providing "strong antibacterial action."

A study to determine the antituberculosis potential of prenylated xanthones isolated from the fruit hulls and edible arils of mangosteen was conducted by the Department of Chemistry, Faculty of Science, Srinakharinwirot University, Thailand. Three xanthones (alpha- and beta-mangostins and garcinone B) showed potent inhibitory action against Mycobacterium tuberculosis. This study is highly relevant to Lyme Disease therapy because tuberculosis, like Lyme Disease, is caused by an adaptable and very hearty bacterium which often does not respond adequately to conventional antibiotic therapy.

CANCER TREATMENT AND PREVENTION

The Department of Microbiology, Faculty of Pharmacy, Mahidol University, Thailand, studied the antiproliferative (growth inhibiting), apoptotic (producing cell death), and antioxidative (protecting against damage from oxidaition) effect of crude methanolic extract from the mangosteen's pericarp on human breast cancer (SKBR3) cells. Results indicated that the xanthone extract has a definite inhibitory effect on breast cancer cells. The authors conclude that, based on their investigation, "the methanolic extract from the pericarp of Garcinia mangostana had strong antiproliferation, potent antioxidation and induction of apoptosis." The report states that "this substance can show different activities and has potential for cancer chemoprevention." A related study compared the ethanolic extracts of nine selected Thai medicinal plants for antiproliferative activity against SKBR3 human breast adenocarcinoma cells. Garcinia mangostana demonstrated the most potent activity of the group

The Ohio State University Division of Medicinal Chemistry and Pharmacognosy, College of Pharmacy, Columbus, Ohio, examined in detail Garcinia mangostana L. "as part of ongoing research on cancer chemopreventive agents from botanical dietary supplements." The researchers looked at 16 known xanthones of the mangosteen and two new highly oxygenated prenylated xanthones which were identified as part of the study. Several of the compounds showed potent antioxidant activities. Particularly effective was alpha-mangostin, which inhibited preneoplastic lesions in a mouse mammary organ culture assay.

The Medical Research and Education Department of the Veterans General Hospital in Taipei, R.O.C., compared the cytotoxic effects of six xanthone compounds from the hulls of mangosteen to several commonly used chemotherapeutic agents in order to determine their potency against hepatocellular (liver) and other carcinomas. The results showed that one of the xanthone derivatives (garcinone E) "has potent cytotoxic effect on all HCC cell lines as well as on the other gastric and lung cancer cell lines included in the study." The researchers "suggest that garcinone E may be potentially useful for the treatment of certain types of cancer."

The Department of Chemistry, Faculty of Science, Srinakharinwirot University, Thailand, in research involving three human cancer cell lines, (mouth, breast, and small cell lung cancer), isolated three new prenylated xanthones and studied them along with 16 known xanthones from mangosteen. Cytotoxic activity was observed against all three malignancies, with alpha-mangostin exhibiting the most potent effect on the breast cancer cells, "an activity greater than the standard drug ellipticine."

In a study which examined the effects of mangosteen components on human leukemia cells, the Gifu International Institute of Biotechnology, Gifu, Japan, discovered that six xanthones found in mangosteen fruit had varying degrees of cell growth inhibitory effects. Alpha-mangostin had complete inhibitory effect on the leukemia cells through induction of apoptosis. A related study showed that mangosteen xanthones cause leukemia cell death by targeting cell mitochondria. The authors state "that alpha-mangostin and its analogs would be candidates for preventive and therapeutic application for cancer treatment."

Another research study from the Gifu Institute in Japan investigated the antiproliferative effects of four mangosteen xanthones on human colon cancer cells. Three of the four substances "strongly inhibited cell growth" and evidenced antitumor activity and apoptosis of the cancer cells. The authors state that "these findings provide a relevant basis for the development of xanthones as an agent for cancer prevention and combination therapy with anti-cancer drugs."

The Faculty of Pharmacy, Silpakorn University, in Nakhonpathom, Thailand, investigated the antioxidative and neuroprotective activities of four Garcinia mangostana xanthone extracts. All four showed antioxidative activity, and two (water and ethanol) were potent free-radical scavengers which were found to be protective against neuroblastoma (a type of brain malignancy) cells. The authors conclude that "the water and 50% ethanol extracts from the fruit hull of GM may be potent neuroprotectants."

The Tumor Pathology Division, Faculty of Medicine, University of the Ryukyus, Okinawa, Japan, performed a study to examine whether crude alpha-mangostin has short-term chemopreventive effects on preneoplastic lesions involved in rat colon carcinogenesis. Although not performed on humans, this study has wider applicability than in vitro studies because it was performed on living animals (rats). Dietary administration of crude alpha-mangostin at various doses was found to inhibit cancer formation and proliferation in the rat colon. The authors of the study go on to conclude, "this finding that crude alpha-mangostin has potent chemopreventive effects in our short-term colon carcinogenesis bioassay system suggests that longer exposure might result in suppression of tumor development."

ANTI-INFLAMMATORY ACTION

The Department of Pharmaceutical Molecular Biology, Graduate School of Pharmaceutical Sciences, Tohoku University, Japan, examined the effects of the gamma-mangostin xanthone purified from the fruit hull of the medicinal plant Garcinia mangostana on various markers of inflammation in rat cells. After noting that the "fruit hull of mangosteen, Garcinia mangostgana L., has been used for many years as a medicine for treatment of skin infection, wounds, and diarrhea," the authors described their results: gamma-mangostin showed "potent inhibitory activity" on cell function and, in particular, on cyclooxgenase (COX), an enzyme responsible for the production of chemical messengers that cause inflammation. Gamma-mangostin "competitively inhibited the activities of both COX-1 and COX-2." The authors note that "this study is a first demonstration that gamma-mangostin, a xanthone derivative, directly inhibits COX activity."

The same graduate institution conducted a follow-up study which demonstrated the anti-inflammatory effect of gamma-mangostin by inhibiting the expression of COX-2, "without affecting the cell viability." The results were derived from several different in vitro experiments as well as an in vivo investigation of the xanthone's inhibitory action on rat paw edema. The results suggest that gamma-mangostin directly prevents COX-2 gene transcription, decreases the inflammatory production in vivo, and "is a new useful lead compound for anti-inflammatory drug development."

A third study by the above named research school conducted a survey of natural compounds (phytochemicals) to identify possible inhibitory actions on several inflammatory responses. The researchers found that another mangosteen xanthone, garcinone B, had potent inhibitory effects, and they concluded that their "results suggest that garcinone B becomes a unique pharmacological tool to investigate intracellular signaling pathways involved in inflammation."

Several studies have investigated possible effects of mangosteen xanthones against histamine receptors. Histamine is a protein involved in many allergic reactions and can cause inflammation directly by increasing permeability of blood vessels or indirectly by causing constriction of smooth muscle tissue. The Department of Pharmaceutical Biology at Tohoku University, Sendai, Japan, demonstrated alpha-mangostin's inhibition of histamine-induced smooth muscle contractions and noted their results suggest that "alpha-mangostin is a novel competitive histamine H1 receptor antagonist in smooth muscle cells." The study also identifies alpha- and gamma-mangostin as "a histaminergic and a serotonergic receptor blocking agent, respectively."

Mangosteen and Lyme Disease

The above summaries describe only a few of the recent medical research projects designed to identify and explore the medicinal attributes of mangosteen. We have focused our attention on the three most widely applicable categories of mangosteen's health benefits (antibacterial, anticarcinogenic, and anti-inflammatory), but additional and very interesting studies have discovered significant antifungal and antiviral (including anti-HIV) activities in the fruit.

Perhaps the most convincing evidence demonstrating the remarkable healing powers of the mangosteen is not the above published studies, but instead, reports from real people with a plethora of health problems who have experienced tremendous improvement by consuming mangosteen or its supplements. In fact, so many people have had positive results that an internet blog was established to chronicle patient stories: www.mangosteenstories.org.

Many people with Lyme Disease are among those who have received benefit. The mangosteen's antibacterial action is the primary property which benefits Lyme Disease sufferers (however, its other healing effects are not minor and are also applicable in treating Lyme Disease). The antibacterial effectiveness of mangosteen fruit has even been sufficient to completely replace pharmaceutical antibiotics for some Lyme Disease patients. Yes, you read that right—mangosteen fruit is, in some cases, equal in effectiveness to pharmaceutical antibiotics. It should be noted, however, that like any antibiotic, results attained by using mangosteen can diminish over time as the elusive and adaptable Lyme Disease bacteria mutate away from susceptibility to the antibacterial properties of this fruit.

Because mangosteen is a strong antibiotic, Lyme Disease sufferers considering its use should be aware that serious herx reactions can occur. Yes, dangerously powerful herx reactions are possible with the consumption of a simple fruit! Because mangosteen can act as an antibiotic, its use should be governed by the same guidelines that apply to use of other types of antibiotics as described in *Lyme Disease and Rife Machines* and in Chapter 1 of this book.

If you are having a difficult time believing that a simple, unmodified fruit can have healing effects comparable to that of pharmaceutical drugs, you are not alone. It is natural to assume that a common fruit simply cannot wield the medicinal power necessary to make a dent in complicated, debilitating disease processes like Lyme Disease. However, let us remember that many unadulterated fruits and vegetables have very powerful medicinal and biological effects, some even to the point of fatality in humans (i.e., poisonous mushrooms). Consider the powerful (albeit unstudied and unpredictable) mercury chelating effects of cilantro or the liver protective properties of milk thistle, both naturally occurring herbs. Many medical disciplines (including much of Eastern and Chinese medicine) rely completely on herbs, fruits, and vegetables to accomplish healing.

Many modern chemotherapeutic agents are derived from plant sources. For example, Taxol, a first line of attack against breast cancer, is derived form the bark of the yew tree; and Vincristine, compounded from the common periwinkle, is used in treatment of a wide variety of hematological malignancies and solid tumors. Additionally, recall that many pharmaceutical drugs are actually nothing more than synthetic (i.e., easy to patent) copycats of biological substances found in fruits and vegetables. Do not let the modern medical paradigm, built around pharmaceutical drugs, brainwash you into thinking that chemicals are powerful and herbs, fruits, and vegetables are weak. Although not all fruits and vegetables have strong biological effects, some most certainly do, and mangosteen is one example.

The most exciting aspect of using mangosteen to treat Lyme Disease is that this powerful medicine is a food, not a drug. One of the basic principles of commonsense medicine is to use foods whenever possible to heal diseases. While some diseases may be beyond reach of healing with simple foods, Lyme Disease has proven to be susceptible to the healing powers of mangosteen. In the current, conventional Lyme Disease treatment climate, in which doctors use large amounts of highly toxic pharmaceutical antibiotics for extended treatment courses, mangosteen is a much needed departure from the norm. Unlike pharmaceutical antibiotics, mangosteen does not suppress the immune system, cause liver toxicity, or create candida infections in the digestive tract. Actually, instead of causing these conditions, it helps them. And as a bonus, mangosteen tastes great and has numerous other health benefits intrinsic to all fruits and vegetables.

One oft asked question is whether mangosteen can cure Lyme Disease. The answer is, probably not alone. As with all antibiotics, the Lyme Disease bacteria can become resistant to the antibacterial action of mangosteen. For this reason, other antibacterial therapies, such as rife machines and the Marshall Protocol, must be utilized throughout the course of a Lyme Disease treatment campaign.

Although mangosteen itself may not be sufficient to eradicate Lyme Disease, it can play a very important role in the recovery process. Ingestion of mangosteen fruit or products can offer non-toxic antibiotic protection while a person takes much-needed breaks from other antibacterial therapies such as rife machine therapy, the Marshall Protocol, or pharmaceutical antibiotics. A break from these therapies offers the body a rest from toxic drug side effects (in the case of antibiotics and the Marshall Protocol), and electromagnetic fields (in the case of rife machine therapy). Taking breaks from these therapies, while very important, is often not possible because the bacterial infection can creep back when antibacterial therapies are not in use. Mangosteen provides a perfect solution.

Mangosteen use may also prove beneficial during business travel or a vacation, when a rife machine is not available and when it is undesirable to use pharmaceutical antibiotics due to unwanted side effects such as diarrhea.

Rotating between various antibacterial treatments, such as the Marshal protocol, pharmaceutical antibiotics, rife machine therapy, and mangosteen fruit, also offers the benefit of increased overall antibacterial action. When treating the evasive and resistant Lyme Disease infection, one of the principles of a successful treatment campaign is simply that rotating antibacterial therapies prevents the infection from developing resistance and ensures continual bacterial load reduction. You will find emphasis on this rotational theme throughout this book.

Evaluating mangosteen products

Several high-profile talking heads in the healthcare industry have leveled criticism at mangosteen products. Although objective evaluation and criticism of any medical treatment is obviously valuable if it advances the interests of medical science and benefits people with health problems, most criticism directed at mangosteen has been less than objective. According to J. Frederic Templeton, M.D., in an editorial written in October of 2005, the majority of the criticism leveled at the medicinal benefits of mangosteen comes from doctors or researchers who have either not studied the available research on mangosteen or admit to having strong biases against using whole foods or alternative medicine to treat serious disease.

Additionally, negative comments about mangosteen products are often directed more at the marketing structure used to promote the products and less at the quality or value of the products themselves. This is because many companies selling mangosteen products use multilevel marketing strategies. Multilevel marketing has gained a very bad reputation over the last several decades as a result of its use by a few corrupt, unethical companies that have employed this business model to swindle consumers. Understandably, many people are skeptical of products being sold under multilevel marketing umbrellas.

While it is rational to take heed when considering the purchase of anything sold through multilevel marketing businesses, a product should not be judged solely by the business model through which it is marketed. Business models themselves are neither good nor evil; instead, they are simply neutral. Good products can be sold through all kinds of business models, as can bad products.

Instead of judging a product by the business model used to promote it, the following three criteria can be used to evaluate the product. These criteria apply to many types of goods—not just health products—including electronics, sports equipment, restaurants, automobiles, and virtually any consumer product.

1. Independent professional reviews. Many physicians and researchers, as part of their professions, regularly publish independent reviews of health products. These reviews can be useful for ascertaining whether or not the production of a given type of product/brand is based on sound science. Physicians have connections in the world of medicine that allow them to see "behind the scenes." If there is no financial relationship between the product and the reviewer, then independent professional reviews can be trusted to be unbiased and objective.

2. Independent user reviews. Probably the most useful way to evaluate a product is to talk with, or read reviews written by, actual consumers who have purchased the product and used it themselves. This information is where the rubber meets the road. Fancy products with expensive marketing may turn out not to help anyone, while simple, affordable products without flashy packaging may in fact be extremely effective. This strategy of product evaluation is becoming more and more popular on the internet. There are hundreds of free online discussion groups in which thousands of people share their experiences with various products.

3. Third-party scientific literature. Many products have generic ingredients about which scientific studies have been conducted. By reviewing these studies, you can determine whether the ingredients

have side effects, are effective for what you need them for, are fairly priced, etc. Avoid products that do not list ingredients or claim to have a "proprietary blend." The scientific studies presented earlier in this chapter relating to mangosteen's biological effects were all conducted by independent reputable research organizations. The studies examined non-commercial samples of mangosteen, without heed to any particular brand or company.

One of the most useful web sites on the internet is the public access point for Pub Med, also known as MEDLINE. Pub Med, an arm of the National Library of Medicine at the National Institutes of Health, indexes published scientific studies from thousands of affiliated research facilities and organizations throughout the world. When you visit this web site you will have at your fingertips the capability to search by keyword through the majority of major and minor scientific studies conducted every year by universities, hospitals, private medical research groups, and other scientific institutions across the globe. Visit www.ncbi.nlm.nih.gov/entrez to access the website. On this web site you can conduct additional research about mangosteen (Garcinia mangostana) and other health-related products you are considering.

I hope that this discussion has given you some tools to use in evaluating health treatments and products. In relation to mangosteen you will not need to do this homework because I have already done it, but you will no doubt be faced with the need or desire to research many other disease-related topics in the future.

Conclusion and product information

Mangosteen should be considered a very valuable treatment for Lyme Disease and other illnesses involving infections, inflammation, and auto-immune disorders.

Based on independent professional reviews, user reports, and scientific literature, the brand of mangosteen fruit (sold as a bottled juice) in which I have the most confidence is Xango. You can learn more about this product at www.xango.com. Generally, the dosing suggestion on the Xango label is appropriate for use in treating Lyme Disease. However, keep in mind that because mangosteen has antibiotic properties, it should be used carefully and treated as an actual antibiotic. Please refer to the guidelines described in *Lyme Disease and Rife Machines* and in Chapter 1 of this book.

Chapter 8:
Lithium Orotate

Protection for your brain

M ost people know of lithium only as a powerful antipsychotic drug used in treating severe psychiatric disease. Lithium is most familiar to the public as a treatment for afflictions such as bipolar disorder, schizophrenia, and depression. You may, therefore, be shocked to see it listed here as one of ten breakthrough therapies for Lyme Disease.

Believe it or not, lithium is not a drug—it is actually a mineral—belonging to the same family of minerals (the alkali metals) that includes sodium and potassium. In fact, some forms of lithium are sold over-the-counter as nutritional supplements and are recommended by physicians for healthy people without any disorder, mental or otherwise. So, pause for a few minutes, take a deep breath, and get ready to learn the truth about lithium. Leave your preconceived notions at the door as we embark on a journey to explore one of the most misunderstood minerals in existence.

It is true that lithium is sold as a prescription drug product for serious mental illnesses like bipolar disorder and schizophrenia. It is also true that the pharmaceutical version of lithium is associated with potentially severe and damaging side effects. Pharmaceutical lithium drugs are comprised of a potent form of lithium (lithium citrate or lithium carbonate) and are given in extremely high doses. Consequently, these drugs often cause side effects in the form of lithium toxicity, which we will examine in a few pages.

What is less well-known is that there is an over-the-counter type of lithium, known as lithium orotate, which is given in smaller doses and is associated with numerous brain-boosting/protecting effects. Lithium orotate can be given in low but still therapeutic doses without imposing the risks associated with prescription lithium. The properties of drug-form lithium at high doses which are responsible for improving symptoms of severe mental illness are the same properties which are at work in lower doses of over-the-counter lithium. Treatment with lithium orotate can lead to improvement in numerous conditions involving less profound forms of brain dysfunction.

This chapter will first examine the beneficial effects of lithium in both its forms, as a prescription drug and as an over-the-counter nutritional supplement. Then we will look at the very important differences between the two types of lithium. We will show how this information is of value to the Lyme Disease sufferer and describe how lithium therapy might be incorporated into a treatment program.

Lithium and neurotoxicity

Although lithium has other effects on the body, its primary beneficial actions are on the brain. These actions are so numerous that it would require the writing of another book to do justice to this powerful mineral. Lithium is so effective in treating illnesses like obsessive-compulsive disorder, bipolar disorder, schizophrenia, and depression that some researchers have postulated that these conditions are actually caused by a lithium deficiency! Lithium's beneficial effects on the brain are a result of its incredible ability to protect the brain from the damaging effects of numerous types of neurotoxins, including, you guessed it, the Lyme Disease neurotoxin.

The neuroprotective effects of lithium were discovered by researchers who set out to identify the mechanism of action behind lithium's ability to stabilize mood and improve symptoms of mental illnesses. These researchers expected to discover that lithium acts on the parts of the brain which control mood and emotions, in much the same way that antidepressant drugs work, by adjusting this or that neurotransmitter in order to create chemical changes in the brain. To their surprise, lithium had no action at all in these areas. Instead, the mood stabilizing effects of lithium were found to be attributed to an entirely unrelated method of action, namely, shielding the brain from neurotoxins. Researchers found that lithium can protect the brain from dozens of different offensive chemicals and toxins, both synthetic and naturally occurring.

The ramifications of this discovery were groundbreaking and have very important implications in several medical disciplines. First, because we now know that lithium's method of action in helping the brain is to protect it from toxins, and because we also know that lithium is incredibly effective in reducing the symptoms of mental illness, we can conclude that numerous serious mental disorders are actually caused by toxic substances that end up in the brain. This finding validates the medical reality that there is a physiological explanation for many psychiatric disorders (such as schizophrenia, depression and manic-depression, multiple personality disorder, and obsessive compulsive disorder) which have long been disparaged as personality problems or character flaws and are sometimes even blamed on the patient. Many mental illnesses are not in fact bizarre personality variances but instead are the result of poisoning with very common toxins found in nature and industrialized society.

The involvement of toxicity in psychiatric and cognitive problems (as is evidenced by their amelioration with a neuroprotective agent like lithium) makes them just as real as cancer or food poisoning. And in the same way that cancer and food poisoning are no fault of the patient, neither are mental disorders. Lyme Disease patients, much like victims of psychiatric disease, are often blamed for behavioral, emotional, and cognitive problems that are actually a direct result of toxic bacterial byproducts in the brain. Thus, an indirect result of lithium research has been to vindicate Lyme Disease patients by enabling them to defeat age-old stereotypes which lead to demoralization, embarrassment, and feelings of hopelessness.

Unfortunately, the discovery that toxins play a role in mental disease is often wholly ignored by the conventional medical community in favor of less accurate, more drug-friendly models of disease. Nevertheless, as we shall see later in the chapter, the availability of an all-natural, over-the-counter supplement to combat mental dysfunction has the potential to empower patients to stop relying solely on medical practitioners and the pharmaceutical industry and to take back control of their own health.

A second important ramification of the discovery that toxins can cause mental dysfunction has been to enhance the ability of medical practitioners to treat mental illnesses more effectively and safely. Instead of masking symptoms with the over-prescribed, dangerous, and side effect-laden anti-depressant/antipsychotic drugs which are so popular in modern medicine, it is now possible to use natural minerals like lithium to actually treat the root cause of the problem and protect the brain. Moreover, when given as over-the-counter lithium orotate, such treatment will save the patient from the ghastly side effects of brain chemistry-altering drugs.

Lithium and Lyme Disease

How does this information about the benefits of lithium relate to Lyme Disease treatment? Since a significant number of Lyme Disease symptoms result from the brain dysfunction caused by Lyme neurotoxins, lithium can play an important role in protecting the brain and minimizing neurological symptoms during the course of Lyme Disease treatment. For some Lyme sufferers, lithium supplementation can replace pharmaceutical treatments for Lyme-related depression, mental confusion, and behavioral instability. Not only can lithium offer increased effectiveness over many prescription antidepressant, antianxiety, and other psychotropic drugs, lithium can be safer and have far fewer side effects.

Lithium can be more effective than pharmaceutical solutions to the cognitive ill-effects of Lyme Disease because, as we have said, lithium actually protects the brain from the harmful toxins causing the problem instead of rearranging brain chemistry to mask the symptoms of toxic poisoning. So profound are the neuroprotective effects of lithium that numerous Lyme Disease sufferers have noticed huge improvements in mood, memory, motivation, aggressive feelings, and other mental functions, simply by adding a very small amount of lithium to their supplementation regimens.

The negative action of Lyme Disease neurotoxins is not limited to behavioral, emotional, and cognitive problems. Many physical symptoms such as fatigue, headaches, vision problems, spatial orientation issues, and vertigo can also be caused by Lyme Disease neurotoxins. Lithium can reduce and even eliminate these symptoms as well.

Lithium supplementation can work synergistically with the detoxification therapies discussed in Chapter 8. Many detoxification therapies send toxins into circulation before they are eliminated. This can cause increased symptoms of toxin circulation as the liver and kidneys and other detoxification pathways work hard to remove the poisons from the bloodstream. Lithium supplementation during this time can greatly reduce symptoms and protect the brain.

Other benefits of lithium

But the story does not end there. Lithium has many other brain boosting and protecting effects. Jonathon V. Wright, M.D., medical director of The Tahoma Clinic in Renton, Washington, is an expert on lithium supplementation. In a two-part article on lithium entitled "The Misunderstood Mineral," he describes some of the many benefits of lithium supplementation. Dr. Wright recommends lithium supplementation not just for disease conditions but also to healthy people for anti-aging and general brain health. Below are some of Dr. Wright's findings and my comments in *italics*:

1. Lithium prevents brain cell death from reduced blood flow after a stroke. Lithium treated rats experienced 56% less cell death and significantly fewer neurologic deficits than control rats in a study which examined potential for lithium to be used as a treatment for stroke. *It is well-known that Lyme Disease causes decreased blood flow to the*

brain. Therefore, lithium may be beneficial in preventing brain cell death in Lyme Disease.

2. Lithium prevents medication-induced toxic side effects. Scientists use the word "robust" to describe the ability of lithium to prevent neurological side effects during treatment with medications which are known to have a negative impact on the brain. *Flagyl (metronidazole), a very effective antibiotic commonly used in treating Lyme Disease, is known to have nasty neurologic side effects. Other medications commonly used in Lyme Disease also have neurologic side effects. Lithium may render Lyme Disease medications safer and more tolerable.*

3. Researchers have suggested that "the use of lithium as a neurotrophic/neuroprotective agent should be considered in the long term treatment of mood disorders, irrespective of the primary treatment modality being used for the condition." *Lyme Disease is known to cause many mood disorders. Research indicates that lithium would be a helpful treatment to combine with any other treatment a Lyme Disease sufferer is using for management of mood disorders.*

4. Lithium can slow progression of, and improve symptoms of, Alzheimer's disease. Lithium may also prevent latent Alzheimer's disease from manifesting. One of the toxins believed to contribute to Alzheimer's disease is the heavy metal aluminum. Lithium's ability to help Alzheimer's disease may be partially a result of its known ability to protect the brain from the negative effects of aluminum. *Recent research has found a possible correlation between Lyme Disease and Alzheimer's disease. Also, aluminum poisoning is known to worsen Lyme Disease. Because aluminum is very difficult (if not impossible) to remove from the brain, lithium's ability to protect the brain from aluminum toxicity is extremely valuable.*

5. 10 years of data accumulated from 27 Texas counties indicate that the incidence of homicide, rape, burglary, drug use, and suicide, as well as other crimes, were significantly lower in counties whose drinking water supplies contain 70 to 170 µg of lithium per liter in comparison with counties with little or no lithium in their water. Researchers conclude "these results suggest that lithium at low dos-

age levels has a generally beneficial effect on human behavior ... increasing human lithium intakes by supplementation or lithiation of drinking water is suggested as a possible means of crime, suicide, and drug-dependency reduction at the individual and community level." *Lyme Disease is very often associated with numerous types of behavioral disorders, ranging from "Lyme rage" and violence to apathy and suicide. Additionally, the Lyme Disease infection has been implicated in other health conditions which involve behavioral disorders, such as autism, Tourette's syndrome, bipolar disorder, obsessive-compulsive disorder, and others. Therefore, lithium may be invaluable in helping Lyme Disease patients who suffer from behavioral disorders.*

6. Lithium has been found to help break addictions to alcohol (and possibly other substances). One article in the British Journal of Addiction found that "both controlled and uncontrolled experiments show that symptoms of both alcoholism and of affective disturbance are reduced in patients treated with lithium." Additionally, Dr. Wright has found that relatives of alcoholics with alcoholism may benefit from taking lithium even if they themselves do not have problems with alcohol. *Although there is no known correlation between alcoholism and Lyme Disease, people with alcohol dependency who suffer from Lyme Disease may find lithium helpful. Additionally, Lyme Disease sufferers are often addicted to sugar and other counterproductive foods as a result of overly acidic pH and other Lyme-related imbalances. Lithium may be helpful in controlling these problems.*

7. Fibromyalgia patients have noticed some helpful effect from lithium treatment. One study which examined three women suffering from fibromyalgia (none of whom had responded to conventional treatment) found that all three noticed a marked reduction in symptoms after lithium was added to their treatment programs. *It is generally accepted that there is a strong correlation between fibromyalgia and Lyme Disease. In some cases, fibromyalgia may actually be caused by Lyme Disease. Therefore, as an added bonus, those who use lithium supplementation to treat neurological symptoms may notice improvement in muscle soreness, fatigue, and other symptoms of fibromyalgia.*

8. Cluster headaches have been found to yield to lithium treatment. One study examined lithium's effect on 19 men with cluster headaches. Eight men experienced rapid improvement in just two weeks. Four individuals had both cluster headaches and psychiatric symptoms—these four had almost complete elimination of their headaches. *This is just another example of lithium's ability to have a profound effect on a wide range of neurological issues.*

9. Viruses, including herpes simplex, adenovirus, Epstein-Barr virus, cytomegalovirus, and the measles virus were found by one study to have inhibited reproductive capabilities when exposed to lithium. Another study demonstrated a "consistent reduction in the number of herpes episodes per month, the average duration of each episode, the total number of infection days per month, and the maximum symptom severity" during lithium treatment. *People suffering from Lyme Disease are also typically affected by co-infection with other bacteria, viruses, protozoa, and parasites. Use of lithium may help control viral co-infections.*

10. Several peer-reviewed studies have shown that lithium has anti-aging effects on the brain including the ability to increase gray matter, stimulate production of new brain cells, and prevent brain shrinkage (which is known to occur as the human brain ages). For example, a study published in the Lancet by the University of Detroit found that eight of 10 people taking lithium experienced a 3% increase in gray matter after just four weeks of supplementation. *This benefit of lithium is self-evident with regard to Lyme Disease: as the body is desperately fighting off the infection, lithium supplementation will help preserve brain function and integrity. Remember, Lyme Disease is primarily a disease of the central nervous system. So, a treatment that can protect the central nervous system is highly valuable.*

The above-listed benefits of lithium add momentum to the already strong argument that lithium deserves a place in the supplement regimens of most Lyme Disease sufferers. Not only does lithium protect the brain from Lyme Disease neurotoxins, it also has many other properties which can reduce symptoms and preserve brain health throughout the recovery process.

Prescription vs. over-the-counter lithium

Now that we have established the benefits of lithium in treating various disorders, including Lyme Disease, we will move on to explore the differences between prescription lithium and over-the-counter lithium. It is important to clarify these differences because prescription lithium often has serious side effects which the Lyme Disease patient will want to avoid at all costs, while over-the-counter lithium (which is therapeutic at low doses) is nontoxic and much safer.

Lithium itself is a mineral. However, as with most minerals, the right amount can be healing but the wrong amount can be dangerous. Prescription lithium drugs contain lithium carbonate or lithium citrate. At low doses, these forms of lithium are harmless. However, the therapeutic benefit of lithium carbonate and lithium citrate is only realized at extremely high doses which come very close to causing lithium toxicity. This is because lithium carbonate and lithium citrate have very low bioavailability (the fraction of a dose of a particular medication that is actively available to the targeted body area). As such, pharmaceutical lithium is formulated to contain mega-doses of lithium and is therefore reserved for treatment of only the most severe of illnesses.

Ward Dean, M.D., describes this phenomenon in an article he released in July, 1999, entitled "The Unique, Safe Mineral with Multiple Uses." Dean's article explains that lithium carbonate and lithium citrate (the drug forms of lithium) require very high doses to have therapeutic effect because these forms of the mineral are poorly absorbed by the body's cells. Because the therapeutic action of lithium takes place inside the cells, acting on intracellular structures like the mitochondria and lysosomes, high doses of pharmaceutical lithium must be taken in order to obtain satisfactory intracellular concentration. Unfortunately, these doses cause blood levels of lithium to be so high that they border on toxic. Thus, people using prescription lithium must be closely monitored for excessive levels of the drug.

Frequent blood tests are necessary to measure both serum lithium and serum creatinine level in order to guard against toxicity.

The toxic effects of high-dose lithium can include frequent urination, thirst, nausea, hand tremors, and vomiting. Extreme toxicity may involve drowsiness, muscular weakness, poor coordination, ringing in the ears, and blurred vision. Kidney damage is also possible. These side effects are listed on the boxes or inserts of prescription lithium medications. Obviously, prescription lithium is no walk in the park. However, because it is so effective in treating certain mental illnesses, people who are debilitated by these disorders are willing to risk the side effects. With these risks and limitations, lithium drugs are not much use to the Lyme Disease sufferer who is interested in protecting the brain but is not willing to endure toxic side effects.

Enter lithium orotate, the non-prescription form of the mineral. Although somewhat similar to lithium carbonate and lithium citrate, lithium orotate differs because it has a much better bioavailability profile, as well as greater intracellular absorbability. Smaller doses of the over-the-counter, orotate form have the same active benefit as much larger doses of prescription lithium. During recent history, several researchers have pointed to lithium orotate as an alternative to lithium carbonate and lithium citrate which offers substantial therapeutic benefit at much lower, much safer doses.

One of the first researchers to study lithium orotate was Hans Nieper, M.D. Dr. Nieper was born in Germany in 1928 and died in 1998. His premedical studies were conducted at Johann Gutenberg University in Mainz and his initial medical training at the University of Freiburg. He received a medical degree from the University of Hamburg.

Hans Nieper was known for his expertise in applying the advanced principles of physics to medical concepts. One of his most significant achievements involved working with mineral supplements as treatments for disease. He and several colleagues identified a series of "mineral transporters," substances that he believed would increase the bioavailability of minerals in tissues and cells. Among the transporters he used were AEP (2-aminoethylphosphonic acid), aspartic acid, arginine, and orotic acid.

According to Nieper, when these transporters are combined with certain minerals, they form organic mineral salts such as magnesium AEP, magnesium aspartame, magnesium arginate, magnesium orotate, and lithium orotate. Of the transporters Nieper worked with, he preferred the orotates because he believed they produced higher bioavailability than other transporters. Consequently, Nieper postulated that lower doses of mineral orotates would have the same therapeutic effect as higher doses of other forms of minerals.

Nieper's work, which began as abstract theory, eventually gained credibility as clinical results followed. Nieper and other physicians have been clinically successful in treating various conditions with low doses of mineral orotates. These conditions include multiple sclerosis, cancer, calcification of bone, coronary heart disease, alcoholism, mood disorders, liver damage, radiation effects, and others. Success has been achieved in these areas even when other forms of mineral dosing/supplementation have failed.

Dr. Ward Dean, whose above-mentioned article described the risks associated with high dose pharmaceutical lithium, went on in that article ("The Unique, Safe Mineral with Multiple Uses") to contrast these drugs with the lithium salt of orotic acid (lithium orotate). In stark contrast to the drug forms of lithium, Dean explains that lithium orotate improves the therapeutic effects of the mineral many fold by increasing lithium bio-utilization. The orotate component of lithium is highly effective in transporting lithium across cell membranes to the mitochondria, lysosomes, and other intracellular structures, Dean says. Because of its superior bioavailability, therapeutic doses of lithium orotate can be much smaller than therapeutic doses of prescription forms of lithium and thereby offer a nontoxic alternative to these drugs.

For example, severe depression can be treated by only 150 mg per day of lithium orotate. In comparison, the same treatment with lithium carbonate or citrate requires 900 to 1800 mg per day. In referring to a study conducted by Hans Nieper, Dean notes that 150 mg per day of lithium orotate is not associated with adverse effects and that there is no need for monitoring blood lithium levels at this low dose. This conclusion agrees with those of Dr. Wright, who has found it unnecessary to monitor his patients when they take low-dose lithium orotate supplements.

The work of doctors Nieper, Dean, and Wright is confirmed by actual experiences of Lyme Disease sufferers, many of whom have taken lithium orotate at low doses and have noticed great benefit without side effect. In fact, many Lyme Literate Medical Doctors (LLMDs) across the United States and abroad include lithium supplementation in their recommended list of supplements. Experience has simply shown that Lyme Disease sufferers receive great benefit from lithium supplementation.

Conclusion and product information

Although very helpful, lithium supplementation is not antibacterial and is thus not a curative treatment for Lyme Disease. Because Lyme Disease is caused by the presence of a bacterial infection, it cannot be cured unless the bacterial infection is eliminated. However, lithium supplementation can reduce symptoms and protect the brain while other antibacterial therapies (such as rife machines, the Marshall Protocol, or antibiotics) are used to eradicate the infection. Considering that healing from Lyme Disease can require two to four years *even if everything is done just right*, it is extremely helpful to utilize available treatments which make that process more tolerable. Lithium orotate is such a treatment.

Dr. Wright recommends 10 to 20 mg of elemental lithium per day in the form of either lithium orotate or lithium aspartate (lithium orotate is more commonly available and has thus been the focus of this book). In some cases, a lower dose is acceptable in the treatment of Lyme Disease—such as 5 to 10 mg. Lithium supplement products sometimes show on their labels quantities of two types of lithium: lithium orotate and elemental lithium. For example, some products contain 5 mg elemental lithium and 120 mg lithium orotate. In these cases, the number upon which to base dosing is the lower number, the elemental lithium content.

Dozens of brands of lithium orotate supplements are available, so the best course of action is to select a brand name that you trust.

Dr. Wright has been recommending lithium supplementation since the 1970s for brain protection and anti-aging. He explains that when he first recommended lithium to his patients, he was exceptionally cautious and asked them to have regular lithium level blood tests and thyroid function tests. However, after a year or so he stopped asking for lithium blood tests because 100% of them came back at very safe levels. Soon after, he stopped asking for thyroid function tests as well, because he rarely found them necessary. However, the decision about whether or not to undergo testing while using lithium supplementation should be made by you and your trusted physician.

Because lithium is cleared by the kidneys, it may not be safe for people with kidney disorders. Some people with Lyme Disease may have unknown kidney disorders or weak kidneys. In these cases, lithium supplementation may not be appropriate. Consult a physician before using lithium. Lithium should not be used by people with certain types of cardiovascular diseases, severe debilitation, dehydration, or sodium depletion, nor by people who are taking diuretics or ACE inhibitors. Consult your doctor before use if you are taking anti-hypertensive drugs, anti-inflammatory drugs, analgesic drugs, or insulin. Lithium should not be used by pregnant women and breast-feeding mothers. Mineral orotates (including lithium orotate) are not FDA approved, and their clinical use remains officially experimental.

Chapter 9:
Coenzyme Q10

What is Coenzyme Q10?

Coenzyme Q10 is a fat soluble, vitamin-like substance found in small amounts in food and synthesized by the human body. Coenzyme Q10 belongs to a family of substances known as ubiquinones and is produced naturally by the majority of aerobic organisms—including bacteria, plants, and animals. In humans, cholesterol and Coenzyme Q10 share a common synthetic pathway.

Coenzyme Q10 is used by the body as an antioxidant and to produce energy for cells. Electron transport and energy production in the mitochondria are the specific functions of coenzyme Q10. The nutrient is necessary for the production of ATP (adenosine troposphere) which fuels all cellular energy. As an antioxidant, Coenzyme Q10 protects cells from damage by certain oxygenated molecules called free radicals, which are highly unstable and reactive compounds that cause cellular damage by chemical chain reactions leading to mutations or cell death. Though all of our body cells produce coenzyme Q10, a higher concentration is contained in the heart, liver, immune system, and muscle tissue.

Coenzyme Q10 was first isolated from beef heart mitochondria in 1957 by Frederick Crane, Ph.D., who is now at Purdue University. Four years later, in 1961, Peter Mitchell, Ph.D., of the University of Edinburgh, found that the coenzyme functions to produce energy at the cellular level. In 1978, Dr. Mitchell was awarded the Nobel Prize in chemistry as a result of this discovery.

Coenzyme Q10 and the heart

In the mid-1960s, Coenzyme Q10 was studied by Japanese researchers who detected its high content in the heart. This finding is logical given coenzyme Q10's involvement in energy production: the heart is among the body's most energetic organs, beating approximately 90,000 times per day. Coenzyme Q10's intimate involvement in cardiac function led to a study by The Institute for Biomechanical Research, at the University of Texas, which looked into a possible role for Coenzyme Q10 in the treatment of heart disease.

The results of this important early study were published in the June, 1985, issue of Proceedings of the National Academy of Sciences of the U.S.A. Coenzyme Q10 supplementation was found to cause "extraordinary clinical improvement" in 19 patients who were expected to die from heart failure. These findings laid the groundwork for establishing coenzyme Q10's role in treating angina, congestive heart failure, and cardiomyopathy. The PDR (Physician's Desk Reference) states that, since this early study, "nearly all of the several placebo-controlled studies investigating Coenzyme Q10's effects on heart muscle function have reported significant positive results." The efficacy of Coenzyme Q10 in treating heart failure appears to be well established in current medical literature.

A well-studied nutrient

Although it is most studied in relation to the cardiac system, Coenzyme Q10 has been found to possess other beneficial effects resulting from its role in energy production and antioxidation. A growing body of research suggests that these functions are not only cardioprotective but also cytoprotective, neuroprotective, and anticarcinogenic. Coenzyme Q10 has been examined in relation to dozens of diseases and health conditions, including malignancies, Parkinson's disease, cystic fibrosis, the aging process, periodontal disease, infectious disease, and inflammation. Deficiencies have been identified in multiple chronic disease states.

Although the therapeutic attributes possessed by coenzyme Q10 are broadly acknowledged in the alternative medicine community, an array of mainstream research has confirmed Coenzyme Q10's impact on maintaining health and countering a variety of unrelated disorders. Examples of this research are the following:

1. The National Cancer Institute found that coenzyme Q10 "helps the immune system work better and makes the body better able to resist certain types of infections and types of cancers." The Institute also cites the protection which Coenzyme Q10 confers against the adverse side effects of certain chemotherapeutic drugs.

2. The Mayo Clinic reports that coenzyme Q10 can be useful in treating high blood pressure and summarizes current research evaluating the substance's impact on a long list of other chronic disease states.

3. In January of 2007, the Duke University Medical Center reviewed Co Q10's "promise as a neuroprotectant." The study described results of several preliminary clinical trials which examined coenzyme Q10's potential role in the treatment of "many neurodegenerative disorders," including Alzheimer's, Parkinson's, and Huntington's disease.

4. Clifford Shults, M.D., of the University of California, San Diego, supervised a phase 2, placebo-controlled clinical trial in which coenzyme Q10 was found to "slow disease progression in patients with early-stage Parkinson's disease." Coenzyme Q10 is being extensively studied to determine its value in treating Parkinson's.

5. According to Biochemical and Biophysical Research Communications, of June 16, 1988, coenzyme Q10 can extend the life span of patients with AIDS. The University of Texas, where the research was performed, subsequently patented the use of Coenzyme Q10 as a treatment for AIDS.

6. Another University of Texas study, conducted at The Institute for Biomedical Research in Austin, found that Coenzyme Q10 supplementation increases blood levels of IgG and T4 lymphocytes, important components of the human immune system. The authors of the study concluded that the coenzyme is clinically important in combating infectious disease. The same researchers have also found that those with allergies and autoimmune disorders are more likely to have a deficiency of coenzyme Q10.

7. Ernie Bliznakov, M.D., of Biomedical Research Consultants in Pompano Beach, Florida, discovered that a single administration of coenzyme Q10 to aged mice was capable of stimulating the host defense system and bolstering immunological responsiveness.

These are just a very few examples of the many published studies looking into the effects on health of coenzyme Q10. The National Library of Medicine has indexed more than 1550 coenzyme Q10 studies, the majority of which (over 1200) were conducted since 1990. You may explore these yourself by searching for "coenzyme Q10" at www.pubmed.com. In addition to individual research studies, more than a dozen books have been written about the beneficial effects of Coenzyme Q10. A useful one is The Coenzyme Q10 Phenomenon by Stephen Sinatra, M.D.

Coenzyme Q10 deficiency in Lyme Disease

Coenzyme Q10 clearly has benefits for a wide spectrum of health problems and it is essential to maintaining health. Although virtually anyone could benefit from Coenzyme Q10 supplementation, Lyme Disease sufferers have a special and urgent need for this nutrient. According to Joseph Burrascano, M.D., arguably the nation's leading Lyme Literate Medical Doctor (LLMD), heart biopsies taken from Lyme Disease sufferers have revealed a significant coenzyme Q10 deficiency. This finding may be one explanation for the many heart-related disease manifestations experienced by Lyme Disease sufferers.

Coenzyme Q10 deficiency, such as occurs in Lyme Disease, has been investigated by numerous scientific institutes. Deficiencies can be attributed to insufficient dietary intake, impairment of coenzyme Q10 biosynthesis, excess utilization of coenzyme Q10 by the body, or the presence of certain disease processes.

Although it is not known exactly why Coenzyme Q10 deficiency occurs in Lyme Disease sufferers, there is no question that it does occur. As a result, those who address this deficiency will notice improvements in a range of symptoms. Additional benefits of Coenzyme Q10 supplementation include increased energy and exercise tolerance, enhanced mental clarity, and even improvement in the quality and quantity of dreams.

It is important to note, before moving on, that if you are being treated for Babesia with Mepron or Malarone, then Coenzyme Q10 supplementation may be contraindicated. Mepron and Malarone actually kill Babesia by decreasing Coenzyme Q10 levels. Check with your doctor.

Conclusion and product information

Since coenzyme Q10 has no known side effects, and has all the beneficial properties discussed in this chapter, there is no good reason for Lyme Disease sufferers not to include this nutrient in their supplementation programs. The only potential issues with supplementation of Coenzyme Q10 are possible interactions with certain pharmaceutical drugs like Warfarin and the cholesterol-lowering statin drugs. As an added precaution, pregnant or nursing women should consult a physician before supplementing Coenzyme Q10.

The most significant factor influencing dosing may be your financial situation. Supplemental coenzyme Q10 is quite expensive. This is unfortunate; however, new manufacturing processes have made the supplement more affordable in an indirect way. Previously available Coenzyme Q10 supplements have shown very poor absorbability, with as little as 40% being absorbed and the other 60% excreted in feces. According to The Life Extension Foundation, a respected nonprofit health studies organization, newer formulations known as emulsified Coenzyme Q10 can greatly increase absorption, meaning that less of the supplement can be taken to obtain the same benefit. Because new research is finding that higher doses are more efficacious, these new products allow maximum leverage of financial expense in obtaining the supplement.

Even highly absorbable Coenzyme Q10 is, however, expensive. There are several steps you can take to reduce cost. First and most importantly, exercise often. Exercise has been proven to dramatically increase production of coenzyme Q10 in the body. The more you exercise, the less need you will have for Coenzyme Q10. Exercise is also beneficial to most other aspects of the Lyme Disease recovery process.

Second, use a high dose of Coenzyme Q10 for only the first couple of weeks or months of supplementation. During this initial period, tissue levels will rise rapidly and return amounts in the body to healthy levels. After this time, supplementation can be cut back to a much smaller maintenance dose. In fact, if you stay on a high dose for too long after healthy levels have been reached, the body may simply begin to eliminate the extra Coenzyme Q10 that is no longer being utilized.

Third, take breaks from coenzyme Q10 supplementation. It is not necessary to use this supplement continuously, all year round.

Coenzyme Q10 supplements are readily available in pharmacies and other retail outlets across the country and online. The Life Extension Foundation has a relatively affordable, highly absorbable Coenzyme Q10 supplement which can be purchased from www.lef.org or by calling 800-766-8433.

Chapter 10: Magnesium

Introduction

Since I published *Lyme Disease and Rife Machines* in 2005, it has become increasingly evident that magnesium plays a critical role in both Lyme Disease pathology and recovery. In fact, even though a section on magnesium supplementation was included in the earlier book, burgeoning evidence has insisted that similar information be included here so that all readers can have access to this crucial data.

How exactly is magnesium significant in Lyme Disease? In my first book I reported that magnesium, a nutritive mineral, was absolutely critical for Lyme Disease sufferers to supplement. Below are some highlights from *Lyme Disease and Rife Machines* which explain why this is the case. After covering these highlights, we will look at several pieces of new information not included in my first book.

Many pathogenic microbes capable of establishing infection in the body have a strong reliance on and can cause a depletion of the body's stores of iron. Malaria is an example of such a microbe; it depends on iron for survival. Lyme Disease researchers were, however, startled to learn that the Lyme Disease bacterium, Borrelia Burgdorferi, is unique in its pathogenesis of disease because it utilizes magnesium instead of iron in its life cycle. This causes a depletion of the body's stores of magnesium. The result is typically a mild to severe magnesium deficiency syndrome that occurs in most, if not all, Lyme Disease sufferers.

Is it possible to "starve" Lyme Disease bacteria?

Because Borrelia Burgdorferi utilizes magnesium as part of its survival mechanism, some people (including doctors) erroneously conclude that withholding magnesium from the bacteria by avoiding supplementation will aid in recovery from the disease. This is known as "starving the bacteria" and is sometimes recommended by doctors despite the fact that magnesium is often in short supply in the bodies of people with Lyme Disease

Although it may seem logical to withhold a nutrient upon which a pathogen relies, the concept of starving Lyme Disease bacteria is completely irrational and very destructive to the healing process. This bacteria can survive being frozen, heated, attacked with antibiotics, and even placed into distilled water. When the bacteria encounter adverse conditions, they simply take on a dormant form and wait for the conditions to improve. If starved, they merely wait until food again becomes available. If deprived of magnesium, they wait and can do so indefinitely. (See *Lyme Disease and Rife Machines* for a more detailed explanation of how and why this occurs).

The human body, on the other hand, cannot do this. The body requires magnesium to survive and for proper immune system function. The body requires magnesium *every single day*. Reducing intake of vitamins, minerals, and other nutrients that feed the bacteria will result in your body only being weakened while the bacteria simply become dormant but no less alive. At some point your immune system will become significantly impaired, and symptoms of nutrient deficiency will begin to appear. When you are forced to resume taking the nutrient in order to avoid getting sick with (or dying from) deficiency and malnutrition, your body will by then be in a state of extreme weakness. But the bacteria will not have lost ground—they are simply biding time. The human body has a much lower tolerance for nutrient depletion than do Lyme Disease bacteria.

The very idea of starving the bacteria is irrational from another perspective as well. Your blood (in order to keep you alive) must always have nutrients circulating. If your blood experienced a large drop in blood sugar or other important nutrients, you would be unconscious and dead soon after. Your circulatory system maintains minimum nutrient supplies as long as they are available in the body. Even if you curtail intake of specific nutrients, there will still be sufficient supply in your blood to keep the bacteria alive and happy while you take a nose dive toward malnutrition. Your body will suffer from the reduction in intake; the bacteria will not.

Instead of "starving" the bacteria, the logical course of action is to actually increase intake of the nutrients the bacteria require to survive because you are most surely deficient in these nutrients—they are being stolen from you by the bacteria on a daily basis. In fact, many symptoms accompanying Lyme Disease are actually symptoms of nutrient deficiency. By increasing intake of these exhausted nutrients, patients are sometimes able to reduce their symptoms significantly, restore their immune systems, and increase their rates of recovery.

Magnesium is a critical nutrient

The rational course of action is for Lyme Disease sufferers to increase magnesium intake in the form of supplements in order to restore the body's optimal magnesium levels and healthy functioning. Increasing intake of the mineral causes three prominent Lyme-related events in the body:

1. Dormant layers of the disease (cyst-form organisms) will activate to retrieve the magnesium which is more readily available in the blood stream due to supplementation. This results in cyst-form organisms converting to spirochetes. Rife machine treatment sessions will typically be more productive (meaning more herx reactions and improvement) as spirochetes are destroyed during magnesium supplementation. Most Lyme patients notice deeper or more productive herx reactions as a result of rife machine therapy while supplementing magnesium.

2. The immune system is restored to optimal functionality with the elimination of a magnesium deficiency. This alone results in the occurrence of herx reactions (even without application of other anti-Lyme therapies) because the immune system is able to fight the infection more effectively. The herx reactions that result from magnesium supplementation are truly productive because they occur as a result of the immune system itself engaging in the battle against Lyme Disease bacteria. The immune system is the body's most effective weapon against the infection, more effective by far than rife machines or antibiotics.

3. Restoration of magnesium levels can also result in a dramatic decrease of symptoms because many common Lyme Disease symptoms are actually caused by magnesium deficiency itself. Examples of symptoms resulting from magnesium deficiency (which overlap with Lyme symptoms) are: cramping, muscle/joint problems, muscle twitching, tremors, depression, bipolar disorder, short-term memory loss, heart dysfunction, appetite problems, vision problems, inflammation, and even syndromes which involve immune system dysfunction. No amount of rife machine therapy, antibiotics, herbs, exercise, or lifestyle changes will help a person who has a severe magnesium deficiency created by the Lyme Disease infection. Only magnesium supplementation can remedy a deficiency.

For these reasons magnesium is one of the most important nutrients for Lyme Disease sufferers to supplement. In fact, even Lyme Disease patients who are doing everything right in other categories of a comprehensive treatment program will eventually reach a plateau in their improvement if magnesium deficiency is not addressed.

Magnesium as an infection fighter

In addition to the above reasons for magnesium supplementation, researchers have found that the mineral is a powerful infection fighter. Both addressing deficiencies and employing magnesium to fight infection can be critical components of the Lyme Disease treatment toolbox.

Magnesium's role in fighting infection was first documented by a French surgeon, Prof. Pierre Delbet, MD. Delbert, having found when treating injured soldiers that traditionally used antiseptics sometimes damaged tissues and even catalyzed infection growth rates, was looking for an improved way to clean wounds. The doctor tested many substances and discovered that a magnesium chloride solution was superior for his purposes. It was harmless to tissues and carried the bonus of greatly increasing leukocyte activity and phagocytosis (destruction of microbes).

Professor Delbet also experimented with the internal use of magnesium chloride and found it to be an impressive immune system stimulator. He noted that phagocytosis increased by more than 300% in some cases. This increased rate of pathogenic microbe destruction was a result of magnesium's ability to increase native immune system responses in the body. These findings opened the door for additional research which eventually documented that magnesium (especially magnesium chloride) is extremely beneficial in health conditions as varied as colitis, gall bladder problems, Parkinson's Disease, tremors and muscle cramps, acne, eczema, psoriasis, warts, itching skin, impotence, prostatic hypertrophy, cerebral and circulatory problems, asthma, hay fever, urticaria, and anaphylactic (allergic) reactions.

New information on magnesium and Lyme Disease

As I neared completion of the book you hold in your hands, I decided to include magnesium as one of the top 5 supplements for treating Lyme Disease. Magnesium supplementation is just too important to leave out of any book on Lyme Disease. Additionally, publication of this book has given me the opportunity to share with you a very important magnesium study not included in my first book.

The study was conducted by Victor Cristea and Monica Crişan, professors of clinical immunology at the University of Medicine and Pharmacy in the city of Cluj-Napoca, northern Romania. The article is entitled (in the English translation) "Lyme Disease with Magnesium Deficiency," and was included in the December, 2003, issue of the *Magnesium Research Journal*, a trade periodical published by John Libbey Eurotext. John Libbey Eurotext, located in Montrouge, France, is an organization that catalogs and distributes medical and scientific journals in Europe.

This article is valuable because it fills in some of the details surrounding the discovery of the role magnesium plays in Lyme Disease. These details are not only fascinating but are also an important framework for future magnesium/Lyme Disease research studies. The fact that magnesium plays a critical role in the disease's pathology is often completely overlooked by modern, conventional medical practitioners. The following information is absolutely critical to a better understanding of Lyme Disease and will lead to better treatment practices and ultimately, faster recovery for Lyme patients.

The article begins with the story of a 26 year-old Romanian man who came to the hospital because he was experiencing pain in both knees, headaches, and a low-grade fever. The patient's family doctor prescribed anti-inflammatory medication and bed rest. His condition did not improve, and he was diagnosed with rheumatoid arthritis and referred to a specialist. Upon examination by the specialist, the man was found to be pale and sweating, with a low-grade fever, elevated white blood cell count, and a slightly enlarged spleen. His medical history also revealed uveitis, a condition of the eye characterized by redness and inflammation. (Sidenote: Many Lyme Disease sufferers [including myself] have experienced uveitis; it is commonly misdiagnosed as either idiopathic or autoimmune in nature when in fact it is a result of the presence of Lyme Disease bacteria in the eyes.) Of particular note also was the laboratory finding of low serum magnesium concentration.

The patient was instructed to continue his anti-inflammatory medication and to begin a seven-day course of antibiotics. However, after another 10 days, the patient returned again, this time complaining of flu-like symptoms and a bull's-eye rash approximately 6 cm in diameter on his thigh. The treating physicians now suspected Lyme Disease. Serum and urine samples were tested using the ELISA technique and the LUAT test. Sure enough, both tests returned positive for Lyme Disease. At this point, more aggressive antibiotic therapy was administered.

The patient was reevaluated at a later time. His condition was somewhat better; however, because he was not completely cured, the doctors decided to administer oral magnesium supplements to address his low serum levels. The article reports that after magnesium supplementation began, the patient's condition became "rapidly favorable." Over the course of just four days, all symptoms and laboratory abnormalities disappeared. The patient returned for a follow-up appointment after six months and again after a year. Clinical manifestations did not reappear.

After relaying the above story, the article then describes several other cases. For example, during the period of April, 2001 to January, 2003, two patients presented with similar symptoms and tested positive (with high titers) for Lyme Disease. In both cases, clinical manifestations were similar to those described above, with shivering, fever, headache, multifaceted pain, bulls-eye rash, and tachycardia. Again, both patients had low serum magnesium, and, again, magnesium supplementation resulted in dramatic clinical improvement—even after aggressive antibiotic therapy yielded only mediocre results. The article goes on to cite statistics from the EUCALB (European Union Concerted Action on Lyme Borreliosis), indicating that, since 1997, three additional cases of Lyme Disease were associated with magnesium deficiency.

The article concludes that "... in certain diseases, magnesium deficiency can cause a decrease in immune response... the appearances of [Lyme Disease relapses] despite adequate antibiotic therapy, which are frequently reported in the literature, could represent an argument for this conclusion... this is why the use of magnesium derivatives in therapy can represent an immuno-stimulating factor... magnesium derivatives have an immediately beneficial effect that was maintained in time." And finally, the concluding sentence: "the presence of magnesium deficiency causes the appearance of a secondary immunodeficiency syndrome which requires the treatment of the patient not only with broad-spectrum antibiotics but also with magnesium in order to obtain efficient results in the long term."

The implications of this article are numerous. Most important, each and every Lyme Disease sufferer should incorporate magnesium supplementation into their treatment programs. It is also interesting to note several key pieces of information in the article: not only is Lyme Disease present in Romania and other parts of Europe (a fact either denied or unbeknownst to most of modern medicine), but, as is the case in the United States, it is also frequently misdiagnosed.

Furthermore, as was illustrated by the Romanian experience, symptoms of Lyme Disease found in patients in the United States are very similar to symptoms found in patients elsewhere in the world. Most Lyme sufferers reading this will recognize, on a personal level, many of the symptoms described in the article. This reality indicates that, although there may be certain differences in Lyme Disease bacteria in various regions across the globe, the disease presentation and clinical manifestations are largely the same. This fact should be both comforting and enlightening to patients and physicians worldwide. Comforting because it means that Lyme Disease sufferers throughout the world are not isolated—their symptoms and experiences are shared by thousands of people on all corners of the earth. And enlightening because Lyme Disease, which was at one time believed to be rare and inconsequential, is actually a rapidly spreading and incomprehensively dangerous infection that should be of primary concern in many nations.

Conclusion and product information

Given that magnesium supplements are essential for Lyme Disease sufferers, which type of magnesium is best and what is the dosage? Magnesium chloride has the best track record as an absorbable form of magnesium and is ideal for modulating and strengthening the immune system against infection. Additional forms of magnesium offer additional advantages and synergism, so many Lyme Disease sufferers take several forms of the mineral, including magnesium citrate, glycinate, taurinate, succinate, aspartate, and several others. They are typically very affordable. Most of these forms of magnesium can be purchased from a local health food store or any large online supplement store. Magnesium chloride can be purchased from www.nutricology.com.

Additional forms of magnesium, including oxide, peroxide, superoxide, and ozonide, reportedly contain oxygen attached to the magnesium atom. When introduced into the body, this kind of magnesium is believed to release singlet oxygen. Homozon is a product containing these ingredients and can be ordered from numerous internet-based supplement stores.

Dosing for magnesium supplements can typically be determined by the product label, however, frequent dosing of magnesium throughout the day (i.e., 2-8 doses per day) is one approach that helps keep the mineral at constant levels in the blood. It is difficult to overdose on magnesium via oral supplementation because if too much is taken, the only adverse event is diarrhea and loose stools as the body fails to absorb excess amounts. Many Lyme Disease sufferers take as much magnesium as possible without creating uncomfortably loose stools and diarrhea. Loose stools caused by magnesium are not necessarily a negative effect, especially during cleansing programs, if a person has a tendency toward constipation.

Because increasing magnesium levels in the body can cause significant herx reactions as the immune system is strengthened and activated, the dose of magnesium should be started at low levels and increased gradually. You may find it difficult to believe that simply supplementing magnesium can cause productive herx reactions, but it can.

Chapter 11:
Building a treatment plan

Putting it all together

N ow that you have been introduced to ten of the most effective Lyme Disease therapies available, the next step is to integrate them into a logical and comprehensive treatment plan.

Before getting started, a note: If you were recently bitten by a tick and/or you are in the early stages of Lyme Disease, put this book down and make an appointment with a Lyme Literate Medical Doctor (LLMD) immediately. In most cases, early stages of Lyme Disease can be successfully treated by aggressive antibiotic therapy. An LLMD who can prescribe appropriate antibiotic therapy can be located through www.lymenet.org or www.lymediseaseassociation.org. If, however, you have chronic Lyme Disease and you were not cured under the care of an LLMD, keep reading—this chapter is for you.

The process of planning a Lyme Disease treatment protocol is highly individual. When I initially wrote this chapter, it was much longer than it is in its current form. However, after reviewing the content, it became obvious that the correct treatment guidelines for one person may be the wrong treatment guidelines for another. For this reason, this chapter is relatively short, leaving the bulk of the work of treatment planning to individual Lyme Disease sufferers who know their unique bodies, circumstances, and needs. You must play an active role in your recovery—you must be willing to experiment with various treatments and determine what your body needs. There is no book or physician that can do this for you. The healing process varies greatly between individuals.

Although he/she cannot solve all your problems, a trusted physician should be enlisted when embarking on the journey of healing Lyme Disease. A physician can order tests if necessary, write prescriptions, monitor the healing process, and provide expert input. No less important, family and friends should also be recruited for logistical and emotional support.

Now let's get started building a treatment plan. Two components are necessary to beat chronic Lyme Disease: time and a multifaceted approach.

Time: No matter how perfect your treatment protocol is, it has been proven over the last 20 years that defeating chronic Lyme Disease can take months or years. So, if you do not get cured overnight, do not despair. And do not overanalyze your treatment protocol. The recovery process is going to be long regardless of what you do. The precise length of recovery depends on how sick you are. The longer you've been sick and the more severe your symptoms, the longer the recovery process. The long recovery process is a result of the fact that Lyme Disease bacteria group together inside your body in dense colonies. The treatments you use will only affect the outer layers of these colonies. It takes time to peel outer layers off and eventually eradicate all of the bacteria. Because of the long recovery process, the most ideal therapies are affordable, convenient, and non-toxic. Therefore, this chapter will not only emphasize effectiveness, but also practicality and sustainability.

Multifaceted approach: Lyme Disease sufferers and practitioners alike have concluded that no single therapy or approach is sufficient to defeat Lyme Disease. Instead, a multifaceted approach must be used that incorporates various antibacterial therapies and supportive measures. As a result, the suggestions in this chapter will draw from a variety of treatment options, each focusing on resolution of a different aspect of the Lyme Disease complex. Remember also that it is not just important to use various treatments in your protocol, but it is also important to use them according to proper timing, combinations, and methodology, as we will see below. The reason these other factors are important is that Lyme Disease bacteria are highly adaptable and survival-oriented. So, eradicating the bacteria from your body requires careful consideration of how the bacteria behave and respond to the treatments you use.

The remainder of this chapter is divided into two sections: antibacterial therapies and supportive therapies. Note that the supportive therapies do not refer only to the 5 supportive supplements discussed in Part II of the book, but instead, to a wide range of modalities that aid the healing process.

Antibacterial therapies

Because Lyme Disease is caused by a bacterial infection, the core of a Lyme Disease treatment protocol is comprised of antibacterial therapies. The most effective antibacterial therapies are pharmaceutical and non-pharmaceutical antibiotics, the Marshall Protocol, and rife machine therapy. At all times during the recovery process, at least one of these three therapies should be in use.

Rife machine therapy will be the foundational antibacterial treatment, used approximately on a weekly basis, throughout the entire recovery process. Rife treatment should be used on a continuous basis, even when other antibacterial therapies are in use. Lyme Disease bacteria cannot become resistant to rife machine therapy as it can to antibiotics, so rife machine therapy will steadily reduce the bacterial load and also ensure that the infection does not get worse. Read *Lyme Disease and Rife Machines* for information about planning a rife treatment schedule.

Some people have recovered completely with rife machine therapy alone. However, using pharmaceutical and non-pharmaceutical antibiotics periodically is beneficial because antibiotics attack the bacterial infection from a different angle, thus accelerating recovery. While rife machine therapy specifically targets spirochetes, antibiotics can target cell-wall-deficient bacteria and cysts. Additionally, when using antibiotics, rife treatments may be taken slightly less frequently, giving the body a break from rife treatment.

Pharmaceutical and non-pharmaceutical antibiotics should be used throughout the recovery process in short courses, with breaks taken between courses, and a different antibiotic used for each course, as described in Chapter 1. Cell wall inhibiting antibiotics should be avoided at all costs, as explained in Chapter 1, to ensure that bacteria do not convert to cell-wall-deficient and cyst forms. A schedule for antibiotic use might look like this: doxycycline might be taken for a week, followed by a one-month break, followed by a week of Samento. Breaks between antibiotic courses are needed because they allow the body to recover from the toxic effects of antibiotics, and they allow rife machine therapy to work more effectively. Although some breaks from antibiotic therapy may be short, at least several of them (in any given year) should be relatively long, for example, 2-6 months—these longer breaks allow rife machine therapy to dig deeper into dormant bacterial colonies, a process described in detail in *Lyme Disease and Rife Machines*.

Rife machine therapy is relied on heavily as the primary antibacterial treatment during breaks from antibiotics, and is also used and relied on while taking antibiotics. This synergistic relationship between rife machine therapy and antibiotic therapy is at the core of the healing process. Antibiotics push, rife pulls, and the right combination of the two greatly weakens the infection. When the two are used together, healing is maximized and side effects are minimized.

Because the Marshall Protocol (Chapter 2) greatly amplifies the effectiveness of pharmaceutical antibiotics, if possible, antibiotic therapy should be used according to and in conjunction with Marshall Protocol guidelines. Remember, the Marshall Protocol addresses aspects of the Lyme Disease complex that no other therapies can touch. This makes the Marshall Protocol invaluable in treating Lyme Disease. Even when antibiotics are omitted from the Marshall Protocol, it still greatly accelerates healing and addresses parts of the Lyme Disease complex that are unreachable by any other therapy. In Chapter 2, I describe some of my own personal experi-

Bacterial forms: characteristics and treatments

	Spirochete	Cell-Wall-Deficient (CWD)	Cyst
Primary bacterial activities and characteristics that facilitate survival	Very mobile. Spiral/drill capable shape allows penetration into dense tissue and bone. Capable of intracellular infection. Rapidly converts to CWD and cyst form when threatened.	Lack of cell wall makes targeting by immune system and antibiotics more difficult. Capable of intracellular infection. Converts Vitamin D to immunosuppressive hormone known as 1,25-D. Causes autoimmunity. Clumps together in dense colonies—inner layers unreachable by antibiotics and immune system.	Dormant form bacteria are not mobile and do not cause symptoms. Can survive antibiotics, starvation, pH changes, hydrogen peroxide, temperature variation, and most other adverse conditions. Converts back to spirochete form when conditions are favorable.
Symptoms	Conventionally recognized Lyme Disease symptoms, i.e., bull's-eye rash, Bell's palsy, flu-like symptoms, fever.	Numerous syndromes and conditions not conventionally attributed to Lyme Disease, i.e., paralysis, multiple sclerosis, mental disorders, chronic fatigue syndrome, "post-Lyme syndrome," many more.	Does not cause symptoms
Common (yet not fully accurate) beliefs	Causative bacteria in Lyme Disease.	Not recognized or acknowledged; insignificant bacterial form.	Not recognized or acknowledged; insignificant bacterial form.
Correct beliefs	Causative bacteria in early-stage Lyme Disease, but not even close to the whole story.	Causative bacteria in many Lyme Disease symptoms and problems. As or more dangerous than spirochete form. Very difficult to treat.	Responsible for "relapsing and remitting" Lyme Disease. Can persist unrecognized and asymptomatic for many years.
Conventional treatment and success rates	Pharmaceutical antibiotics. Sometimes successful if infection is caught early. Often causes conversion to CWD and cyst form.	Often misdiagnosed as autoimmune or psychiatric disorders and mistreated with steroids, painkillers, antidepressants. Symptoms are often deemed idiopathic. Very low success rate.	Asymptomatic so conventionally not treated with anything. Frusteration and confusion experienced by patient and practitioner upon inevitable relapses due to cysts.
Proper treatment (as described in this book) and success rates	Rife machine therapy is the preferred treatment, and is the only known treatment that kills spirochetes and does not induce conversion to CWD and cyst form. Highly successful.	Marshall Protocol is preferred treatment and is typically successful, often leading to remission of "incurable" diseases, ranging from autoimmune diseases to mental disorders to chronic fatigue syndrome.	Cyst form antibiotics (5-nitroimidazoles) are somewhat successful. Avoidance of cell wall inhibiting antibiotics (e.g. Rocephin) and use of a rife machine (to kill spirochetes that emerge from cysts) is highly successful.

-ences with the Marshall Protocol which may be helpful to you as you plan your own treatment program. The Marshall Protocol is only appropriate for use under the close supervision of a licensed, Marshall Protocol-literate physician.

This book bases its antibacterial methodology on the assumption that Lyme Disease bacteria come in three forms: spirochete form, cell-wall-deficient form (also known as variant, or L-form), and cyst form. How much of each form is in the body at any given time is a function of many different factors. Ultimately, though, to effectively eradicate Lyme Disease, all three of these forms must be addressed. Here is a summary of how this can be accomplished:

1. The Marshall Protocol and protein synthesis inhibiting antibiotics provide antibacterial action against the cell-wall-deficient form of Lyme Disease.

2. Rife machine therapy provides antibacterial action against the spirochete form of Lyme Disease.

3. Breaks from antibiotic therapy during which time cysts are allowed to activate into spirochetes (and are then killed by rife machine therapy) provides antibacterial action against the cyst form of Lyme Disease. Cyst form antibiotics are also helpful in treating the cyst form.

The precise schedule and methodology by which these approaches should be used will differ between different individuals. Trial and error will help you fine-tune your treatment plan. Because of individual differences, certain antibacterial therapies may work better for you than others. For example, some people find the Marshall Protocol to be extremely helpful, while other people notice that the Salt / Vitamin C protocol is more beneficial, and visa versa. Some people even find that systemic enzyme supplementation provides optimal antibacterial action. Do not force yourself to use a one-size-fits-all treatment plan. Instead, stay flexible and only use therapies that help you. The above three approaches should be considered a rough guideline only, not inflexible instructions.

As the healing process progresses and the bacterial load decreases, rife treatments may be needed less often and breaks between antibiotic courses can be lengthened. Because the recovery process is long, patience is needed. If you measure your progress from day to day or week to week, you will be disappointed. Instead, progress should be measured from month to month and year to year. The recovery process can take between six months and 5 years, depending on severity of the infection and other factors such as lifestyle choices and general health.

Supportive therapies

Now that we have looked at antibacterial therapies, lets move on to examine other facets of a Lyme Disease treatment plan. The reality is that the Lyme Disease complex causes problems and symptoms which require treatment beyond mere antibacterial therapies. Supportive therapies should be used throughout the recovery process to address these problems.

Lithium can be used to protect the brain from circulating neurotoxins. Systemic enzyme supplementation helps reduce inflammation, increase blood and nutrient supply to cells, and break down harmful debris throughout the body. The Marshall Protocol (which also happens to be antibacterial) corrects hormonal imbalances and allows the immune system to function properly. Detoxification and aerobic exercise (both discussed later in this Chapter) promote accelerated removal of neurotoxins and dramatic symptom relief.

Unlike antibacterial therapies, which are needed at all times during the recovery process, most supportive therapies are needed only part of the time. Determining whether or not a specific supportive therapy should be used continuously or intermittently is more of an art than a science. You will need to fine-tune your use of supportive therapies according to your individual responses.

Use of various types of supplements is one example of a supportive treatment that is typically most beneficial when used intermittently, not continuously. The length of time you should take a given supplement can vary depending on your financial situation and how much benefit you feel you are getting from the supplement. Some people discover that taking a given supplement for an extended period of time is beneficial, but the vast majority of people find that improvement gleaned from a supplement diminishes with time. In most cases, a given supplement should be used for only several months of each year—for example, you could take coenzyme Q10 January through March of each year, and use systemic enzyme supplementation from April to June of each year. In the same way that pulsing antibacterial therapies provides optimum effectiveness with minimum side effects, pulsing supplements can offer the same benefit. You should listen to your body and use a given supplement as much or as little as you feel is beneficial. If you find that taking a given supplement continuously, without breaks, is most beneficial, then do that. Most supplements can be combined—but they should be added to your protocol one-at-a-time so you can recognize and isolate both the benefits and the side effects of each one.

Remember that some supplements have significant antibacterial action (such as systemic enzyme supplements and mangosteen juice). During use of these types of supplements, rife machine therapy will be much less effective, so it is important to take breaks from use of supplements with antibacterial activity in the same way that it is important to take breaks from any other type of antibiotic. See *Lyme Disease and Rife Machines* for further discussion of this topic.

Although the vast majority of supportive therapies are most helpful when used intermittently, there are some supportive therapies that may be most beneficial when used continuously. Detoxification therapies, for example, should be utilized on an ongoing basis throughout the entire recovery process. Because of individual differences, some detoxification therapies will work better than others for a particular person. For example, some people take a sauna every other day, while other people feel better using a liver flush every couple of weeks. Listen to your body and use the treatment/frequency which yields the best results. Do not force yourself to use a detoxification therapy that makes you worse. Reactions to cleansing therapies are normal but they should not be overwhelming or debilitating. The right detoxification therapy for your individual needs will provide relief and symptom improvement, so it will become natural and easy to settle into a routine—doing so will simply help you feel better. Because Lyme Disease bacteria continuously secrete neurotoxins during normal life processes and during herx reactions, continual detoxification provides both symptom reduction and accelerated healing.

Similarly, aerobic exercise should also be used throughout the recovery process without breaks, as it strengthens the body and facilitates healing. An aerobic exercise program is mandatory, not optional. Exercise should not be done to the point of exhaustion or a severe crash, but should be done to challenge the body. If a short walk is all that can be tolerated, it is still beneficial. Exercise serves many purposes in the recovery process and can lead to rapid symptom improvement. Exercise is among the most effective detoxification therapies because it cleanses the lymphatic system, oxygenates tissues, and accelerates waste removal from the kidneys and gut. Do not miss this point: exercise is not just recommended, it is mandatory.

Dietary and lifestyle considerations are another example of a supportive measure that should be used continuously. Poor diet and lifestyle choices will lead to a prolonged or even indefinitely delayed recovery process. Mandatory to the recovery process are a nutritious diet and avoidance of bad habits like smoking, excessive alcohol and caffeine consumption, recreational drug use, poor sleep, etc.

Because chronic Lyme Disease and mercury poisoning are often companions that come hand-in-hand, a large number of Lyme Disease sufferers need to undertake the complicated and unpleasant task of mercury detoxification. Mercury detoxification is not a short-term project but instead, a long-term, involved process. The mercury detoxification approach discussed in Chapter 4 is most effective and has the least side effects. Mercury detoxification often requires months or years, so it should be incorporated into the foundation of a treatment plan. Do not ignore mercury toxicity as a possible reason for chronic infection.

What to expect

Be ready to endure some intense herx reactions. Because the Lyme Disease complex successfully evades the human immune system and maintains an elusive and entrenched position in the body, when you successfully attack it, and the immune system wakes up, symptoms of inflammation and immune system activation will inevitably increase. Herx reactions are both uncomfortable and necessary for recovery. Although necessary, herx reactions should be induced in controlled moderation. Antibacterial therapies must be initiated slowly and moderately ramped up in intensity to avoid out of control herx reactions. If an overwhelming herx reaction is encountered, therapy should be paused until the reaction completely subsides.

During certain times of the year, especially spring and fall, the infection is more active and symptoms are more severe, and both rife and antibiotic treatment schedules may need to be intensified. These will also be the times when the most progress is made and significant steps toward recovery are taken. You may also notice flareups during or after other illness, stressful events, lack of sleep, or other occurrences that can put undue burden on the body. These heightened periods of infective activity will diminish with each additional year of treatment.

When traveling, expect symptom flareups. Lyme Disease is always more active when you are changing environments or traveling through different climates. Bring a non-pharmaceutical antibiotic with you on your trips, such as mangosteen juice or Samento—these can be real life savers during a flareup. Pharmaceutical antibiotics are not ideal for traveling because they can cause more significant side effects, including diarrhea. If you travel to the same place often and have storage space, consider keeping a rife machine there to have handy if necessary. See Chapter 5 for more information about traveling.

Keeping a treatment diary can help you log your progress and identify helpful or harmful patterns in your treatments. It can also show you that despite your frustration, you really are getting better. Do not feel the need to write a book of a diary—putting that expectation on yourself will just cause frustration. Instead, write only short entries occasionally when you feel something significant has occurred.

As your treatment program progresses and you begin to feel better and better, you can slowly reduce the frequency/doses/intensity of your various treatments. Keep in mind, however, that you will probably need to use various Lyme Disease therapies for quite a long time. Even after you get the majority of Lyme Disease bacteria out of your body, it can take additional months or years to eradicate 100% of the small amount of remaining bacteria. Do not discontinue treatment too early or else a small remaining population of bacteria might grow back into a full-blown Lyme Disease infection.

New treatments, supplements, protocols, and information will most certainly become available as you recover. Be flexible and curious and always investigate new treatment options. Be ready to do away with old treatments that are not helping you as much anymore in favor of newer treatments which might offer a better solution. It is very helpful to communicate with other Lyme Disease sufferers and learn about what they are doing, as well as share what you are doing. Lyme Community Forums, an online discussion group, is an excellent place to communicate with Lyme Disease sufferers. Access to the group is easy and free. Visit the group at www.lymecommunity.com.

Successfully treating Lyme Disease requires a paradigm shift from the quick-fix philosophy often used by Western medicine, to an approach of slow, steady, plodding progress. Recovering from Lyme Disease is a marathon, not a sprint. If you view recovery as a sprint you actually won't get better but you will certainly experience scary herx reactions and undue frustration. If you view recovery as a marathon, slow and steady, you will get better and you will avoid discomfort, scary reactions, and frustration.

Ultimately, the protocol you end up with will be determined in large part by your intuition and knowledge of your own body. Stay away from physicians who have a "one-size-fits-all" program. View this book as a toolbox from which you can select tools that meet your needs. This book is only valuable when you, the reader, play an active part in analyzing and applying its content to your unique situation. If you find that other treatment practices work better than those described in this book, trust your experience, instinct, and analysis. The book is not a final answer for you but instead a platform upon which you can build a solid foundation of your own.

If you have chronic Lyme Disease, you can get better, and even return to a normal, healthy lifestyle. Chronic Lyme Disease is considered incurable in modern times only because the treatment paradigm which happens to govern American medicine in the 21st century is not conducive to the comprehensive, long-term healing of chronic diseases. Instead, it is conducive to putting quick-fix band-aids on health problems. If you adopt a paradigm shift and treat your chronic Lyme Disease with a carefully planned, comprehensive, multifaceted approach, and if you are patient, recovery is possible. Remember, beating Lyme Disease requires permanent lifestyle changes and discipline—it does not happen overnight.

Appendices

Appendix A: Are herx/healing reactions necessary to get well?

The herx reaction occurs when Lyme Disease bacteria are killed by antibacterial therapies or the immune system. This reaction is characterized by symptoms of discomfort caused by neurotoxin release and inflammation, as bacteria die. This book will not present a comprehensive explanation of the herx reaction—see *Lyme Disease and Rife Machines* to further elucidate these concepts.

In *Lyme Disease and Rife Machines*, it was stated that herx reactions are not only necessary to get well, but that they also occur throughout the entire healing process if you are using a treatment that actually works. My position on this issue has not changed since that book was published—I still believe that, regardless of which antibacterial therapy is in use, herx reactions are a reliable indicator of successful therapy.

THE DEBATE

In recent months, there has been some debate about the accuracy of this position. Opponents have stated that reactions can be avoided if the body is properly balanced and detoxified. While I agree that such steps can ameliorate these reactions, I do not believe they can completely eliminate them. Although my position is admittedly investigational, and not 100% proven, I believe it is the most logical conclusion given the available data. Following is a discussion that further explores the issue. Hopefully, this information, combined with that in *Lyme Disease and Rife Machines*, will give you the tools to come to your own conclusion.

While it may be true that some abnormal situations involve healing without herx reactions, most people who successfully recover from Lyme Disease report that herx reactions did indeed mark their road to recovery.

In *Lyme Disease and Rife Machines*, Chapter 4, the two primary physiological reasons for the herx reaction were described: neurotoxin circulation and inflammation, both occurring as a result of bacterial die off subsequent to antibacterial therapy such as a rife machine treatment or antibiotic use. It is recommended that you review Chapter 4 in *Lyme Disease and Rife Machines*.

During the recovery process, as the bacterial load is reduced and bacteria are killed, there is simply no logical reason that bacterial toxin release and associated inflammation would cease—that is, until the infection is completely gone. For this reason, it is logical to conclude that herx reactions characterized by symptoms of toxin circulation and inflammation will occur throughout the entire healing process. These reactions may be diminished by detoxification therapies, but not completely eliminated.

WHAT IS A HEALING REACTION?

In addition to classic herx reactions involving neurotoxin circulation and inflammation resulting from dying bacteria, there are other aspects of recovery that also point to the necessity of various types of healing reactions. These other reactions are not herx reactions by their technical definition but, instead, should be thought of as healing reactions, detoxification reactions, or simply the process by which the body adjusts to a new, healthier equilibrium. Whether you call these herx reactions or not, they are similar to herx reactions in that they are both uncomfortable and completely necessary to the healing process.

What exactly are these other reactions and why must they occur?

A healthy person's body is in equilibrium when they are healthy, and out of equilibrium when they are acutely sick (for example, with a cold or flu). The immune system's struggle to return to equilibrium (health) is ultimately why people who get a cold do not stay sick forever. In scientific observation, whether of the human body or of nature, living systems always try to stay in equilibrium. Everything that happens in the ecosystem on planet Earth yields to equilibrium. For a human being, being out of equilibrium feels bad. Thirsty people are experiencing disequilibrium. Hungry people are out of equilibrium. Acutely ill people are out of equilibrium.

The discomfort involved in these conditions is a result of the body's natural struggle to return to equilibrium. This is the proper way a body should function. It is normal to feel uncomfortable during periods of disequilibrium. In the worst-case scenario, if the body did not struggle to return to equilibrium, you would eventually die. The discomfort compels you to do something about the situation. Thirsty people experiencing the disequilibrium of thirst will do something to correct their situation—they will drink water. If thirst was not actually felt as discomfort, the person may never be compelled to drink, and death would result. So, the lesson here is simply that a state of disequilibrium is typically experienced as discomfort.

A chronically ill person's body is the opposite of a healthy person's body: frighteningly, the body of a chronically ill person has reluctantly adopted a *sick status* as a state of equilibrium. Most chronic illnesses began with an acute struggle during which time the body desperately attempted to return to a healthy equilibrium. This initial struggle is often experienced as acute discomfort and illness. If this struggle is lost, the body must accept the illness as a new state of equilibrium. There is really no choice in the matter. For the body to keep fighting a losing battle in an attempt to get back to a healthy equilibrium would simply require too much energy. Accepting a diseased state is the body's way of compromising to survive. A perfect example is chronic Lyme Disease, in which a state of sick (but not quite fatal) equilibrium has been reluctantly adopted. This new sick state of equilibrium can be thought of as a state of "pseudo-equilibrium."

What differentiates an acute illness from which the body can recover, from a chronic illness which the body accepts, is the severity of the disease. The body has enough resources to recover from some afflictions but not others. The common cold or flu is an example of an affliction which the body can handle on its own. In some cases, people with compromised immune systems remain sick with the common cold for weeks or months, perhaps as a result of lack of sleep, poor diet, stress, or other weaknesses.

However, with most people, colds and flus are eventually defeated and healthy equilibrium is again attained.

In contrast, chronic Lyme Disease is an affliction in response to which the body does not have adequate resources. Thus, acute Lyme Disease often becomes chronic as the body gives up the fight and learns to live with the disease. When this happens, equilibrium becomes sickness instead of health. The sick state, or pseudo-equilibrium, becomes the norm.

All this to explain why healing reactions are necessary throughout the entire process of recovering from chronic Lyme Disease: in the treatment of chronic Lyme Disease, each time we initiate a new therapy, whether it be exercise, antibiotics, rife machine therapy, herbs, or detoxification, we are pushing the body out of a state of unhealthy pseudo-equilibrium (sickness) and into a state of healthier equilibrium. Remember, chronically ill people are in equilibrium (or pseudo-equilibrium) when they are *sick*, so returning to health requires asking, even forcing, the body to leave sick equilibrium and move back to a state of *healthy* equilibrium. The body will not undergo this shift on its own (as it would with a cold or flu) because it has actually accepted the presence of the illness.

Just as fighting a cold or flu is uncomfortable and energy consuming, so is fighting Lyme Disease. The difference is that when fighting a cold or flu, the body does the work and you just hang on for the ride. With chronic Lyme Disease, the body is not capable of crawling out of the hole it is in, so we must help it with therapies such as those discussed in this book. As we do this, we experience the discomfort of moving from pseudo-equilibrium healthy equilibrium. This discomfort is defined as a healing reaction. It is similar to the discomfort experienced when fighting a cold or flu. The discomfort is mandatory to recovering. There is simply no feasible way to shift from a state of sick, pseudo-equilibrium to a state of healthy equilibrium without experiencing discomfort; thus, the necessity of uncomfortable reactions.

THE CONCLUSION

The conclusion to these concepts is that getting better is hard work and uncomfortable at the same time. Both herx reactions (caused by neurotoxin release and inflammation) and healing reactions (caused by moving from sick equilibrium to healthy equilibrium) are experienced as discomfort. But more than merely uncomfortable, recovery from chronic Lyme Disease is also hard work and is more difficult than recovering from the flu. In chronic Lyme Disease, not only must you experience the inevitable discomfort of shifting equilibriums (similar to fighting the flu), you must also be the one to poke and prod your body into action by thinking about, deciding on, and ultimately implementing therapies which are not much fun at all.

Additionally, these concepts teach us that there is no "quick fix" for most people with chronic illness. Chronic illness is a very entrenched physiological state. It is very deep-rooted in the body—it becomes the new equilibrium. Recovering from chronic illness requires slow, consistent, intentional adjustments to coerce the body back into healthy equilibrium. The process of recovering is generally anywhere from six months to 5 years, depending on the severity of the illness and how long a person has been sick. A long and difficult recovery process is the norm for most chronic illnesses, not just Lyme Disease. It is simply difficult to cajole the body out of a sick equilibrium into a healthy equilibrium. This is the defining feature of chronic disease in comparison with acute disease.

As a result of the extended process by which recovery happens, most "quick fix" therapies do not lead to permanent improvement. Examples of such therapies include expensive, special clinics in Mexico, Germany, Switzerland, and other places. While the therapies practiced at these clinics are often excellent, backed by sound science, the problem is that you only get two or three weeks at the clinic. In most cases, nothing short of a magic wand can restore equilibrium to a chronically ill body in a time period as short as two or three weeks. The body is simply incapable of such drastic changes in such a short period of time. Healthy equilibrium may be reestablished briefly, but when you leave the clinic, your body will rapidly return to sick equilibrium.

Because it takes the body a long time to slowly shift back to healthy equilibrium, it makes sense to try to formulate a treatment protocol that is affordable, convenient, can be done at home, is non-toxic, and is not time-consuming. In other words, if you need to commit to a treatment protocol for months or years to slowly move back to healthy equilibrium, that treatment protocol had better be sustainable. If a protocol is developed in this way, the long recovery period is not miserable, but instead tolerable and realistic. Yes, this theme has been repeated multiple times in this book. However, the repetition is intended to ensure that this principle is not missed—it is perhaps the most important principle governing Lyme Disease recovery.

Presenting to you such a sustainable protocol is why this book was written. The therapies described in this book were chosen because they fit well into a sustainable, long-term treatment protocol. The treatments are not quick-fix band-aids. If you are not fond of the treatments this book presents and you want to go find your own innovative therapies, just remember to take into consideration the long recovery process, and the necessity of sustainability, when selecting treatments.

With regard to the original question of whether or not herx reactions and healing reactions are necessary during the recovery process, it is my hope that this discussion has at least helped you formulate your own opinion. While the discussion may not have provided the final answer, I hope it has fueled the discussion.

Appendix B: Reinforcing the importance of avoiding processed sugar

Because the study of diet, nutrition, and supplementation is so broad and interdisciplinary, this book does not offer a complete nutritional guide. Instead, this section will center on one aspect of diet and nutrition which has focused application in the treatment of chronic Lyme Disease: avoidance of processed sugar.

PROCESSED SUGAR: A HISTORICAL PERSPECTIVE

To understand why avoiding processed sugar when healing from Lyme Disease is so important, let's examine a different, more common health problem in which bacteria and sugar are known to cause problems: tooth decay. The difference between a mouthful of cavities and a healthy mouth can be, among other factors, a result of how much processed sugar someone consumes. When reporting to a NIH (National Institute of Health) panel, Professor Brian Burt, B.D.S., Ph.D., M.P.H., of the University of Michigan, said "avoiding consumption of excess sugar is a justifiable part of [cavity] prevention."

Dr. Weston Price, an Ohio dentist who left private practice to travel the world in search of a better understanding of dentistry, found numerous tribes that, though having never used a toothbrush, had no cavities and a healthy mouth. One of the reasons for this, he determined, was that these people had never eaten processed foods (and sugars). Sure enough, he also found that in just one generation of consumption of modern, processed foods and sugars, the dental health of uncivilized tribes deteriorated rapidly. These observations were confirmed by Vilhjalmur Stefansson, an Arctic explorer who observed Eskimo tribes in the early 1900s. Not only did he find that ancient skulls in Iceland had no signs of tooth decay, he also found many uncivilized peoples throughout the world who had perfect mouths and teeth despite not having any modern dental health care.

Because bacteria living in the mouth and between the teeth eat away at tooth enamel to cause cavities, and because processed sugar feeds bacteria, it is generally accepted in modern medicine that consumption of processed sugar is a causative factor in tooth decay. When I was growing up, on Halloween, my dentist's office would always have chewy caramel candies out for unsuspecting children to snack on. Although this was not what I would call an ethical practice for a dental professional, it is a clear illustration that dentists know what needs to happen for them to keep their jobs! Simply stated, the difference between those with tooth decay and those with healthy mouths is, in large part, the amount of processed sugar consumed.

Lyme Disease bacteria, although different from bacteria that cause tooth decay, also feed on processed sugar. In the same way that oral bacteria thrive and destroy your teeth when they have lots of processed sugar to feed on, Lyme Disease bacteria thrive and destroy your body when they have lots of processed sugar to feed on. In the same way that sugar consumption can destroy your mouth, it can also completely halt your Lyme Disease recovery process.

OTHER DAMAGING EFFECTS OF PROCESSED SUGAR

In addition to rotting your teeth and worsening your Lyme Disease infection, processed sugar causes many other problems. The human body was simply not designed to deal with large amounts of simple, processed sugars and associated blood sugar spikes. This type of sugar does a massive amount of damage to even healthy people who are not suffering from any disease. Consider the earlier examples detailing how the dental health of ancient people was so much better before processed foods were introduced.

To understand the negative effects of sugar elsewhere in the body, we must look at the pancreas and how it reacts to sugar consumption. The pancreas is a small gland located close to the stomach. It has two functions: first, it secretes insulin and glucagon, two endocrine hormones which control blood sugar levels; and second, it plays an important role in food digestion by secreting enzymes that break down fat, starch, and proteins.

In this discussion, we are most concerned with the first function. When a meal high in processed sugar is consumed, considerable strain is placed on the pancreas as it is forced to rapidly manufacture and secrete insulin to lower blood sugar levels. High blood sugar levels (hyperglycemia) are toxic and the body works hard to lower them quickly. Similar to all hormones, insulin has many effects on the body. Most doctors only pay attention to insulin's primary function of facilitating glucose (sugar) transportation from the blood to the cells.

New research shows that insulin also encourages the body to store up calories as fat, promotes arterial damage, and possibly even accelerates the growth rate of tumors. Additionally, frequent outbursts of insulin from the pancreas may cause cells to decrease their sensitivity to insulin. This is known as insulin resistance and is associated with abnormalities of blood fats, high blood pressure, adult onset diabetes, cardiovascular disease, and even difficult cases of obesity which do not respond to diet and exercise. In fact, the negative effects of insulin are quite possibly at the root of many modern health problems which did not exist prior to manufacture and consumption of processed sugars.

Because consumption of processed sugar causes blood sugar spikes, it is associated with the above negative health effects. Insulin levels increase dramatically—far beyond healthy levels—after processed sugar is consumed. Additionally, processed sugar has also been found to:

1. Suppress the immune system and impair defenses against infections.

2. Cause mineral imbalances.

3. Cause hyperactivity, anxiety, and difficulty concentrating.

4. Produce a significant rise in total cholesterol.

5. Be associated with cancer of the breast, ovaries, prostate, rectum, pancreas, biliary tract, lung, gallbladder, and stomach.

6.   Increase fasting levels of glucose and cause reactive hypoglycemia.

7.   Cause problems with the gastrointestinal tract including an acidic digestive tract, indigestion, and imbalances which include candida and other pathogenic microorganisms.

8.   Cause food allergies.

9.   Lower the ability of enzymes to function.

10.   Increase your body's fluid retention.

11.   Increase your risk of Alzheimer's disease.

12.   Cause hormonal imbalances such as: increasing estrogen in men, exacerbating PMS, and decreasing growth hormone.

13.   Increase platelet adhesion.

14.   Be addictive.

15.   Increase emotional instability.

16.   Cause 2 to 5 times more fat storage than starch.

17.   Promote excessive food intake in obese subjects.

18.   Slow down the ability of your adrenal glands to function.

19.   Cause a significant increase in antisocial behavior in juvenile rehabilitation camps.

WHAT TO DO?

Unfortunately, you cannot starve Lyme Disease bacteria by eliminating sugar from your body because your brain also happens to require sugar to survive. Your body always maintains a level of sugar in the blood (quantified by a medical term called "blood sugar"). If this level drops too low, you'll be unconscious and eventually dead. For the purpose of feeding your brain, your body converts all foods—proteins, fats, and carbohydrates—into sugar. Diabetics are people whose bodies cannot regulate their blood sugar and when it drops too low, they pass out. If they do not get sugar into them they can go into insulin shock and die.

So, avoiding all sugar is impossible because sugar is in the bloodstream at all times. However, although your brain does need sugar, it actually prefers a relatively low, steady supply of it. Too little sugar will starve your brain, but too much sugar will over-stimulate and weaken it. Coincidentally, growth and replication of Lyme Disease bacteria is also greatly (although not completely) slowed when blood sugar levels are kept in a moderate range. In this way, your brain will be most happy, and your Lyme Disease bacteria will have the most difficult time hurting you, if you are careful about how much sugar you eat. This is actually not a small consideration in treating Lyme Disease. It is a very big consideration and can make or break treatment.

So, the goal is not to reduce blood sugar levels to zero (this would kill you), but instead, to keep blood sugar levels moderate and steady. The key to accomplishing this is to avoid processed foods and sugars that cause spikes in blood sugar. These spikes cause accelerated growth and replication of Lyme Disease bacteria and also directly weaken the immune system. In this way, spikes in blood sugar have a 1-2 punch effect: they both increase the strength of the infection and decrease the strength of your defenses. Avoiding processed sugars and, instead, reaching for healthier foods will not completely eliminate sugar from your blood, but it will keep your blood sugar levels in a moderate, healthy zone.

The glycemic index is one tool established to measure whether or not a particular food will cause a spike in blood sugar. Although beyond the scope of this book, it would be valuable for you to learn about the glycemic index and identify foods which you like that have a low glycemic index.

GOOD NEWS FOR SUGAR ADDICTS

If you are beginning to panic because you have a love affair with processed sugar goodies and can't imagine giving them up, you'll be happy to know that there are many sweet and tasty foods which you can still eat. One example of a tasty, sweet food with a low glycemic index is whole fruit, including, for example, blueberries, strawberries, raspberries, oranges, peaches, nectarines, pears, bananas, plums, mangoes, etc. Due to its fiber content and natural, unprocessed state, whole fruit is an acceptable food for people with Lyme Disease to consume.

The important distinction to make is that of processed sugar versus natural sugar. Processed sugar is detrimental to health while natural sugar is helpful to health. It is absolutely essential to stay away from processed sugar, including that found in sugar cereal, sodas and soft drinks, cakes and desserts, candy, etc. When your friends or family are reaching for a piece of birthday cake or a cinnamon roll, you do not have to miss out on the fun—simply grab a peach or a mango and enjoy!

Whole fruits, while permissible, should be consumed in moderation. Two to three moderate sized servings per day is a good rule of thumb. Some people are even able to get away with more. The key is to watch for how you respond to fruit consumption and to note any reactions you might have. Fortunately, of all the mistakes you can make when treating Lyme Disease, consumption of too much sugar is one that will make itself known to you: the increased inflammation and bacterial activity resulting from excess sugar consumption results in a perceptible, acute increase in symptoms. Because of this, it is often very easy to tell when you have overdone it. By this logic, you should be able to increase or decrease your whole fruit consumption based on your personal tolerance.

Fruit juices should be avoided because they separate out the fiber content of fruit. Without intact fiber, the sugar in the fruit juice is rapidly absorbed and causes spikes in blood sugar levels. Fruit juices containing the whole fruit (including pulp) should be approached with caution—it is simply best to eat unaltered, whole fruit.

If you miss drinking sodas, here is a sugar-free, chemical free, great tasting alternative: mix a squirt of 100% lime juice (available at most grocery stores) into a glass of carbonated club soda. The result is a refreshing drink, similar to a Sprite or 7up, which can take the place of sugar sodas (or sugar free sodas that are still off-limits because they contain the toxic, health damaging artificial sweetener known as aspartame). If you have a real sweet tooth, add 3 tablespoons of pomegranate juice to the beverage to give it an exotic, zingy flavor. This drink has become known as a Pom-Yummy in my house, and while it was originally intended for Lymies with limited menus, it quickly became a favorite even with people who indulge in real soda pops.

Appendix C: Interview with Willy Burgdorfer, Ph.D., discoverer of Lyme Disease

Reprinted with permission from:
VECTOR-BORNE AND ZOONOTIC DISEASES
Volume 6, Number 4, 2006
© Mary Ann Liebert, Inc.

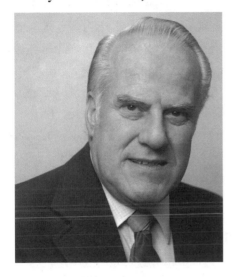

ABOUT WILLY BURGDORFER, PH.D.

Born and Educated in Basel, Switzerland, Willy Burgdorfer earned his Ph.D. in zoology, parasitology, and bacteriology from the University of Basel and from the Swiss Tropical Institute in Basel. As a research subject for his thesis he chose to study the development of the African relapsing fever spirochete, Borrelia duttonii, in its tick vector, Ornitnodoros moubata, and to evaluate this tick's efficiency in transmitting spirochetes during feeding on animal hosts. During his college years, he was a member of a research team investigating outbreaks of Q fever in various parts of Switzerland and became interested in similar research activities carried out at the Rocky Mountain Laboratories (RML) in Hamilton, Montana.

Burgdorfer joined RML in 1952, as a Research Fellow, and later became a Research Associate in the U.S. Public Health Service (U.S.P.H.S.) Visiting Scientist Program. In 1957, he became a U.S. citizen, and shortly thereafter he joined the RML staff as a Medical Entomologist. Throughout his career, Dr. Burgdorfer participated in a number of World Health Organization (WHO) and other health organization-sponsored seminars and congresses. From 1967 to 1972, he served as Associate Member on the Rickettsial Commission of the Armed Forces Epidemiology Board. For several years (1968–1971) he was also Co-Project Officer of the PL 480-

sponsored Research Project on Rickettsial Zoonoses in Egypt and adjacent areas, and from 1979 to 1986, he directed the WHO-sponsored Reference Center for Rickettsial Diseases at RML.

Although retired since 1986, Dr. Burgdorfer continues his association with RML's Laboratory of Human Bacterial Pathogenesis as Scientist Emeritus. Throughout his career, Dr. Burgdorfer has received honors and special recognition for his scientific contributions, including the following: the Schaudinn-Hoffman Plaque (1985, German Society of Dermatologist), Robert Koch Gold Medal (1988, Berlin, Germany), Bristol Award (1989, Infectious Diseases Society of America), Walter Reed Medal (1990, American Society of Tropical Medicine and Hygiene), Doctor Medicina Honoris Causa (1986, University Bern, Switzerland and 1991, University of Marseilles, France).

INTERVIEW BY VICKI GLASER

Dr. Burgdorfer, in 1981, you discovered the tick-borne spirochete that causes Lyme Disease, which was subsequently named Borrelia Burgdorferi. Please describe for our readers the events that led up to that discovery and some of the main challenges and successes in the field and in the laboratory that enabled you to identify this microorganism and describe its lifecycle and mechanism of transmission.

The serendipitous discovery of the Lyme Disease spirochete, now known as Borrelia Burgdorferi, was closely connected with studies on the natural history of spotted fever rickettsiae on Long Island, New York, where, during 1971–1975, a total of 124 cases of spotted fever with eight deaths occurred. Dr. Jorge Benach from the New York State Health Department and I were primarily interested in obtaining a strain of virulent Rickettsia rickettsii from ticks collected near the homes of these patients. Although 6% of Dermacentor variabilis were positive for spotted fever group rickettsiae, none harbored the virulent type of R. rickettsii. They all had R. montana, a rickettsia non-pathogenic for humans. We then speculated that possibly other tick species such as the black-legged deer tick Ixodes dammini, which occurs abundantly on Long Island and its offshore islands, may have had an as yet unestablished role in the ecology of spotted fever. Consequently, hundreds of these ticks were collected and examined by hemolymph testing. Again, none proved infected with virulent R. rickettsii.

In the fall of 1981, Dr. Benach supplied us with additional ticks from Shelter Island. Again, none of 414 males and females had rickettsiae, but the hemolymph of two female ticks contained several microfilariae that were recognized as Dipetalonema rugosicauda, a microfilaria of deer. To determine whether this nematode was also present in other tissues, I dissected both ticks and prepared smears of all their tissues including midgut. No additional microfilariae were found; instead, I encountered poorly stained, rather long, irregularly coiled spirochetes. Dark-field microscopy of additional midgut diverticula confirmed the nature of the organism. Tissues of all other glands (salivary glands, malpighian tubes, ovary, and central ganglion) from both female ticks were free of spirochetes. The antigenic relationship and relatedness of the I. dammini spirochete to the etiological agent of Lyme Disease was established by indirect immunofluorescence and by Western blot of sera from patients recovered from Lyme Disease.

The discovery of this spirochete as the long-sought agent of Lyme Disease and other related disorders was hailed as an important breakthrough that led to a reconnaissance of research on other spirochetal diseases. It soon became clear that spirochetes closely related to B. burgdorferi occur throughout the temperate zone where they are maintained and transmitted by ixodid ticks of the genus Ixodes.

Treatment of Lyme Disease remains problematic. Early Lyme is treatable with antibiotics, whereas late stages require intravenous treatment and long-term applications.

What were your thoughts when you found the spirochete?

I recalled the 1949/1950 discussion by Dr. Hellerström from the Karolinska Institute in Stockholm on the unknown cause of the skin order Erythema chronicum migrans. He pointed out that spirochetes transmitted by the bite(s) of the deer tick Ixodes ricinus may be involved, and he suggested that microbiologists and/or entomologists concentrate their research on the tick digestive system. Nobody followed his suggestion; it took 30 years until we found that midgut tissues of the tick vectors are the principal tissues for the development of the Lyme Disease spirochetes.

Your research on tick-borne bacterial diseases dates back to your Ph.D. dissertation on the development of the African relapsing fever spirochete, Borrelia duttonii and its tick vector, Ornitnodoros moubata. And in Switzerland you were a member of a research team investigating outbreaks of Q fever. What led you to your interest in infectious and, specifically, tick-borne diseases and how did you first become involved in this research area?

As a graduate student, I had the opportunity to join a team of physicians to investigate two cases of Q fever on a farm in the eastern part of Switzerland. My role was to search the patients' premises for ticks and other arthropods and to examine them for Coxiella burnetii, the causative agent of Q fever. Even though I did not find any ticks, I enjoyed playing a part in the study.

How did your earlier doctoral training on relapsing fever borreliae position you to be able to make such an epochal discovery?

My first experience with tick-borne pathogens happened during Professor Rudolf Geigy's study on tick-borne relapsing fever in Tanzania. Interested in the epidemiology of relapsing fever, Geigy undertook several safaris and collected thousands of Ornithodoros moubata, a soft-shelled tick known since the beginning of the century as the vector of Borrelia duttonii, the spirochetal cause of relapsing fever in Africa. Geigy's collections were shipped to the Swiss Tropical Institute in Basel, CH for analysis by the hemolymph test. This test, which I developed, is based on the fact that certain microorganisms like rickettsiae, spirochetes, protozoa, etc., develop in the hemolymph of their vectors. Therefore, a small drop of hemolymph obtained by amputation of a tick's most distant portion of one or more legs smeared on a clean slide and examined by dark-field microscopy may readily reveal the presence of germs, especially spirochetes and rickettsie. The hemolymph test has been a fast, economical, and dependable technique. If applied with care, the test can be performed repeatedly on the same specimen.

Did you ever imagine that your discovery of the Lyme Disease spirochete ultimately would lead to the detection of so many other previously unrecognized tick-borne zoonotic pathogens (e.g., Ehrlichiae, Anaplasma)?

In 1935, French scientists Donatien and Lestoguard described in the blood of dogs a rickettsia-like obligate, intracellular microorganism that initially was named Rickettsia canis and renamed Ehrlichia canis (in honor of the German Microbiologist Dr. Paul Ehrlich) and was recognized as the cause of canine ehrlichiosis.

Today, the genus Ehrlichiosis contains at least eight species pathogenic for domestic animals such as dogs, horses, and cattle. Three species, E. sennetsu, E. ehaffeensis, and phagocytophila are pathogenic for humans.

All species known so far are tick-borne and occur in cycles including ixodid ticks and their hosts. Ecological and epidemiologic studies have named the deer tick Amblyomma americanum as the vector of Ehrlichia chaffeensis, whereas granulocytic ehrlichiosis is maintained and disseminated by the black-legged deer tick Ixodes scapularis and Dermacentor andersoni as well as Ixodes persulcatus in California. As yet no detailed studies have been made on the development of ehrlichiae in these tick species.

Dr. Burgdorfer, looking back on your long and distinguished career, what would you highlight as some of your key discoveries and accomplishments?

The majority of my 227 scientific publications deal with the ecology of arthropod-borne diseases and with the vector/pathogen relationship such as development and transmission of pathogens to their hosts. A list of key discoveries and accomplishments would include the following:

- Analyse des Infektionsverlaufes bei Ornithodoros moubata (Murray), und der Berücksichtigung der naturlichen Ubertragung von Spirochaeta duttoni [in German]. Acta Trop. 1951;8:193–262.

- Isolation of the Colorado tick fever virus from ticks (Dermacentor andersoni) and hosts. Published in: Studies on the ecology of Colorado tick fever virus in western Montana. Am. J. Hyg. 1959;69:127–137.

- Fluorescent microscopy successfully applied to other bacterial and viral agents. Published in: Identification of Rickettsia rickettsii in the wood tick, Dermacentor andersoni, by means of fluorescent antibody. J. Infect. Dis. 1960; 107:241–244.

- First isolation from a host other than humans; led to ecological studies of this virus in mosquitoes. Published in: Isolation of California encephalitis virus from the blood of a snowshoe hare (Lepus americanus) in western Montana. Am. J. Hyg. 1961;73:344–349.

- First isolation from mammals west of the Mississippi. Published in: Ecology of Rocky Mountain spotted fever in western Montana. I. Isolation of Rickettsia rickettsii from wild mammals. Am. J. Hyg. 1962;76:293–301.

- Investigation of "transovarial transmission" of Rickettsia rickettsii in the wood tick, Dermacentor andersoni. Exp Parasitol. 1963;14: 152–159.

- Very important finding and most popular paper. Published in: Transstadial and transovarial development of disease agents in arthropods. In: Smith RF, Mittler TE, eds. Annual Review of Entomology. Palo Alto, CA: Annual Reviews, Inc., 1967;12:347–376.

- Very popular paper describing the hemolymph test. Published in: Hemolymph test. A technique for detection of rickettsiae in ticks. Am. J. Trop. Med. 1970;19:1010–1014.

- Rocky Mountain spotted fever (tick-borne typhus) in South Carolina: an educational program and tick/rickettsial survey in 1973 and 1974. Am. J. Trop. Med. Hyg. 1975;24: 866–872.

- Microimmunofluorescence test for the serological study of Rocky Mountain spotted fever and typhus. J. Clin. Microbiol. 1976;3: 51–61.

- Lyme Disease—a tick-borne spirochetosis? Science 1982;216:1317–1319.

- Discovery of the Lyme Disease spirochete and its relation to tick vectors. Yale J. Biol. Med. 1984;57:515–520.

- How the discovery of Borrelia Burgdorferi came about. Clin. Dermatol. 1993;11:335–338.

- Arthropod-borne spirochetoses: a historical perspective [Editorial]. Eur. J. Clin. Microbiol.Infect. Dis. 2001;20:5.

What experiences and events led you to join Rocky Mountain Laboratories (RML) and to come to the United States to pursue your research interests?

During most of the last century, RML has enjoyed a worldwide reputation as the center for vector-borne pathogens, primarily rickettsiae, spirochetes, and tick-borne viruses. Having the opportunity to conduct research in one of RML's units or in the field was the dream of many young European medical entomologists. This dream came true for me when, in 1951, I was awarded a U.S. Public Health Service Visiting Fellowship to join RML's Dr. Gordon E. Davis in a study on the taxonomy of relapsing fever spirochetes.

Years came and years went, but after 52 years of research on multiple scientific problems and 227 publications, I am still associated with RML as a Scientist Emeritus, trying to understand the complex vector-pathogen relationship of human and animal diseases.

Who were some of your mentors and key collaborators during your career?

The most important mentors and supporters of my research included (but are not limited to) the following individuals:

- Professor Rudolf Geigy, Director, Swiss Tropical Institute, Basel, CH

- Professor T. Tomesik, Director, Hygiene Institute, Basel, Switzerland

- Professor H. Mooser, Director, Hygiene Institute, Zurich, Switzerland

- Dr. H. Baltazard, Institute Pasteur, Teheran, Iran

- Dr. Gordon E. Davis, Rocky Mountain Labs

- Dr. C.B. Philip, Rocky Mountain Labs

- Dr. C. Eklund, Rocky Mountain Labs

- Dr. J. Smadell, Rocky Mountain Labs/NIAID

- Dr. J. Benatch, New York State Health Department

- Dr. R.N. Philip, Rocky Mountain Labs

There is a tick genome project ongoing at present. What are the key areas that will benefit from this work, and how will this influence our understanding of tick-borne pathogens?

The genome of ticks has been established, and a defense protein ("Defensin") has been isolated. It is being evaluated as to its effect on the development of tick-borne pathogens in Ixodes dammini and Dermacentor variabilis.

The Rocky Mountain laboratories are undergoing major construction at the moment. What types of research will be conducted there in the future and how will this address the RML's mission of developing diagnostics, vaccines and therapeutics for tick-borne pathogens?

The B-4 level unit at RML nears completion. As yet no information on projects planned is available.

Appendix D: Bibliography

The following are books I relied on in the writing of this book. I highly recommend these books as further resources.

Alkalize or Die
Dr. Theadore A. Baroody
ISBN: 0961959533
Published by Holographic Health Press

Amalgam Illness: Diagnosis and Treatment
Andrew Hall Cutler, Ph.D.
ISBN: 0967616808
Published by Andrew Hall Cutler, Ph.D.

Angel of the Northwoods
J.A.N.
ISBN: Not Available

Antibiotic Prescribing Guide
ISBN: Not Available
Published by PDR

Cancer Cure That Worked!, The
Barry Lynes
ISBN: 0919951309
Published by Marcus Books

Chitosan: The Ultimate Health Builder
Akira Matsunaga, M.D., Ph.D.
ISBN: 0533126290
Published by Vantage Press

Coyote Medicine
Lewis Mehl-Madrona, M.D.
ISBN: 0684839970
Published by Fireside/Simon and Schuster

Detoxify or Die
Sherry A. Rogers, M.D.
ISBN: 1887202048
Published by Sand Key Company

Diagnosis and Treatment of Babesia, The
James Schaller, M.D.
ISBN: 0978747372
Published by Hope Academic Press

Eating Well for Optimum Health
Andrew Weil, M.D.
ISBN: 0375407545
Published by Alfred A. Knopf

Hair Test Interpretation: Finding Hidden Toxicities
Andrew Hall Cutler, Ph.D.
ISBN: 0967616816
Published by Andrew Hall Cutler, Ph.D.

Handbook of Rife Frequency Healing, The
Nenah Sylver, Ph.D.
ISBN: 0966835239
Published by The Center for Frequency

Healing Lyme
Stephen Buhner
ISBN: 0970869630
Published by Raven Press

Holistic Handbook of Sauna Therapy, The
Nenah Sylver, Ph.D.
ISBN: 0967249171
Published by The Center for Frequency

Hydrogen Peroxide: Medical Miracle
William Campbell Douglass, M.D.
ISBN: 1885236077
Published by Second Opinion Publishing

Microbiology and Infectious Diseases
Gabriel Virella
ISBN: 0683062352
Published by Williams & Wilkins

Mold Illness and Mold Remediation Made Simple
James Schaller, M.D. and Gary Rosen, Ph.D.
ISBN: 0978747364
Published by Hope Academic Press

Mucusless Diet Healing System
Arnold Ehret
ISBN: 0879040041
Published by Beneficial Books

Nutritional Balancing and Hair Mineral Analysis
Lawrence Wilson, M.D.
ISBN: 0962865745
Published by L.D. Wilson Consultants

Outsmart Your Cancer
Tanya Harter Pierce
ISBN: 0972886737
Published by Thoughtworks Publishing

Owner's Manual for the Human Body, The
Saul Pressman, DCh
ISBN: Not Available
Published by Plasmafire International

PDR for Nutritional Supplements
ISBN: 1563633647
Published by Medical Economics/Thomson
Healthcare

PDR for Herbal Medicines
ISBN: 1563633612
Published by Medical Economics/Thomson
Healthcare

Pharmacology, 2nd Edition
M. Mycek, R. Harvey and P. Champe
ISBN: 0397515677
Published by Lippincott-Raven

Prescription for Nutritional Healing

James F. Balch, M.D. and Phyllis A. Balch,
C.N.C.
ISBN: 0895297272
Published by Avery

Rational Fasting
Arnold Ehret
ISBN: 087904005X
Published by Beneficial Books

Sauna Therapy
Lawrence Wilson, M.D.
ISBN: 0962865761
Published by L.D. Wilson Consultants

Therapeutic Manual
Ed Smith
ISBN: Not Available
Published by Ed Smith

Tired So Tired and the Yeast Connection
William G. Crook, M.D.
ISBN: 0933278259
Published by Professional Books

Training Manual for the Ozone Hyperthermic
Technician
Saul Pressman, DCh
ISBN: Not Available
Published by Plasmafire International

Understanding Nutrition
Eleanor N. Whitney and Sharon R. Rolfes
ISBN: 0534546129
Published by West/Wadsworth

Appendix E: Web sites listed by topic

EDUCATIONAL BOOKS, VIDEOS AND DVDS

Lymebook.com/catalog—Publishers of the book you hold in your hands, Lymebook.com also offers other Lyme Disease educational resources, including books, videos, and software. This is the Lymebook.com Online Store. Lymebook.com is a subsidiary of BioMed Publishing Group.

Lymebook.com—Learn more about rife machine therapy in the treatment of Lyme Disease.

Lymebook.com/conference—DVD containing video of Bryan Rosner's presentation at the 2006 Rife International Health Conference in Seattle, WA. Also contains video of Bryan Rosner's interview with Doug MacLean at the same conference. Doug is the "father" of modern rife technology as used to fight Lyme Disease; he was the first person ever to use a rife machine for this purpose. In fact, he invented the first modern rife machine used for Lyme Disease: the Coil Machine. You can read Doug's story in *Lyme Disease and Rife Machines.* Visit www.lymebook.com/conference to learn more about the DVD and see pictures from the conference.

Lymebook.com/babesia—Book entitled *The Diagnosis and Treatment of Babesia: Lyme's Cruel Cousin—The Other Tick-Borne Infection,* written by James Schaller, M.D., on the diagnosis and treatment of Babesia, with which one of his own children suffered.

Lymebook.com/mercury—Book entitled *Amalgam Illness: Diagnosis and Treatment.* The book focuses on diagnosing and treating mercury poisoning. It was written by Andrew Cutler, Ph.D., a chemical engineer who himself had mercury poisoning, figured out how to get well, and wrote this book to help others do the same.

Lymebook.com/hair—Also by Andrew Cutler, Ph.D., this book is entitled *Hair Test Interpretation, Finding Hidden Toxicities,* and was written to help patients interpret their hair tests to look for a variety of potential toxicities and dysregulations.

Lymebook.com/rifehandbook—Written by Nenah Sylver, Ph.D., this book is entitled *The Handbook of Rife Frequency Healing*, and is considered to be the authoritative textbook on principles of rife frequency healing. Weighing over 2lbs, this large book is thorough and comprehensive.

Lymebook.com/marshallprotocol—4 DVD set with a wealth of information on the Marshall Protocol (see Chapter 2 of this book), including video of Dr. Trevor Marshall explaining the protocol, and panel sessions with patients describing their experiences.

Lymebook.com/powerpoint—Microsoft PowerPoint presentation on CD with instructions for building a Coil Machine, which is the machine invented by Doug MacLean (see Chapter 5). The Coil Machine is believed to be the most helpful rife machine for fighting Lyme Disease.

Lymebook.com/sauna.htm—*Sauna Therapy*, written by Lawrence Wilson, M.D., is an excellent book on how to use a sauna for detoxification and healing.

Lymebook.com/cancercure—Investigative journalism at its best. Barry Lynes, author of *The Cancer Cure That Worked,* takes readers on an exciting and mysterious journey into the life work of Royal Raymond Rife, inventor of the rife machine. This book reveals the history and healing power of energy medicine. An excellent complementary book to go along with *Lyme Disease and Rife Machines.*

Lymebook.com/rifevideo—The Rife Research Group of Canada is the producer of this excellent, informative and objective 2-part video documentary on the history, life work, and relationships of Royal Raymond Rife.

Lymebook.com/top10book—Website for the book you hold in your hands—read excerpts and order the book.

INTERNET MESSAGE BOARDS

Lymecommunity.com—The central hub for discussion of Lyme-related topics. Visit this site first. Also includes a blog written by a former nurse and member of the Lyme community. Lots of helpful features and resources.

Lymenet.org—The Lyme Disease Network of New Jersey, one of the internet's largest Lyme Disease resource web sites, including lots of information and a very active internet discussion group (10,000+ members).

Groups.yahoo.com—Search for internet discussion groups using keywords. Helpful for finding online Lyme support groups in your area, or any other group you may be interested in.

Lymebook.com/resources—From this page you can access the Lyme-and-rife Yahoo! discussion group, which has over 2,000 members. The group focuses on discussion of rife machine therapy but also covers numerous related topics. This page also provides access to several other discussion groups and internet-based resources. One of the groups you will have access to is the "frequent-dose-chelation" group, which examines various ways to remove mercury from the body, including the method invented by Andrew Cutler, Ph.D. (see www.lymebook.com/mercury).

INDIVIDUAL TREATMENTS

Marshallprotocol.com—One of the most effective Lyme Disease treatment protocols. This web site includes a free online discussion group with more than 3000 people, free instructions for using the protocol, and referrals to doctors who understand the protocol and are willing to prescribe it to patients.

Lymephotos.com—This is the original web site documenting the Salt / Vitamin C treatment for Lyme Disease. The web site chronicles both patient experiences and scientific information substantiating the protocol.

There are many interesting photos documenting various bacteria and parasites.

RIFE MACHINE THERAPY

Lymebook.com/resources—Access the Lyme-and-rife internet discussion forum here. This discussion group has more than 2,000 members and is the primary hub for discussing and learning about rife machine therapy as a treatment for Lyme Disease.

Lymebook.com/machinesources—Website with contact information for manufacturers of the rife devices discussed in *Lyme Disease and Rife Machines*.

Rifeconference.com—Website for the *Annual Rife International Health Conference*, coordinated by Richard Lloyd, Ph.D. This conference is typically held in October in the Seattle area and includes a product expo and numerous highly qualified speakers. Past speakers have included Hulda Clark, Nenah Sylver, Ph.D., Richard Lloyd, Ph.D., Henry Lai, Ph.D., and other experts in the field.

Royalrife.com—The website of Richard Loyd, Ph.D., a nutritionist and rife therapy expert in Seattle, WA. This website has numerous useful resources, including a used rife equipment for-sale board. This is one of the best and most accurate sources of information on rife treatments for many diseases.

Info.lymebook.com/listings—Dozens of personal stories from people using rife machines to fight Lyme Disease.

MISCELLANEOUS WEBSITES

Ilads.org—International Lyme and Associated Diseases Society. One of the largest Lyme Disease organizations in the world, this group offers dozens of resources for patients and practitioners. This is one of the most important Lyme Disease organizations, and many LLMDs are members.

Lyme.org—The Lyme Disease Foundation.

Canlyme.com—Canadian Lyme Disease Foundation.

Tiquatac.org—French Lyme Disease organization.

Lymediseaseaction.org.uk—UK Lyme Disease organization.

Lyme.org/resources/dr_ref.html—Obtain a referral to a Lyme Literate Medical Doctor (LLMD).

Lymedisease.org—California Lyme Disease Association.

Future-drugs.com—Discover new antibiotics and other drugs on the horizon.

Lymediseaseaudio.com—Excellent collection of Lyme-related audio clips.

Lymebook.com/lymelinks—Thousands of organized Lyme-related links.

Lymeinfo.net—One of the most complete, accurate and user-friendly databases of Lyme Disease information. Don't miss this site!

Lymeinfo.net/lymefiles.html—Organized summaries of dozens of Lyme Disease research studies.

Publichealthalert.org—Recently launched, printed Lyme Disease newsletter, with excellent and relevant content. The newsletter is printed once a month, and you can mail order issues for just the cost of shipping.

Lymebook.com/lymenews—Get free, up-to-the-minute Lyme Disease news headlines from newspapers across the country. This site is updated continuously so each time you visit, there will be fresh information.

Lymebook.com/mercurynews—Get free, up-to-the-minute mercury poisoning news headlines from newspapers across the country. This site is updated continuously so each time you visit, there will be fresh information.

www.ncbi.nlm.nih.gov/entrez/—One of the most useful web sites on the internet, this is the public access point for Pub Med, also known as MEDLINE, which indexes thousands of published scientific studies conducted by The National Library of Medicine, National Institutes Of Health, and affiliated research organizations throughout the world. When you visit this web site you will have at your fingertips the capability to search by keyword through the majority of major and minor scientific studies conducted by universities, private medical research groups, and other scientific institutions across the globe.

Betterhealthguy.com—This web site is run by a Lyme Disease sufferer who is engaged in advanced research into products and protocols benefiting Lyme Disease sufferers. The web site is a clearinghouse for excellent information. There is a free monthly e-mail newsletter which includes updated research and new findings.

Nenahsylver.com—Website of Nenah Sylver, Ph.D., author of two excellent books: *The Holistic Handbook of Sauna Therapy* and *The Handbook of Rife Frequency Healing.*

Npjulie.com—Website of Julie Anderson, ARNP, a nurse practitioner in Seattle, WA, who offers high-quality and knowledgeable healthcare services to patients with complex illnesses such as Lyme Disease and mercury poisoning.

Igenex.com—One of the more advanced and accurate Lyme Disease testing laboratories.

Lymebook.com/resources—This is the information repository for Lymebook.com. It offers numerous links to a vast array of Lyme-related sites.

Lymebook.com/newsletter—Subscribe to the email newsletter that is edited by Bryan Rosner! Also, view past newsletters in .html format.

Plasmafire.com—Manufacturer of high-quality ozone saunas.

Ozonegenerator.com—Manufacturer of high-quality ozone equipment.

Iherb.com—one of the internet's most affordable retailers of nutritional supplements.

Personalconsult.com—Website of James Schaller, M.D., writer of the Foreword of this book, and a prolific Lyme Disease author and LLMD.

Neuraltherapy.com—Website of Dietrich Klinghardt, M.D., Ph.D., Lyme Disease expert and physician located in the Seattle area.

Doctorsdata.com—Company that provides interpretation of toxic element hair tests. Many people with Lyme Disease have toxic levels of dangerous minerals in their bodies, such as mercury, cadmium, lead, and arsenic. This company offers hair tests that look for these dangerous elements. See www.lymebook.com/hair for more information on interpreting theses tests.

Greatplainslaboratory.com—Company that provides interpretation of toxic elements hair tests. Many people with Lyme Disease have toxic levels of dangerous minerals in their bodies, such as mercury, cadnium, lead and arsenic. This company offers hair tests that look for these dangerous elements. See www.lymebook.com/hair for more information on interpreting theses tests.

Remedyfind.com—This website has user ratings of dozens of different remedies for numerous health conditions. The site is well-organized and user-friendly. It was founded by a sufferer of chronic disease.

Lymememorial.org—A website dedicated to people who have died as a result of tick-borne infections (and associated complications). More than just a memorial, this site offers scientific documentation (journal citations, articles, and autopsy reports) of cases in which Lyme Disease and its co-infections were actually responsible for fatalities. This information is invaluable to show to friends, families, and physicians, especially those who may be unfamiliar with the severity of Lyme Disease or, worse, belittle the disease as an inconsequential health problem. Don't miss this site!

LEF.org—founded in 1980, the Life Extension Foundation provides information and high-quality supplements. Their web site offers a vast array of cutting-edge articles and studies examining numerous health related issues, with special focus on "radical extension of the healthy human life-span" (their mission statement). A nonprofit organization, Life Extension Foundation is unbiased and reliable.

Their homepage features daily news, summaries of breakthrough research, consumer action alerts, and tidbits of information useful to anyone who wants to stay healthy. Particularly valuable is their shrewd and objective perspective on the FDA, the pharmaceutical industry, and other entities which wield power in the arena of medicine.

One of the most valuable components of their web site is the Innovative Doctors Directory, which offers free referrals to physicians in your local area who practice rational and holistic medicine. This information can be invaluable to someone looking for a health care practitioner who can provide flexible, integrative medical care.

Also incredibly useful is LEF's Innovative Clinic Directory, which provides a description of and contact information for dozens of the best alternative health clinics throughout the world. This resource is valuable for several reasons. First, many of these international clinics offer types of therapies that are not available in the United States due to U.S. government regulations. Second, a significant number of clinics located outside the United States are nearly impossible to discover without a direct referral because these clinics often keep a low profile. Many of them also do not have web sites, so internet searches do not reveal them.

The web site's free "E Adviser" allows you to view specific treatment protocols for a number of different health conditions. These articles offer background information about the condition, suggested supplements, recommended reading, and safety caveats (supplements or activities to be avoided).

Two professional advisory boards, one scientific and one medical, are employed by the Life Extension Foundation. Experts on these boards include numerous MDs and Ph.D.s who offer guidance in researching and producing new products and articles.

The Life Extension Foundation also publishes an excellent monthly magazine. Unlike some other, free alternative health magazines, this one is not just an advertising vehicle in disguise—a regular subscription costs $40 per year, and the magazine's content is accurate and informative. If you become a member of the Life Extension Foundation, a subscription is included. Membership costs $75/year and comes with numerous benefits including access to a toll-free health advisory phone number, a significant discount on supplements, a 1665 page reference book called *Disease Prevention and Treatment*, and other benefits. Because the Life Extension Foundation is a nonprofit organization, a significant portion of your membership dues are fed directly into various research projects. Life Extension Foundation projects have had great success in the past—dozens of scientific breakthroughs which we take for granted today were actually made possible by research funded by the Life Extension Foundation.

Appendix F: Websites listed by chapter

Browse this list to ensure that you have visited the websites you are interested in. Instead of scanning the entire book for websites to visit, this list provides a handy shortcut for seeing the websites discussed in the book. If you are interested in additional websites not included in the content of the book, see the Appendix section immediately previous to this one.

FOREWORD BY JAMES SCHALLER, M.D.

www.personalconsult.com—Website of James Schaller, M.D.

INFORMATION FOR THE READER

www.lymecommunity.com—Internet discussion forum
www.lymenet.org—Internet discussion forum
www.google.com—Search engine
www.wikipedia.com—Encyclopedia with entries for rare words/phrases
www.lymebook.com/resources—Books, videos, links related to this book

CHAPTER 1: THE ANTIBIOTIC ROTATION PROTOCOL

www.thefallspharmacy.com—Compounding pharmacy in Seattle, WA
www.silvermedicine.org—Further information on colloidal silver
www.silver-colloids.com—Further information on colloidal silver
silverlist.org—Colloidal silver discussion forum
health.groups.yahoo.com/group/colloidalsilver—Discussion forum
health.groups.yahoo.com/group/colloidalsilver2—Discussion forum
www.nutramedix.com—Learn about and purchase Samento
www.nutricology.com—Allergy Research Group
www.ameriden.com—Learn about and purchase olive leaf extract
www.eastparkresearch.com—Learn about and purchase olive leaf extract
www.jeansgreens.com—Learn about and purchase Sarsaparilla
www.sourcenaturals.com—Many vitamins and supplements
www.nutriteam.com—Learn about and purchase grapefruit seed extract
www.lauricidin.com—Learn about and purchase lauric acid (from coconut)

CHAPTER 2: THE MARSHALL PROTOCOL

www.marshallprotocol.com—Learn about and discuss the protocol
www.lymeinfo.net—Repository of dozens of Lyme-related scientific studies

CHAPTER 3: THE SALT / VITAMIN C PROTOCOL

www.lymephotos.com—Learn about the Salt / Vitamin C protocol
www.lymebook.com/resources—Salt/C discussion group and E-book
www.realsalt.com—Learn about and purchase natural, healthy salt

CHAPTER 4: DETOXIFICATION

www.drcranton.com—Pioneering alternative M.D., clinic in Yelm, WA
www.rifeconference.com—Annual Rife International Health Conference
www.curezone.com—Many discussion forums and info about liver cleanse
www.chronicneurotoxins.com—Dr. Shoemaker's website
www.ncbi.nlm.nih.gov/entrez—Search thousands of scientific studies
www.traceminerals.com—Learn about and purchase ConcenTrace minerals

CHAPTER 5: ELECTROMEDICINE (RIFE MACHINE THERAPY)

www.lymebook.com—Learn about and purchase Rosner's first book
www.lymebook.com/conference—DVD of the 2006 Rife Conference
www.lymebook.com/resources—Links and resources related to this book
www.amazon.com—Online bookseller

CHAPTER 6: SYSTEMIC ENZYMES

www.ncbi.nlm.nih.gov/entrez—Search thousands of scientific studies
www.renewlife.com—Digestive enzymes and digestive support

CHAPTER 7: MANGOSTEEN

www.mangosteenstories.org—Mangosteen user reports
www.ncbi.nlm.nih.gov/entrez—Search thousands of scientific studies

www.xango.com—Learn about and purchase mangosteen juice

CHAPTER 9: COENZYME Q-10

www.pubmed.com—Search thousands of scientific studies
www.LEF.org—Life Extension Foundation

CHAPTER 10: MAGNESIUM

www.nutricology.com—Learn about and purchase magnesium chloride
www.lymecommunity.com—Online discussion group

CHAPTER 11: BUILDING A TREATMENT PLAN

www.lymenet.org—Discussion forum with over 10,000 members
www.lymebook.com/resources—Links and resources related to this book
www.lymecommunity.com—Online discussion group

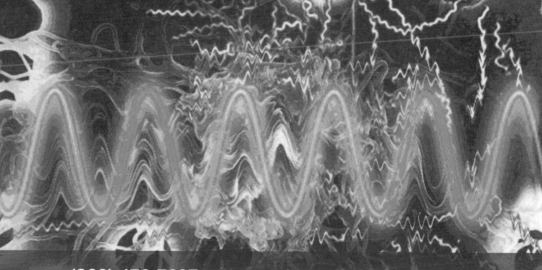

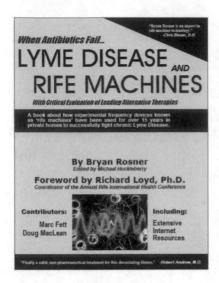

Book • $35

When Antibiotics Fail: Lyme Disease And Rife Machines, With Critical Evaluation Of Leading Alternative Therapies

By Bryan Rosner
Foreword by Richard Loyd, Ph.D.

There are enough books and websites about what Lyme Disease is and which ticks carry it. But there is very little useful information for people who actually have a case of Lyme Disease that is not responding to conventional antibiotic treatment. Lyme Disease sufferers need to know how to get better, not how to identify a tick.

This book describes how electromagnetic frequency devices known as rife machines have been used for over 15 years in private homes to successfully fight Lyme Disease. Also included are evaluations of more than 20 conventional and alternative Lyme Disease therapies, including:

- Homeopathy
- IV and oral antibiotics
- Mercury detox.
- Hyperthermia / saunas
- Ozone and oxygen
- Samento®
- Colloidal Silver
- Bacterial die-off detox.
- Colostrum
- Magnesium supplementation
- Hyperbaric oxygen chamber (HBOC)
- ICHT Italian treatment
- Non-pharmaceutical antibiotics
- Exercise, diet and candida protocols
- Cyst-targeting antibiotics
- The Marshall Protocol®

Many Lyme Disease sufferers have heard of rife machines, some have used them. But until now there has not been a concise and reliable source to explain how and why they work, and how and why other therapies fail. In the book you will learn that rife machine therapy offers numerous advantages over antibiotic therapy, including sustained effectiveness, affordability, convenience, autonomy from the medical establishment, and avoidance of candida complications.

The Foreword for the book is by Richard Loyd, Ph.D., coordinator of the annual Rife International Health Conference. The book takes a practical, down-to-earth approach which allows you to learn about:

> "This book provides life-saving insights for Lyme Disease patients."
>
> **- Richard Loyd, Ph.D.**

- Why rife machines work after other therapies fail, with analysis of antibiotics.
- Rife machine treatment schedules and sessions.
- The most effective rife machines: High Power Magnetic Pulser, EMEM Machine, Coil Machine, and AC Contact Machine.
- Explanation of the "herx reaction" and why it indicates progress.
- Evaluation of leading alternative therapies.
- Antibiotic categories and classifications, and which antibiotics are most efficacious.
- What it feels like to use rife machines – discover the steps to healing!

Paperback book, 8.5 x 11", 203 pages, $35

To order, click www.LymeBookStore.com or call (801) 925-2411
NOTE: Website and phone number are for ordering only, not medical advice.

The Top 10 Lyme Disease Treatments: Defeat Lyme Disease With The Best Of Conventional And Alternative Medicine

By Bryan Rosner
Foreword by James Schaller, M.D.

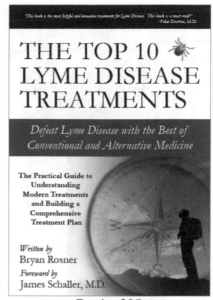

Published in 2007, Rosner's newest book identifies ten cutting-edge conventional and alternative Lyme Disease treatments and gives practical guidance on integrating them into a comprehensive treatment plan that maximizes therapeutic benefit while minimizing side effects.

This book was not written to replace Bryan Rosner's first book (*Lyme Disease and Rife Machines*). Instead, it was written to complement that book, offering Lyme sufferers many new foundational and supportive treatments to use during the recovery process. New treatments and information in this book include:

Book • $35

- Systemic enzyme therapy, which helps detoxify tissues and blood, reduce inflammation, stimulate the immune system, and kill Lyme Disease bacteria.
- Lithium orotate, a powerful yet all-natural mineral (belonging to the same mineral group as sodium and potassium) capable of profound neuroprotective activity.
- Thorough and extensive coverage of a complete Lyme Disease detoxification program, including discussion of both liver and skin detoxification pathways. Specific detoxification therapies such as liver cleanses, bowel cleanses, the Shoemaker Neurotoxin Elimination Protocol, sauna therapy, mineral baths, mineral supplementation, milk thistle, and many others. How to reduce and control herx reactions.
- Tips and clinical research from James Schaller, M.D.
- A detailed look at how to properly utilize antibiotics during a rife machine treatment campaign.
- Wide coverage of the Marshall Protocol, including an in-depth description of its mechanism of action in relation to Lyme Disease pathology. Also, coverage of Vitamin D and the debate surrounding this unique, fat-soluble vitamin.
- An explanation of and new information about the Salt / Vitamin C protocol.
- Hot-off-the-press information on mangosteen fruit (not to be confused with mango) and its many benefits, including antibacterial, anti-inflammatory, and anti-cancer properties.
- New guidelines for combining all the therapies discussed in both of Rosner's books into a complete treatment plan. Brief and articulate with step-by-step instructions for healing.
- Also includes updates on rife therapy, cutting-edge supplements, new political challenges, an exclusive interview with Willy Burgdorfer (who discovered Lyme), and so much more!

"Bryan Rosner thinks big and this new book offers big solutions."
- James Schaller, M.D.

"Another ground-breaking Lyme Disease book."
- Jeff Mittelman, moderator of the Lyme-and-rife group

"Brilliant and thorough."
- Nenah Sylver, Ph.D.

Do not miss this top Lyme Disease resource. Discover new healing tools today!

Paperback book, 7 x 10", 367 pages, $35

To order, click www.LymeBookStore.com or call (801) 925-2411
NOTE: Website and phone number are for ordering only, not medical advice.

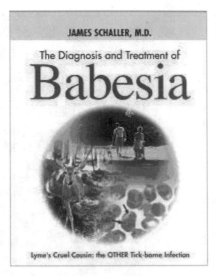

Book • $35

The Diagnosis and Treatment of Babesia: Lyme's Cruel Cousin – The Other Tick-Borne Infection

By James Schaller, M.D.

Do you or a loved one experience excess fatigue? Have you ever had unusually high fevers, chills, or sweats? You may have Babesia, a very common tick-borne infection. Babesia is often found with Lyme Disease and, like all tick-borne infections, is rarely diagnosed and reported accurately.

The deer tick which carries Lyme Disease and Babesia may be as small as a poppy seed and injects a painkiller, an antihistamine, and an anticoagulant to avoid detection. As a result, many people have Babesia and do not know it. Numerous forms of Babesia are carried by ticks - this book introduces patients and health care workers to the various species that infect humans and are not routinely tested for by sincere physicians.

Dr. Schaller, who practices medicine in Florida, first became interested in Babesia after one of his own children was infected with it. None of the elite pediatricians or child specialists could help. No one tested for Babesia or considered it a possible diagnosis. His child suffered from just two of these typical Babesia symptoms:

- Significant Fatigue
- Coughing
- Dizziness
- Trouble Thinking
- Fevers
- Memory Loss

- Chills
- Air Hunger
- Headache
- Sweats
- Unresponsiveness to Lyme Treatment

With 396 pages, this book is the most current and comprehensive book on Babesia in the English language. It reviews thousands of articles and presents the results of interviews with world experts on the subject. It offers you top information and broad treatment options, presented in a clear and simple manner. All treatments are explained thoroughly, including their possible side effects, drug interactions, various dosing strategies, pros/cons, and physician experiences.

"Once again Dr. Schaller has provided us with a much-needed and practical resource. This book gave me exactly what I was looking for."

- Thomas W.

Finally, the book also addresses many other aspects of practical medical care often overlooked in this infection, such as treatment options for managing fatigue. Plainly stated, this book is a must-have for patients and health care providers who deal with Lyme Disease and its co-infections. Dr. Schaller's many years in clinical practice give the book a practical angle that many other similar books lack. Don't miss this user-friendly resource!

Paperback book, 7 x 10", 374 pages, $35

To order, click www.LymeBookStore.com or call (801) 925-2411
NOTE: Website and phone number are for ordering only, not medical advice.

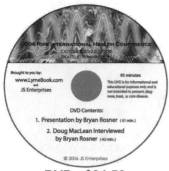

DVD • $24.50

2006 Annual Rife International Health Conference DVD (93 Minutes)

Bryan Rosner's Presentation and Interview with Doug MacLean

Conf. Dates: October 20-22, 2006
Conf. Location: Seattle, WA, USA

If you were unable to attend the 2006 Rife Conference, this DVD is your opportunity to catch up on two of the presentations that took place at the conference:

Presentation #1: Bryan Rosner's Sunday morning talk entitled *Lyme Disease: New Paradigms in Diagnosis and Treatment - the Myths, the Reality, and the Road Back to Health.* (51 minutes)

Presentation #2: Bryan Rosner's interview with Doug MacLean, in which Doug talked about his experiences with Lyme Disease, including the incredible journey he undertook to invent the first modern rife machine used to fight Lyme Disease. Although Doug's journey as a Lyme Disease pioneer took place 20 years ago, this was the first time Doug has ever accepted an invitation to appear in public. This is the only video available where you can see Doug talk about what it was like to be the first person ever to use rife technology as a treatment for Lyme Disease. Now you can see how it all began. Own this DVD and own a piece of history! (42 minutes)

Lymebook.com has secured a special licensing agreement with JS Enterprises, the Canadian producer of the Rife Conference videos, to bring this product to you at the special low price of $24.50. Total DVD viewing time: 1 hour, 33 minutes. We have DVDs in stock, shipped to you within 3 business days.

Price Comparison (should you get the DVD?)

Cost of attending the 2006 Rife Conference (2 people):
Hotel Room, 3 Nights = $400
Registration = $340
Food = $150
Airfare = $600
Total = $1,490

Cost of the DVD, which you can view as many times as you want, and show to family and friends:
DVD = $24.50

Bryan Rosner
Presenting on
Sunday Morning

DVD
93 Minutes
$24.50

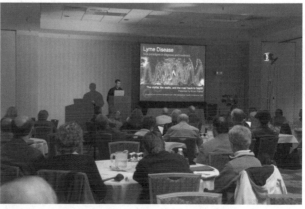

To order, click www.LymeBookStore.com or call (801) 925-2411
NOTE: Website and phone number are for ordering only, not medical advice.

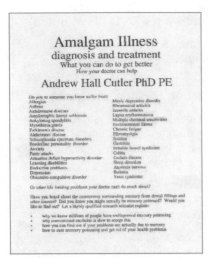

Book • $35

Amalgam Illness, Diagnosis and Treatment: What You Can Do to Get Better, How Your Doctor Can Help

By Andrew Cutler, PhD

This book was written by a chemical engineer who himself got mercury poisoning from his amalgam dental fillings. He found that there was no suitable educational material for either the patient or the physician. Knowing how much people can suffer from this condition, he wrote this book to help them get well. With a PhD in chemistry from Princeton University and extensive study in biochemistry and medicine, Andrew Cutler uses layman's terms to explain how people become mercury poisoned and what to do about it.

Mercury poisoning can easily be cured with over-the-counter oral chelators – this book explains how.

In the book you will find practical guidance on how to tell if you really have chronic mercury poisoning or some other problem. Proper diagnostic procedures are provided so that sick people can decide what is wrong rather than trying random treatments. If mercury poisoning is your problem, the book tells you how to get the mercury out of your body, and how to feel good while you do that. The treatment section gives step-by-step directions to figure out exactly what mercury is doing to you and how to fix it.

"Dr. Cutler uses his background in chemistry to explain the safest approach to treat mercury poisoning. I am a physician and am personally using his protocol on myself."

- Melissa Myers, M.D.

Sections also explain how the scientific literature shows many people must be getting poisoned by their amalgam fillings, why such a regulatory blunder occurred, and how the debate between "mainstream" and "alternative" medicine makes it more difficult for you to get the medical help you need.

This down-to-earth book lets patients take care of themselves. It also lets doctors who are not familiar with chronic mercury intoxication treat it. The book is a practical guide to getting well. Sample sections from the book:

- Why worry about mercury poisoning?
- What mercury does to you – symptoms, test irregularities, diagnostic checklist.
- How to treat mercury poisoning easily with oral chelators.
- Dealing with other metals including copper, arsenic, lead, cadmium.
- Dietary and supplement guidelines.
- Balancing hormones during the recovery process.
- How to feel good while you are chelating the metals out.
- How heavy metals cause infections to thrive in the body.
- Politics and mercury.

This is the world's most authoritative, accurate book on mercury poisoning.

Paperback book, 8.5 x 11", 226 pages, $35

To order, click www.LymeBookStore.com or call (801) 925-2411
NOTE: Website and phone number are for ordering only, not medical advice.

Hair Test Interpretation: Finding Hidden Toxicities

By Andrew Cutler, PhD

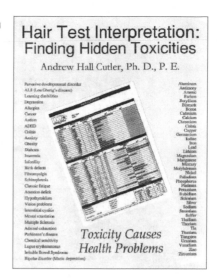

Hair tests are worth doing because a surprising number of people diagnosed with incurable chronic health conditions actually turn out to have a heavy metal problem; quite often, mercury poisoning. Heavy metal problems are easy to correct. Hair testing allows the underlying problem to be identified – and the chronic health condition often disappears with proper detoxification.

Hair Test Interpretation: Finding Hidden Toxicities is a practical book that explains how to interpret Doctor's Data, Inc. and Great Plains Laboratory hair tests. A step-by-step discussion is provided, with figures to illustrate the process and make it easy. The book gives examples using actual hair test results from real people.

Book • $35

One of the problems with hair testing is that both conventional and alternative health care providers do not know how to interpret these tests. Interpretation is not as simple as looking at the results and assuming that any mineral out of the reference range is a problem mineral.

Interpretation is complicated because heavy metal toxicity, especially mercury poisoning, interferes with mineral transport throughout the body. Ironically, if someone is mercury poisoned, hair test mercury is often low and other minerals may be elevated or take on unusual values. For example, mercury often causes retention of arsenic, antimony, tin, titanium, zirconium, and aluminum. An inexperienced health care provider may wrongfully assume that one of these other minerals is the culprit, when in reality mercury is the true toxicity.

"This new book of Andrew's is the definitive guide in the confusing world of heavy metal poisoning diagnosis and treatment. I'm a practicing physician, 20 years now, specializing in detoxification programs for treatment of resistant conditions. It was fairly difficult to diagnose these heavy metal conditions before I met Andrew Cutler and developed a close relationship with him while reading his books. In this book I found his usual painful attention to detail gave a solid framework for understanding the complexity of mercury toxicity as well as the less common exposures. You really couldn't ask for a better reference book on a subject most researchers and physicians are still fumbling in the dark about."
- Dr. Rick Marschall

So, as you can see, getting a hair test is only the first step. The second step is figuring out what the hair test means. Andrew Cutler, PhD, is a registered professional chemical engineer with years of experience in biochemical and healthcare research. This clear and concise book makes hair test interpretation easy, so that you know which toxicities are causing your health problems.

Paperback book, 8.5 x 11", 298 pages, $35

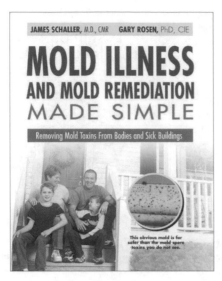

Book • $26.50

Mold Illness and Mold Remediation Made Simple: Removing Mold Toxins from Bodies and Sick Buildings

By James Schaller, M.D. and Gary Rosen, Ph.D.

Indoor mold toxins are much more dangerous and prevalent than most people realize. Visible mold in and around your house is far less dangerous than the mold you cannot see. Indoor mold toxicity, in addition to causing its own unique set of health problems and symptoms, also greatly contributes to the severity of most chronic illnesses.

In this book, a top physician and experienced contractor team up to help you quickly recover from indoor mold exposure. This book is easy to read with many color photographs and illustrations.

Dr. Schaller is a practicing physician in Florida who has written more than 15 books. He is one of the few physicians in the United States successfully treating mold toxin illness in children and adults.

Dr. Rosen is a biochemist with training under a Nobel Prize winning researcher at UCLA. He has written several books and is an expert in the mold remediation of homes. Dr. Rosen and his family are sensitive to mold toxins so he writes not only from professional experience, but also from personal experience.

Together, the two authors have certification in mold testing, mold remediation, and indoor environmental health. This book is one of the most complete on the subject, and includes discussion of the following topics:

- Potential mold problems encountered in new homes, schools, and jobs.
- Diagnosing mold illness.
- Mold as it relates to dryness and humidity.
- Mold toxins and cancer treatment.
- Mold toxins and relationships.
- Crawlspaces, basements, attics, home cleaning techniques, and vacuums.
- Training your eyes to discern indoor mold.
- Leptin and obesity.
- Appropriate/inappropriate air filters and cleaners.
- How to handle old, musty products, materials and books, and how to safely sterilize them.
- A description of various types of molds, images of them, and their relative toxicity.
- Blood testing and how to use it to find hidden health problems.
- The book is written in a friendly, casual tone that allows easy comprehension and information retention.

> "A concise, practical guide on dealing with mold toxins and their effects."
>
> **- Bryan Rosner**

Many people are affected by mold toxins. Are you? If you can find a smarter or clearer book on this subject, buy it!

Paperback book, 8.5 x 11", 140 pages, $26.50

To order, click www.LymeBookStore.com or call (801) 925-2411
NOTE: Website and phone number are for ordering only, not medical advice.

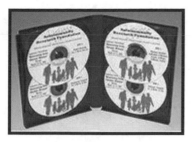

4-DVD Set • $45

Marshall Protocol 4-DVD Set

2005 Chicago Conference:
"Recovering from Chronic Disease"
2005 Hartford Conference:
"30th Anniversary of Lyme"

The Marshall Protocol is not just important, but critical in Lyme Disease recovery. It addresses a part of the Lyme Disease complex that no other treatment, protocol, diet, or supplement can even come close to touching: infection with cell-wall-deficient bacteria.

Borrelia Burgdorferi, the causative bacteria in Lyme Disease, comes in three forms: spirochete, cyst, and cell-wall-deficient. All forms must be addressed to achieve a complete recovery. Spirochetes are successfully killed by rife technology. Cysts can be killed by certain antibiotics (including 5-nitromidizoles and hydroxychloroquine). Cysts can also be exposed and killed by rife therapy with proper treatment timing and planning. However, until the Marshall Protocol, there was not an effective treatment for cell-wall-deficient bacteria.

Conventionally, doctors have tried to use certain types of antibiotics to kill cell-wall-deficient bacteria. Top choices include protein synthesis inhibitors such as the macrolides (Zithromax and Biaxin), the ketolides (Ketek), and the tetracyclines (tetracycline, doxycycline, and minocycline).

> "The Marshall Protocol – especially when combined with rife therapy – fills an important gap in existing Lyme treatment."
> **- Bryan Rosner**

Unfortunately, these antibiotics have been ineffective at worst and only moderately effective at best. According to new research and user reports, the Marshall Protocol successfully targets and kills these cell-wall-deficient bacteria.

This 4-DVD set is exclusively offered by lymebook.com. It was assembled for lymebook.com by the founder of the Autoimmunity Research Foundation, Trevor Marshall, PhD, who also invented the protocol. The DVD set includes video recordings from two conferences of particular interest to Lyme sufferers:

- DVD 1: 30th Anniversary of Lyme – Hartford, Connecticut, May 7, 2005
- DVD 2-4: Recovering from Chronic Disease – Chicago, Illinois, March 12-13, 2005

James P Kiley, PhD   **Leonard Jason, PhD**   **Lida H Mattman, PhD**   **Janet Whitley, PhD**

Researching the Marshall Protocol is an Essential part of Your Lyme Disease Education!

Conference Speakers

Andrew Wright, MD   **Trevor G Marshall, PhD**   **Meg Mangin, RN**

4-DVD Set

12+ hours of viewing

Coverage of two Conferences

$45

To order, click www.LymeBookStore.com or call (801) 925-2411
NOTE: Website and phone number are for ordering only, not medical advice.

Physicians Desk Reference (PDR) Books

Most people have heard of *Physicians Desk Reference* (PDR) because, for over 60 years, physicians and researchers have turned to PDR for the latest word on prescription drugs. Today, PDR is considered the standard prescription drug reference and can be found in virtually every physician's office, hospital, and pharmacy in the United States. In fact, nine out of 10 doctors consider PDR their most important drug information reference source. The current edition is over 3,500 pages long (with a full color directory) and weighs more than 5 lbs. It includes comprehensive and up-to-date information on more than 4,000 FDA-approved drugs.

It is less well known that Thomson Healthcare, publisher of PDR, offers PDR reference books not only for drugs, but also for herbal and nutritional supplements. No other available books come even close to the amount of information provided in these PDRs—*PDR for Herbal Medicines* weighs 5 lbs and has over 900 pages, and *PDR for Nutritional Supplements* weighs over 3 lbs and has more than 500 pages.

THOMSON

Lymebook.com carries all three PDRs: *PDR for Prescription Drugs*, *PDR for Herbal Medicines*, and *PDR for Nutritional Supplements*. Although PDR books are typically used by healthcare practitioners, we feel that these resources are also essential for people interested in or recovering from chronic disease. Ownership of PDR books allows you to have at your fingertips information that has historically not been available to the public. Health decisions are always made based on information, and we want you to have the most complete information available.

Would you like to be able to look up all the details of the treatments you are using (or planning to use)? PDR reference books offer the following data on thousands of herbs, supplements and drugs:

- Description and method of action
- Pharmacology
- Available trade names / brands
- Indications and usage
- Research summaries, with recent scientific studies and clinical results
- Contraindications, precautions, adverse reactions
- How supplied
- Scientific literature overviews
- Dosage and administration
- History of use
- Biochemistry and metabolism
- Pharmacokinetics
- Cross references to other helpful data relating to the drug or herb discussed

The PDRs organize the supplements, herbs, and medicines in numerous ways, so you can quickly and easily find the information you need. Multiple color-coded, photo-supported indexes are provided. Supplements and drugs are categorized according to type, name, and health condition, among other differentiators.

"I relied heavily on the PDRs during the research phase of writing my books. Without these books, I'm not sure I could have pulled together the information I needed."

- Bryan Rosner

In addition to information about individual herbs, supplements, and drugs, the PDRs also provide high-level comprehensive health resources such as breakthroughs in the treatment of specific health conditions, anti-aging science, cancer studies, sports medicine, nutrition, and much more.

If you are a doctor, nurse, holistic healthcare provider, or simply a patient wishing to do your own research, these books are must-have resources. They pay for themselves many times over after years of use as reliable reference guides.   (See next page for PDSs).

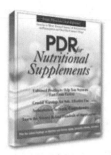

PDR for Nutritional Supplements

This PDR focuses on the following types of supplements:

- Vitamins
- Minerals
- Amino acids
- Hormones
- Lipids
- Glyconutrients
- Probiotics
- Proteins
- Many more!

Book • $69.50

"In a part of the health field not known for its devotion to rigorous science, [this book] brings to the practitioner and the curious patient a wealth of hard facts."

- Roger Guillemin, M.D., Ph.D., Nobel Laureate in Physiology and Medicine

The book also suggests supplements that can help reduce prescription drug side effects, has full-color photographs of various popular commercial formulations (and contact information for the associated suppliers), and so much more! Become educated instead of guessing which supplements to take.

Hardcover book, 11 x 9.3", 575 pages, $69.50

PDR for Herbal Medicines

PDR for Herbal Medicines is very well organized and presents information on hundreds of common and uncommon herbs and herbal preparations. Indications and usage are examined with regard to homeopathy, Indian and Chinese medicine, and unproven (yet popular) applications.

In an area of healthcare so unstudied and vulnerable to hearsay and hype, this scientifically referenced book allows you to find out the real story behind the herbs lining the walls of your local health food store.

Use this reference before spending money on herbal products!

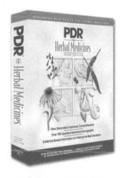

Book • $69.50

Hardcover book, 11 x 9.3", 988 pages, $69.50

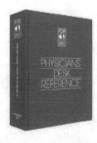

PDR for Prescription Drugs

With more than 3,500 pages, this is the most comprehensive and respected book in the world on over 4,000 drugs. Drugs are indexed by both brand and generic name (in the same convenient index) and also by manufacturer and product category. This PDR provides usage information and warnings, drug interactions, plus a detailed, full-color directory with descriptions and cross references for the drugs. A new format allows dramatically improved readability and easier access to the information you need now.

Book • $99.50

Hardcover book, 12.5 x 9.5", 3533 pages, $99.50

To order, click 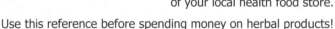www.LymeBookStore.com or call (801) 925-2411
NOTE: Website and phone number are for ordering only, not medical advice.

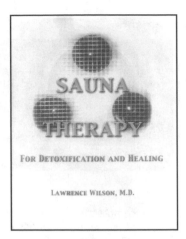

Book • $19.95

Sauna Therapy for Detoxification and Healing

By Lawrence Wilson, MD

This book is the single most authoritative source on sauna therapy. It includes construction plans for a low-cost electric light sauna. The book is well referenced with an extensive bibliography.

Sauna therapy, especially with an electric light sauna, is one of the most powerful, safe and cost-effective methods of natural healing. It is especially important today due to extensive exposure to toxic metals and chemicals.

Fifteen chapters cover sauna benefits, physiological effects, protocols, cautions, healing reactions, and many other aspects of sauna therapy.

Dr. Wilson is an instructor of Biochemistry, Hair Mineral Analysis, Sauna Therapy and Jurisprudence at various colleges and universities including Yamuni Institute of the Healing Arts (Maurice, LA), University of Natural Medicine (Santa Fe, NM), Natural Healers Academy (Morristown, NJ), and Westbrook University (West Virginia). His books are used as textbooks at East-West School of Herbology and Ohio College of Natural Health.

Paperback book, 8.5 x 11", 167 pages, $19.95

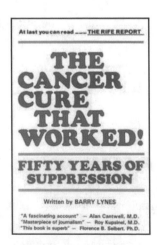

Book • $19.95

The Cancer Cure That Worked: Fifty Years of Suppression

At Last You Can Read... The Rife Report

By Barry Lynes

Investigative journalism at its best. Barry Lynes takes readers on an exciting and revealing journey into the life work of Royal Raymond Rife, inventor of the rife machine. This book reveals the history and healing power of energy medicine.

"A fascinating account..." -Alan Cantwell, MD

"This book is superb." -Florence B. Seibert, PhD

"Barry Lynes is one of the greatest health reporters in our country. With the assistance of John Crane, longtime friend and associate of Roy Rife, Barry has produced a masterpiece..." -Roy Kupsinel, M.D., editor of *Health Consciousness Journal*

Paperback book, 5 x 8", 169 pages, $19.95

To order, click www.LymeBookStore.com or call (801) 925-2411
NOTE: Website and phone number are for ordering only, not medical advice.

Rife Technology Video Documentary
2-Part VHS Video Set, 145 Minutes
Produced by *Zero Zero Two Productions*

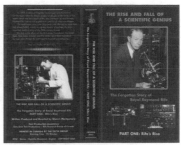

Part I: Rife's Rise

PART I: Rife's Rise (74 min, VHS)

In 1999, a stack of forgotten audio tapes was discovered. On the tapes were the voices of several people at the center of the events which are the subject of this documentary: a revolutionary treatment for cancer and a practical cure for all infectious disease.

The audio tapes were over 40 years old. The voices on them had almost faded, nearly losing key details of perhaps the most important medical story of the 20th Century.

But due to the efforts of the Kinnaman Foundation, the faded tapes have been restored and the voices on them recovered. So now, even though the participants have all passed away...

...they can finally tell their story.

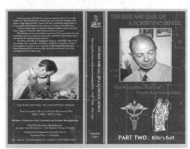

Part II: Rife's Fall

VHS Video Set • $53.95

"These videos are great. We show them at the Annual Rife International Health Conference."
-Richard Loyd, Ph.D.

"A mind-shifting experience for those of us indoctrinated with a conventional view of biology."
-Townsend Letter for Doctors and Patients

PART II: Rife's Fall (71 min, VHS)

In the summer of 1934 at a special medical clinic in La Jolla, California, sixteen patients withering from terminal disease were given a new lease on life. It was the first controlled application of a new electronic treatment for cancer: the Beam Ray Machine.

Within ninety days all sixteen patients walked away from the clinic, signed-off by the attending doctors as cured.

What followed the incredible success of this revolutionary treatment was not a welcoming by the scientific community, but a sad tale of its ultimate suppression.

The Rise and Fall of a Scientific Genius - Part II: Rife's Fall documents the scientific ignorance, official corruption, and personal greed directed at the inventor of the Beam Ray Machine, Royal Raymond Rife, forcing him and his inventions out of the spotlight and into obscurity.

Do not miss this opportunity to educate yourself about the history of rife technology!

2 VHS video cassettes, 145 min., $53.95

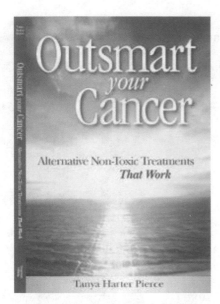

Book and Audio CD • $24.95

**Outsmart Your Cancer:
Alternative Non-Toxic
Treatments That Work**

By Tanya Harter Pierce

Although Lymebook.com primarily focuses on books and resources for Lyme Disease, we know that cancer affects many of our customers. Consequently, we offer this excellent book/audio CD set on alternative cancer therapy.

Publisher's Remarks:

Why BLUDGEON cancer to death with common conventional treatments that can be toxic and harmful to your entire body?

When you OUTSMART your cancer, only the cancer cells die — NOT your healthy cells!

OUTSMART YOUR CANCER: Alternative Non-Toxic Treatments That Work is an easy guide to successful non-toxic treatments for cancer that you can obtain right now! In it, you will read real-life stories of people who have completely recovered from their advanced or late-stage lung cancer, breast cancer, prostate cancer, kidney cancer, brain cancer, childhood leukemia, and other types of cancer using effective non-toxic approaches.

"As a doctor practicing alternative medicine, I recommend this book to anyone that is involved with cancer."
- Dr. L. Durrett

This book explains the successful approaches these people used. It also gives you the resources to obtain these treatments right now, including a list of phone numbers and answers to questions about financial cost.

You will also learn other valuable information, such as:

• The unique characteristics of cancer cells that can be exploited to "outsmart" cancer.
• How to evaluate mainstream conventional treatments and what questions to ask your doctor.
• What women need to know about their hormones and cancer.
• How to alkalize your body and why this matters, both for prevention and treatment of cancer.
• Many of the causes of cancer that are increasingly common in our modern world.
• How and why many of the best alternative treatments for cancer have been suppressed.
• How to cope with the fear that comes with a cancer diagnosis.

Plus, *OUTSMART YOUR CANCER* is one of the few books in print today that gives a complete description of the amazing formula called "Protocel," which has produced incredible cancer recoveries over the past 20 years! A supporting audio CD is included with this book. Pricing = $19.95 book + $5.00 CD.

Paperback book, 6 x 9", 437 pages, with audio CD, $24.95

To order, click www.LymeBookStore.com or call (801) 925-2411
NOTE: Website and phone number are for ordering only, not medical advice.

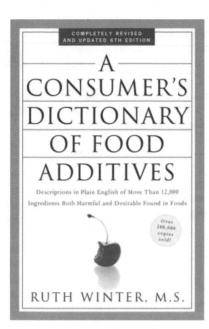

Book • $16.95

A Consumer's Dictionary of Food Additives (6th Edition): Descriptions in Plain English of More Than 12,000 Ingredients, Both Harmful and Desirable, Found In Foods

By Ruth Winter, M.S.

Have you ever wondered about those impossible-to-pronounce ingredients in your food and supplements? Now you can find out *exactly* what you are putting in your body!

In an updated sixth edition, this valuable reference gives you all the facts about the relative safety and side effects of more than 12,000 ingredients that end up in your food as a result of processing and curing, including preservatives, food-tainting pesticides, and animal drugs.

In addition to food and supplement additives, the book covers other relevant information. Included are startling statistics about the large amount of dollars spent on certain additives ($1.4 billion on flavorings and flavor enhancers alone) and descriptions of resistant strains of bacteria which develop as a consequence of antibiotic additives in animal feed.

A Consumer's Dictionary of Food Additives is a precise tool that will tell you exactly what to leave on supermarket shelves as a reminder to manufacturers that you know what the labels mean and which products are safe to bring home to your family.

Ruth Winter, M.S., is an award-winning science writer who is nationally known for her many books and magazine articles in *Family Circle*, *Woman's Day*, *Good Housekeeping*, and *Reader's Digest*. She is also the author of *A Consumer's Dictionary of Cosmetic Ingredients*, *A Consumer's Dictionary of Medicines: Prescription, Over-the-Counter, Homeopathic, and Herbal*, and *Poisons in Your Food*.

If you are concerned about the food and supplement products you purchase and use, this book can help you make better, more educated decisions.

> I found this book (and Winter's other books) to be thoroughly researched, well written, and intuitive to use. I appreciated the clear language and detailed references. By providing both the scientific terminology and the vernacular language, the author educates her audience on the many ways in which consumers may be getting MORE than they bargained for when they are selecting foods (and cosmetics).
>
> **- Marie Tangondoro**

Paperback book, 5.3 x 8", 592 pages, $16.95

To order, click www.LymeBookStore.com or call (801) 925-2411
NOTE: Website and phone number are for ordering only, not medical advice.

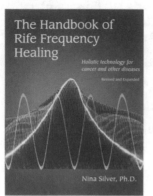

The Handbook of Rife Frequency Healing: Holistic Technology for Cancer and Other Diseases

By Nenah Sylver, PhD

This is the most complete, authoritative Rife technology handbook in the world. Weighing over 2 lbs., and 448 pages long, a broad range of topics are covered:

- Little-known differences between allopathic (Western) medicine and holistic health care
- Royal Raymond Rife's life, inventions, ideas and relationships
- Frequently Asked Questions about Rife sessions and equipment, with extensive session information
- Ground-breaking information on strengthening and supporting the body, based on decades of research by the author
- A 200-page, cross-referenced Frequency Directory including hundreds of health conditions
- Bibliography, Three Appendices, Historical Photos, **and MUCH MORE!**

Book • $60

Paperback book, 8.5 x 11", 430 pages, $60

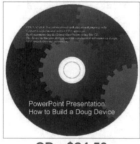

CD • $24.50

PowerPoint Presentation on CD
How to Build a Coil Machine

Of all rife machines used to fight Lyme Disease, the Coil Machine (also known as the Doug Device or QSC1850HD Device) has the longest and most established track record. This PowerPoint presentation was put together by the husband of a Lyme Disease sufferer who built the machine for his wife. It provides construction information, parts sourcing, and a detailed schematic. Now you can build your own Coil Machine!

Microsoft PowerPoint Presentation on CD, $24.50

Ordering Options

- **(866) 476-7637**
- **www.LymeBookStore.com**

Call today to place an order or request additional catalogs. Detailed product information and online ordering is available on our website.

Join Lyme Community Forums (www.lymecommunity.com), a new online discussion group, to communicate for FREE with fellow Lyme sufferers!

DISCLAIMER: Our products are for informational and educational purposes only. They are not intended to prevent, diagnose, treat, or cure disease. Statements in this catalog have not been evaluated by the FDA. Do not consult our products or catalog for medical advice – see a physician.

To order, click www.LymeBookStore.com or call (801) 925-2411
NOTE: Website and phone number are for ordering only, not medical advice.

About the Author

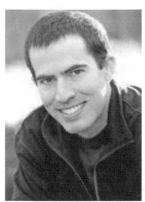

Bryan Rosner

Bryan Rosner is an internationally recognized author, educator and speaker. His articles and books on Lyme Disease have received critical acclaim from patients and physicians in more than 15 countries. Bryan's first book, *Lyme Disease and Rife Machines*, has earned bestselling status in the United States, Europe, and elsewhere in the world.

Bryan's work goes beyond merely educating the world about Lyme Disease—he is also active in the Lyme Disease community itself. In 2003, Bryan founded the Electromedicine and Lyme Disease Research Forum (also known as the Lyme-and-Rife group), which, at the time of this book's publication, had more than 2,000 participating members. In 2006, he founded Lyme Community Forums, a hub for Lyme Disease communication and education. You can access both groups by visiting www.lymebook.com/resources.

The research substantiating Bryan's work is derived from numerous sources, including his personal experience with Lyme Disease, input from hundreds of other Lyme Sufferers, clinical and laboratory studies, and collaboration with leading physicians on several continents.

Bryan's books are known to include not only treatments popular in the United States, but also successful healing modalities found throughout the world. In fact, Bryan communicates with researchers and physicians world-wide, and many of the treatments found in his books are unpublished and unknown to the public in the United States. In this way, his writing is balanced and broad, offering readers a wide array of treatment options from which to choose.

Bryan has spoken at numerous Lyme-related conventions and events, including, of particular note, the Annual Rife International Health Conference (www.lymebook.com/conference). He is available on a limited basis for speaking engagements. Bryan Rosner works as a journalist in the health-care industry and lives in the mountains of Northern California with his wife Leila.

Bryan Rosner is a journalist, not a doctor or health care provider. His writing is intended for informational purposes only, not as medical advice.

-B-

-C-

-D-

Pollen 32, 104
Post-Lyme Syndrome 37
Powdered Vitamin C 152
Prednisone 196
Pregnancy 34, 273, 279
Prescription
  antidepressant 264
  laxatives 152
  lithium drugs 269, 270
Processed sugar 309-311, 313, 314
Progress, recovery
  continuous 123, 209
  forward 19
  long-term 47
  plodding 301
  slowed 199
  stagnated 91, 197
Propioni-bacterium acnes 250
Prostate 176, 229, 285, 311
Protease
  enzymes 230, 233, 234, 236, 238,
    240, 242, 243
  inhibitors 243
Protein synthesis inhibiting antibiotics
  83, 101, 119
Proteolytic enzymes 230, 235
Protozoa 268, 318
Pseudo-equilibrium 305, 306
Psychiatric disease 1, 25, 26, 37,
  147, 190, 239, 240, 261, 263,
  268, 295
Publichealthalert.org 329
Pulsing (taking breaks from) the
  Marshall Protocol 127

-Q-

QSC1850HD Machine (another name
  for the Coil Machine or Doug
  Device) 218
Quercetin 196
Quinovic acid glycosides 91

-R-

Rages (see also Lyme rage) 2, 147
Ranch dressing 116
Rash, itchy, caused by ozone sauna
  170
Rats, lithium treated 265

Reactions, herx (see also herx reactions)
  out-of-control 194, 195
  scary 301
  strong 125
  uncomfortable 306
Reasoning abilities 2, 147
Recovery
  accelerating 293
  complete 3, 104, 210
  process
    long 51, 53, 292, 308
    stagnates 46
  speedy 53
  time frame 53
Rectal insufflation of ozone, as a
  treatment 168
Red-coated Wobenzym tablets 245
Red meat 178
Rejuvenated feeling 154
Relapses 38, 65, 67, 135, 295
Remission 51, 67, 113, 135, 204,
  209, 295
Resistance, bacterial 41, 66, 70, 71,
  74, 75, 84, 85, 91, 256, 257, 293
Rickettsia
  canis 319
  spotted fever 316-318, 320, 321
Rife International Health Conference
  153,
  Watch Doug MacLean interviewed at
    205
Rife machine 17-19, 41, 57, 74, 91,
  100-102, 128, 132, 199-203, 205,
  206, 208-212, 216-221, 255-257,
  281, 282, 293-295, 303, 304
  manufacturer contact information
    220
  ownership 220
  principles, basic 203, 212
  therapy 17, 41, 44, 60, 61, 73-76,
    82, 101, 102, 128, 131, 135, 173,
    199-222, 256, 257, 283, 284,
    293-296
  treatment
    campaign 218
    schedule 128, 212, 213, 293
    sessions 283
  treatments 92, 177, 213, 215-217,
    304
  updated user tips 200, 212